Dedicated to
THE NEW PHYSICIAN

CLINICAL SYMPOSIA
ANTHOLOGY

CLINICAL SYMPOSIA ANTHOLOGY

J. HAROLD WALTON, M.D., *Editor Emeritus* 1948-1971

RICHARD H. ROBERTS, M.D., *Editor* 1971-1972

ROBERT K. SHAPTER, M.D., C.M., *Editor* 1973-

FRANK H. NETTER, M.D., *Illustrator*

CIBA PHARMACEUTICAL COMPANY

DIVISION OF CIBA-GEIGY CORPORATION

SUMMIT, NEW JERSEY

C I B A

5 P/5147

FOREWORD

This anthology contains six of the most popular issues of CLINICAL SYMPOSIA published during the past several years.

CIBA Pharmaceutical Company publishes CLINICAL SYMPOSIA as a service to the medical profession. Each issue contains one or more articles of clinical significance in medicine and surgery.

Texts are authored by leading authorities. Accompanying illustrations, most of them in full color, are by the renowned medical illustrator Frank H. Netter, M.D.

Some of the illustrations appear in THE CIBA COLLECTION OF MEDICAL ILLUSTRATIONS, a continuing series of atlases that portrays normal and pathologic anatomy—including surgical and manipulative technics—involving all the systems of the human organism.

CONTENTS

SECTION A

CIBA

THE TREATMENT OF HEAD INJURIES
Commander Frederick E. Jackson, MC, USN

THE TREATMENT OF HEAD INJURIES

COMMANDER FREDERICK E. JACKSON, MC, USN

J. HAROLD WALTON, M.D., *Editor*

FRANK H. NETTER, M.D., *Illustrator*

MARY LOU GRAVES, *Editorial Assistant*

CIBA PHARMACEUTICAL COMPANY

SUMMIT, NEW JERSEY 07901

THE TREATMENT OF HEAD INJURIES

COMMANDER FREDERICK E. JACKSON, MC, USN

Department of Neurosurgery
United States Naval Hospital
Charleston, South Carolina

In a previous article* we have emphasized the structural relationships which predispose certain portions of the brain to injury, the susceptibility of the neuron to metabolic damage, and the importance of intracranial hemorrhage as a cause of persistent morbidity and early fatality.

In this issue we shall attempt to outline those aspects of medical and surgical management which have proved most important in our own experience, from first aid to final discharge.

FIRST AID TREATMENT

The head-injured patient presents a few special problems in first aid. He is often unconscious and may suffer additional neuronal damage or even die of asphyxia unless very careful attention is given the airway. Also, associated injuries of the neck are commonly encountered. Thus, the following points are of greatest importance. The priority given each will vary with circumstances (Plate I).

1. *Clear the airway, keep it clear, and assure adequate ventilation.* Make sure

---

*The Pathophysiology of Head Injuries, CLINICAL SYMPOSIA, Volume 18: Number 3, 1966.

the tongue or loose dentures have not fallen back in the throat. Keep the throat and mouth clear of blood and vomitus. Nothing is more lethal to head-injured patients than aspiration pneumonia caused by gastric content, particularly when it contains alcohol. To decrease the possibility of aspiration, the patient should be on his side, the face downward — but care must be exercised in obtaining this position (see below). Also, as soon as possible the stomach should be aspirated.

A good way to improve the airway is to pull upward and forward on the posterior angles of the jaw. This will also help maintain traction on a possibly injured neck.

Even with a clear airway, ventilation may be inadequate because of coincidental chest injury. To assure adequate respiratory exchange, first aid personnel should be trained in the use of a mechanical device, such as the Ambu respirator.

2. *Don't let the head flop around on the trunk.* The blow which injured the head may have fractured or dislocated a verte-

---

The opinions or assertions contained in this paper are those of the author and are not to be construed as official or reflecting the views of the Navy Department or the Naval Service at large.

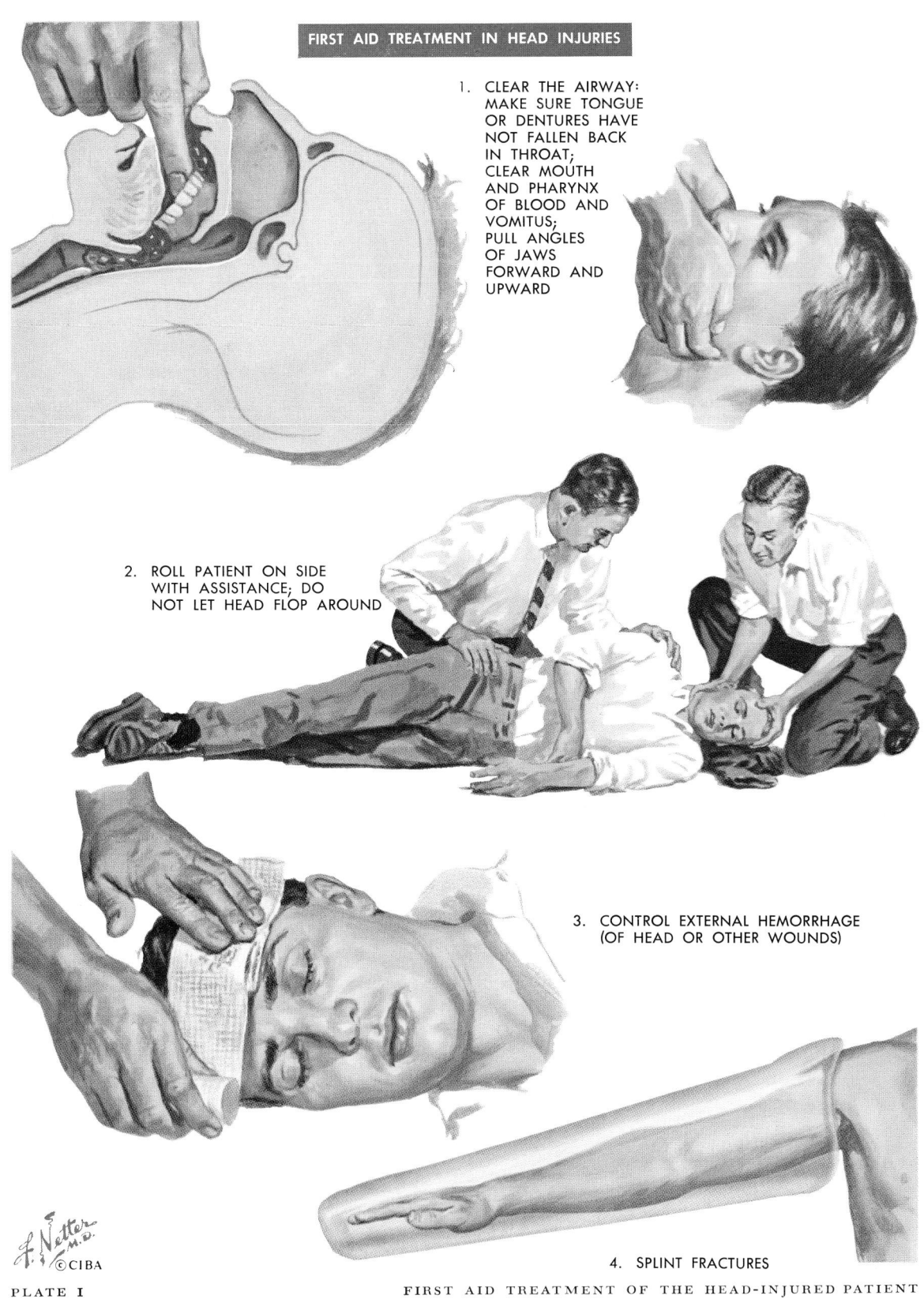

1. CLEAR THE AIRWAY: MAKE SURE TONGUE OR DENTURES HAVE NOT FALLEN BACK IN THROAT; CLEAR MOUTH AND PHARYNX OF BLOOD AND VOMITUS; PULL ANGLES OF JAWS FORWARD AND UPWARD

2. ROLL PATIENT ON SIDE WITH ASSISTANCE; DO NOT LET HEAD FLOP AROUND

3. CONTROL EXTERNAL HEMORRHAGE (OF HEAD OR OTHER WOUNDS)

4. SPLINT FRACTURES

PLATE I

FIRST AID TREATMENT OF THE HEAD-INJURED PATIENT

bra, and rough handling may convert a minimal compression of the spinal cord into a permanent quadriplegia. When moving the patient, "roll him like a log" so that head, trunk, and extremities maintain the same relative position, particularly the head and trunk. This requires several people. Usually, one person alone should wait for help.

3. *Stop external hemorrhage.* The best blood for the patient is his own! A profusely bleeding scalp wound can be controlled by external pressure. If a pressure dressing is applied, be careful of the neck.

4. *Splint all broken extremities.* The hypotension of shock due to a broken leg may reduce circulation to the injured brain past the point of no return.

INITIAL MEDICAL MANAGEMENT

(PLATE II)

In these days of high-speed transportation, it is not unusual for several people to become involved in the same accident. When faced with a number of patients, some with multiple injuries, the *first* duty of the physician is to conduct a *rapid triage.* This consists of quickly evaluating the seriousness and manageability of the various injuries suffered, deciding which can be cared for by assistants, nurses, or even laymen, which must receive personal attention, and the order in which the problems must be attacked.

In these first "golden moments" when every move is important and every mistake may be catastrophic, the physician cannot afford to spend time suturing a laceration while another patient is in need of an airway!

In the initial medical management of the head-injured patient, a system must be followed that puts first things first. While no rigid rule can apply to every set of circumstances, experience has proved the relative importance of the following clinical priorities:

1. *Establish a clear airway.* In any head injury, cerebral circulation may be impaired by edema, cerebral vascular spasm and, not infrequently, by increased intracranial pressure. If, added to this, respiratory function is impaired, blood that does reach the brain is poorly oxygenated, further compromising damaged neurons and threatening others. Indeed, *the damage caused by cerebral anoxia may be worse than that produced by the initial injury.*

The first necessity is *suction* to clear the oropharynx and nasopharynx of blood, secretions, and foreign material. When necessary, and if the patient is comatose, an endotracheal tube may be inserted. However, this device will not be tolerated by one who is partly conscious.

One of the greatest advances in treatment has been early *tracheostomy,* which is particularly indicated in injuries causing bleeding from the nose or mouth. Early tracheostomy using a *cuff-type* tracheostomy tube, as shown in Plate III, has the following advantages:

A. It prevents the aspiration of blood and vomitus, thus greatly reducing the incidence of aspiration pneumonia.

B. When provided with an inflatable cuff between tube and tracheal wall, intermittent positive pressure can be used to assist breathing. This will help keep the patient ventilated, oxygenated and pink, and reduce the incidence of atelectasis and hypostatic pneumonia.

C. Suction can be applied to remove accumulated secretions.

D. Anesthesia, when necessary, can be given without additional intubation.

E. It reduces dead space, which consumes such a large portion of the total respiratory volume, particularly when breathing is rapid and shallow.

F. It allows the physician to forget this aspect of treatment and concentrate on the patient's other urgent needs.

The value of tracheostomy is aptly summarized by the dictum: *"The time to do a tracheostomy is the first time you think it may become necessary."*

2. *Treat shock.* An adequate blood pressure and satisfactory hematocrit is as essential for survival of cerebral tissues as is a clear airway. While the question of vasoconstrictors versus adrenolytics may be controversial, there can be no argument about the importance of expanding blood volume. To assure adequate tissue perfusion and avoid cerebral anoxia, a start must be made promptly. While waiting for blood-typing and crossmatching, the patient should be started on lactated Ringer's solution, dextran, or human serum albumin. One of these solutions is started intravenously, and a switch is made to blood as soon as available.

To avoid overloading the vascular compartment, it is wise to monitor the central venous pressure in elderly patients in hypovolemic shock, when there is no way of estimating amount of blood loss. Central venous pressure can be determined by inserting a catheter into the jugular vein, to which both a manometer and source of blood are attached by a three-way stopcock. A central venous pressure of more than 150 mm above the level of the right atrium is an indication of circulatory overloading, and the administration of intravenous fluid should be stopped or continued very slowly.

Where shock persists after central venous pressure has become elevated, myocardial insufficiency should be suspected and digitalization considered.

In estimating the probable volume of blood replacement required, it may be helpful to recall that shock rarely occurs from acute blood loss that is less than 30 percent of total blood volume.

A person's blood represents approximately 7 percent of the total body weight. For example, a 70 kg man will have about 5 liters of blood ($70{,}000 \text{ Gm} \times 0.07 = 4{,}900 \text{ Gm}$ or ml). If in shock, a man of this weight may be presumed to have lost about 30 percent of 5 liters, or 1,500 ml. Also, if hemorrhage continues during the administration of blood, probably an additional 10 percent blood volume replacement will be needed to make up the deficit.

A useful index of the adequacy of perfusion is the rate of urine flow. As soon as a Foley catheter has been inserted, urine flow should be measured at hourly intervals. In general, a urinary output of less than 25 ml per hour (or 600 ml per day) is evidence that more fluid is required.

One of the more important innovations in the treatment of shock has been the use of adrenal corticoids in extremely large doses. Indeed, dosage of hydrocortisone as high as 50 mg/kg has been recommended, as has 3 to 4 Gm per day of methylprednisolone. It has been our own practice to utilize as an initial dose 10 to 20 mg of dexamethasone phosphate or 250 mg of methylprednisolone succinate intravenously. One-half this dose is then given at intervals of 4 to 6 hours until circulatory stability has been established. In head-injured patients, the use of adrenal corticoids has the additional advantage of decreasing cerebral edema, and it has been our impression that not only is recovery from shock hastened, but also reaction to subsequent operation is improved.

It is our opinion that the Trendelenburg position is contraindicated in head-injured patients because of its tendency to increase cerebral venous stasis and intracranial pressure. Also, cardiac and respiratory function may be embarrassed by pressure of abdominal viscera upward on the diaphragm.

When *only* the head is injured, the blood pressure, as a rule, is amazingly well maintained. Indeed, shock that lasts longer than 1 or 2 hours is definitely *not* due to the head injury, and a careful search must be made elsewhere, particularly in the chest and upper abdomen.

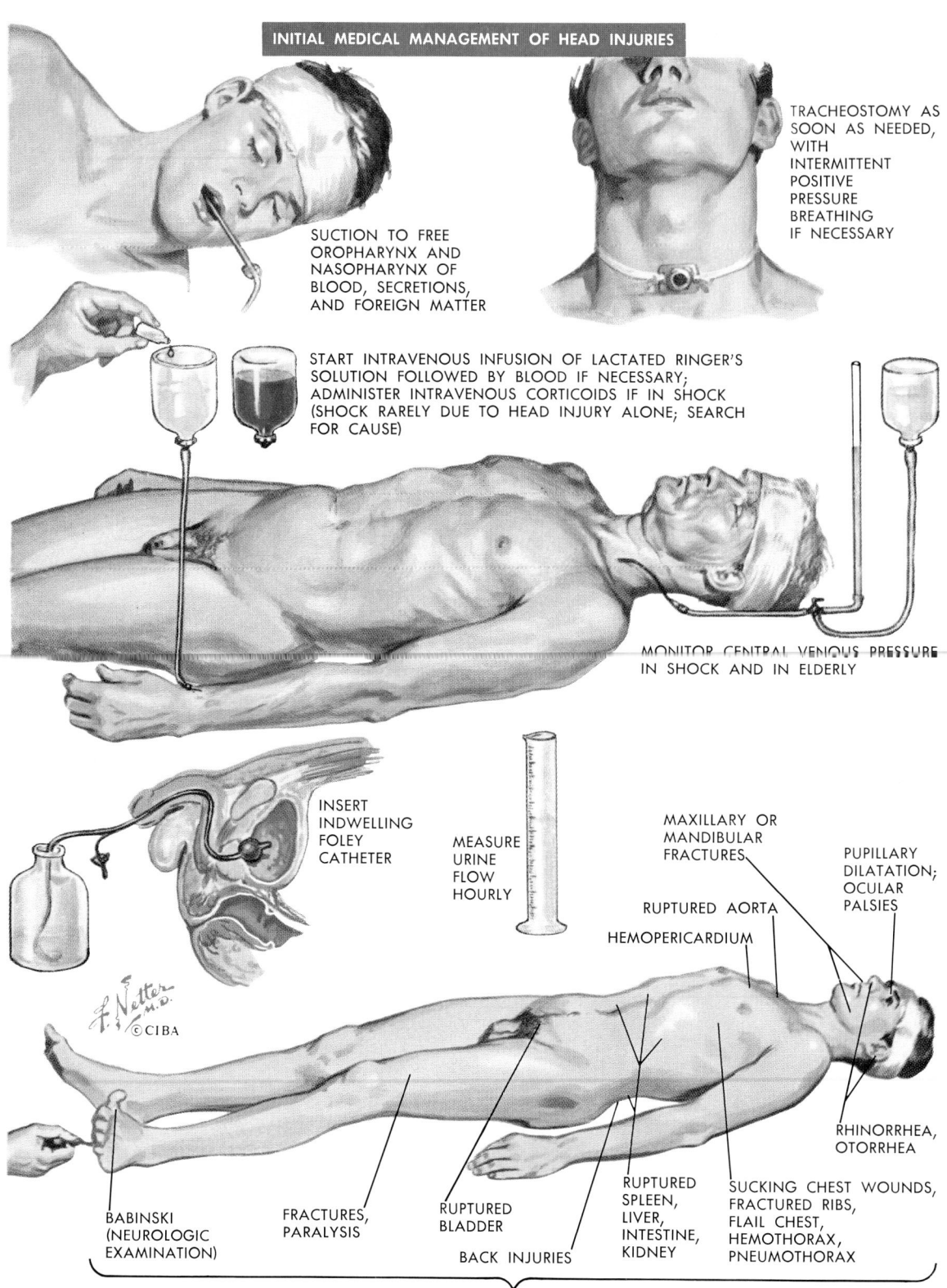

TRACHEOSTOMY AS SOON AS NEEDED, WITH INTERMITTENT POSITIVE PRESSURE BREATHING IF NECESSARY

SUCTION TO FREE OROPHARYNX AND NASOPHARYNX OF BLOOD, SECRETIONS, AND FOREIGN MATTER

START INTRAVENOUS INFUSION OF LACTATED RINGER'S SOLUTION FOLLOWED BY BLOOD IF NECESSARY; ADMINISTER INTRAVENOUS CORTICOIDS IF IN SHOCK (SHOCK RARELY DUE TO HEAD INJURY ALONE; SEARCH FOR CAUSE)

MONITOR CENTRAL VENOUS PRESSURE IN SHOCK AND IN ELDERLY

INSERT INDWELLING FOLEY CATHETER

MEASURE URINE FLOW HOURLY

MAXILLARY OR MANDIBULAR FRACTURES

PUPILLARY DILATATION; OCULAR PALSIES

RUPTURED AORTA

HEMOPERICARDIUM

RHINORRHEA, OTORRHEA

BABINSKI (NEUROLOGIC EXAMINATION)

FRACTURES, PARALYSIS

RUPTURED BLADDER

BACK INJURIES

RUPTURED SPLEEN, LIVER, INTESTINE, KIDNEY

SUCKING CHEST WOUNDS, FRACTURED RIBS, FLAIL CHEST, HEMOTHORAX, PNEUMOTHORAX

CONDUCT COMPLETE PHYSICAL EXAMINATION AND REPEAT PERIODICALLY

PLATE II　　　　　　　　　　INITIAL MEDICAL MANAGEMENT OF HEAD INJURIES

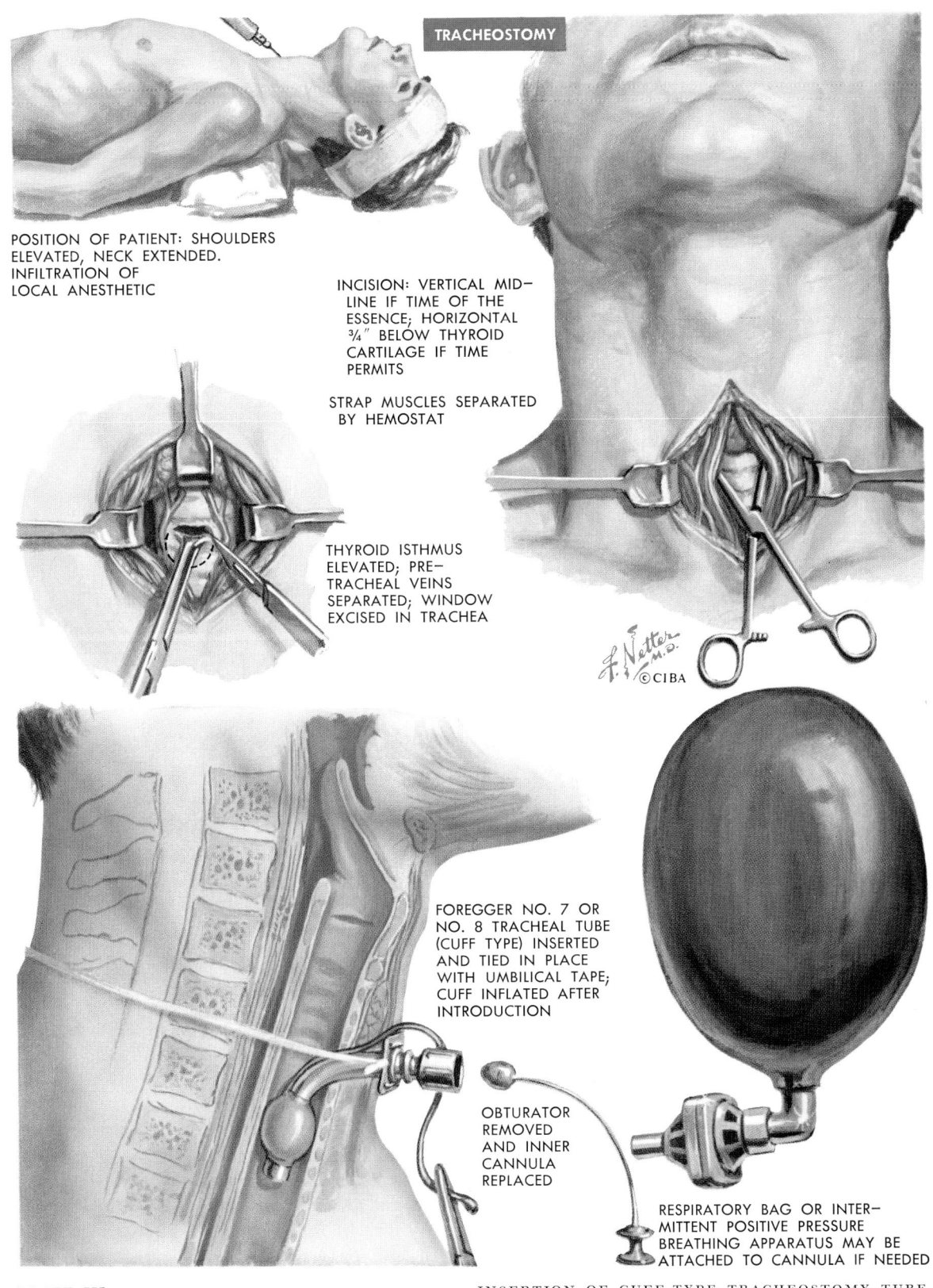

TRACHEOSTOMY

POSITION OF PATIENT: SHOULDERS ELEVATED, NECK EXTENDED. INFILTRATION OF LOCAL ANESTHETIC

INCISION: VERTICAL MID-LINE IF TIME OF THE ESSENCE; HORIZONTAL ¾" BELOW THYROID CARTILAGE IF TIME PERMITS

STRAP MUSCLES SEPARATED BY HEMOSTAT

THYROID ISTHMUS ELEVATED; PRE-TRACHEAL VEINS SEPARATED; WINDOW EXCISED IN TRACHEA

FOREGGER NO. 7 OR NO. 8 TRACHEAL TUBE (CUFF TYPE) INSERTED AND TIED IN PLACE WITH UMBILICAL TAPE; CUFF INFLATED AFTER INTRODUCTION

OBTURATOR REMOVED AND INNER CANNULA REPLACED

RESPIRATORY BAG OR INTER-MITTENT POSITIVE PRESSURE BREATHING APPARATUS MAY BE ATTACHED TO CANNULA IF NEEDED

PLATE III   INSERTION OF CUFF-TYPE TRACHEOSTOMY TUBE

3. *Conduct a complete physical examination.* This serves two purposes. First, it may uncover life-threatening complications contributing to shock, such as flail chest or ruptured spleen. Second, it will provide a baseline with which to relate subsequent findings.

Complicating Injuries

In the chest, search should be made, especially for correctable conditions which may threaten life. These include sucking wounds (which may be occluded by sterile vaseline and a dressing), flail chest (corrected by appropriate rib traction), hemothorax, pneumothorax, and hemopericardium with tamponade (paracentesis).

Especially where there has been a steering wheel injury, one should be alert for the possibility of intimal tear of the aorta. This is suggested by a widening of the superior mediastinum on x-ray, transient harsh murmurs in the aortic area, complaint of pain in that area, an otherwise unexplained falling hematocrit, and blood pressure higher in the arms than in the legs.

Injuries to *the upper abdomen* not infrequently are the cause of hemorrhage and shock due to ruptured spleen or liver. Rupture of intestines, while uncommon, can occur from the shearing stress of an automobile seat belt.

In examining the abdomen, we must remember that a head injury does *not* cause abdominal rigidity. Where intra-abdominal bleeding has occurred, acute tenderness may be elicited by rectal palpation of the rectovesical pouch. When in doubt, one should not hesitate to do an abdominal paracentesis or even exploratory laparotomy.

The most frequent injury to *the lower abdomen* is rupture of the bladder. This can be determined by catheterization followed by instillation of 90 ml of 50% Hypaque or other water-soluble radio-paque compound. X-ray will reveal extravasation of the opaque material if bladder rupture has occurred. In addition, a Foley catheter will prevent overdistention of the bladder, permit accurate monitoring of urinary output, and assure the unconscious patient of a dry bed.

Careful search should be made for possible fractures. A broken rib may splint the chest of an unconscious patient and lead to atelectasis. A fractured femur may extravasate a pint or two of blood into adjacent tissues. Even the pain of an unsplinted fractured digit may contribute to shock.

Later, when the excitement has passed, repeated *complete* examinations of the patient are essential. Even the best and most methodical of physicians can miss an important finding under the stress of an emergency situation.

NEUROLOGIC EVALUATION

State of Consciousness

The many gradations between complete coma and alert normalcy have been given various names — semicoma, stupor, delirium, confusion, and others which may not have precisely the same meaning for everyone. So that there can be no misunderstanding, it is better to record exactly the patient's actions and his level of consciousness. Do the pupils react to light? Does he move his limbs spontaneously? Will they be withdrawn on painful stimulation? Will he react to sudden noise? In general, a deepening of coma is an indication for consideration of angiography and possible surgical intervention.

Vital Signs

In the absence of shock, the *pulse rate* may be full, slow, and bounding initially and become faster as improvement occurs. Indeed, a pulse rate as low as 40 or 50 may be found in some patients who have apparently suffered only minor head injury. However, where the pulse rate is relatively normal or rapid on admission and later a bradycardia develops with or without other evidence of increased intracranial pressure, an expanding intracranial lesion requiring surgery is to be strongly suspected. If intracranial hypertension is not relieved surgically, the heart rate may increase over a period of minutes to hours and become very rapid (120–180). This is usually a preterminal phenomenon.

Respiration may be entirely normal. Accelerated rates are more often than not due to thoracic difficulties, such as pulmonary edema, atelectasis, or pneumonia. Irregular respiration (Cheyne-Stokes or Kussmaul), which is frequently due to cerebral anoxia, gives a poor prognosis and is an indication for positive-pressure assisted breathing. Slow, deep respiration, especially when associated with increasing stupor and a decreasing pulse rate, are strong indications of an expanding intracranial hemorrhage.

Temperature is usually moderately elevated, ranging from 100° to 101° F. Since each degree of temperature elevation increases cellular metabolism, measures should be taken to reduce it to normal (see page 26). Blood in the spinal fluid will raise the temperature moderately. Brain stem injury affecting the heat regulatory center can cause fever of 104° F and even higher. This elevation, too, must be combated.

One must not forget that dehydration and infection are also important causes of fever. Therefore, a continuing fever is always an indication for careful search for infection, particularly in the urinary tract if the patient has been catheterized.

Blood pressure is usually well sustained near normal levels in the head-injured patient unless there are extracranial causes of shock. A rising blood pressure with a slowing of pulse and respiration is an indication of a dynamically increasing hematoma.

The vital signs are not infallible. There are many instances in which one of these vital signs is altered without the others and, not infrequently, there is little correlation between any of them and the intracranial pressure which may itself be normal in the presence of an enlarging hematoma.

This is particularly true of elderly people and alcoholics, whose brains have become atrophic, leaving considerable space inside the skull in which a hematoma can accumulate without increasing the intracranial pressure. In contrast, children and young adults will quickly show a marked elevation of pressure following a relatively small intracranial collection of blood.

Thus, the vital signs are *only* signs. They are never absolutely pathognomonic, but taken together with the state of consciousness (which is the most reliable index of the neurologic status), they do serve to alert the physician to the need for angiography or surgical exploration.

Neurologic Examination

The usual neurologic findings in an injury involving cranial nerves are listed in the chart on pages 18 and 19. The Babinski reflex indicating involvement of the pyramidal tract is elicited by lightly stroking the lateral portion of the sole of the foot. It is present when the great toe goes into dorsiflexion. For Hoffmann's sign, one flexes or taps the fingernail of the middle finger. When positive, flexion of the terminal phalanx of the thumb and adduction of the thumb occurs.

DIAGNOSTIC TESTS AND PROCEDURES

In head injury, an order for a laboratory test or even an x-ray is *not* a substitute for careful, complete physical examination and expert clinical judgment. Thus, we

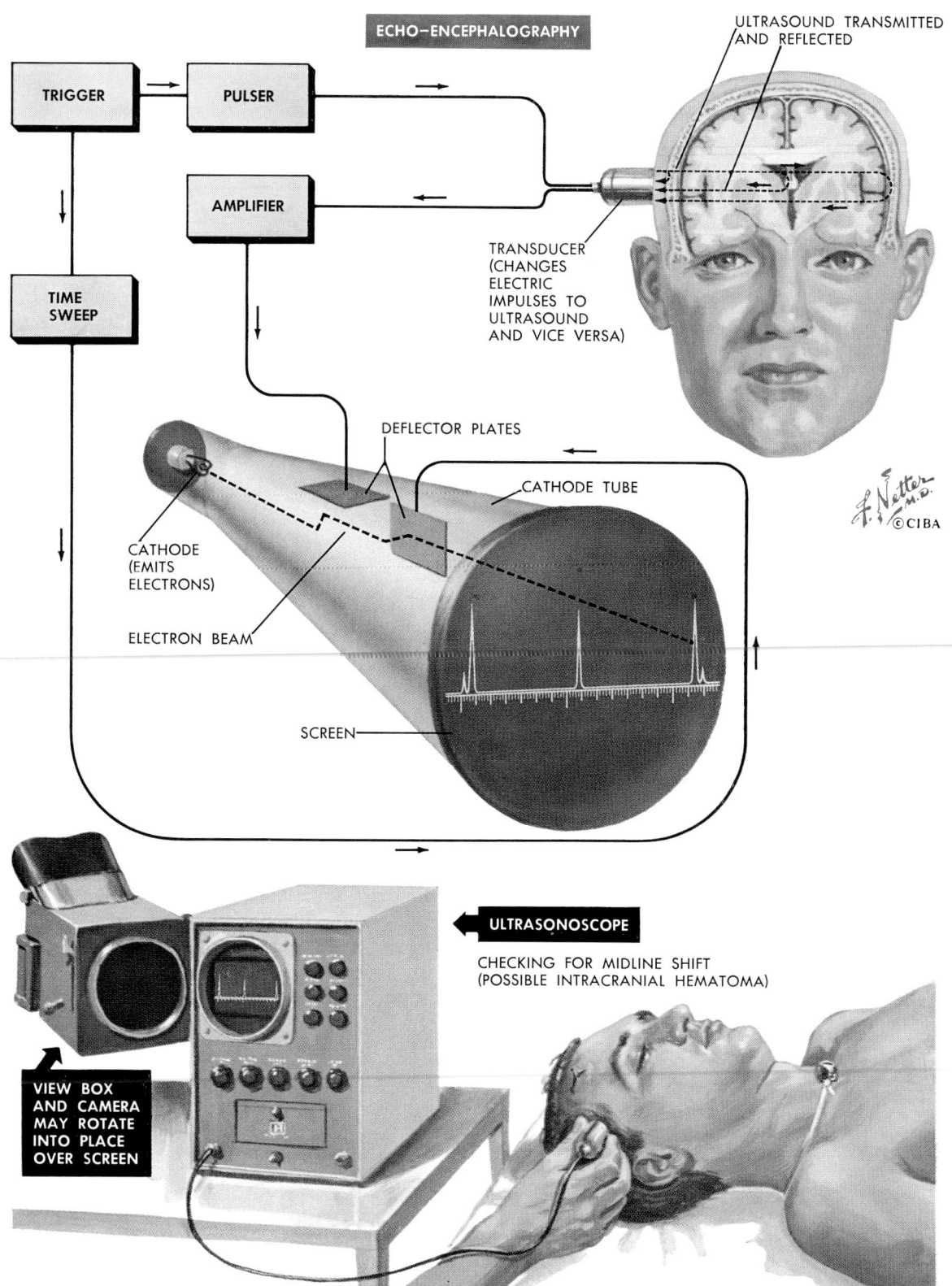

ECHO–ENCEPHALOGRAPHY

TRIGGER → PULSER

AMPLIFIER

TIME SWEEP

ULTRASOUND TRANSMITTED AND REFLECTED

TRANSDUCER (CHANGES ELECTRIC IMPULSES TO ULTRASOUND AND VICE VERSA)

DEFLECTOR PLATES

CATHODE TUBE

CATHODE (EMITS ELECTRONS)

ELECTRON BEAM

SCREEN

ULTRASONOSCOPE

CHECKING FOR MIDLINE SHIFT (POSSIBLE INTRACRANIAL HEMATOMA)

VIEW BOX AND CAMERA MAY ROTATE INTO PLACE OVER SCREEN

F. Netter M.D.
©CIBA

PLATE IV

ECHO–ENCEPHALOGRAPHY FOR DETERMINATION OF MIDLINE SHIFT

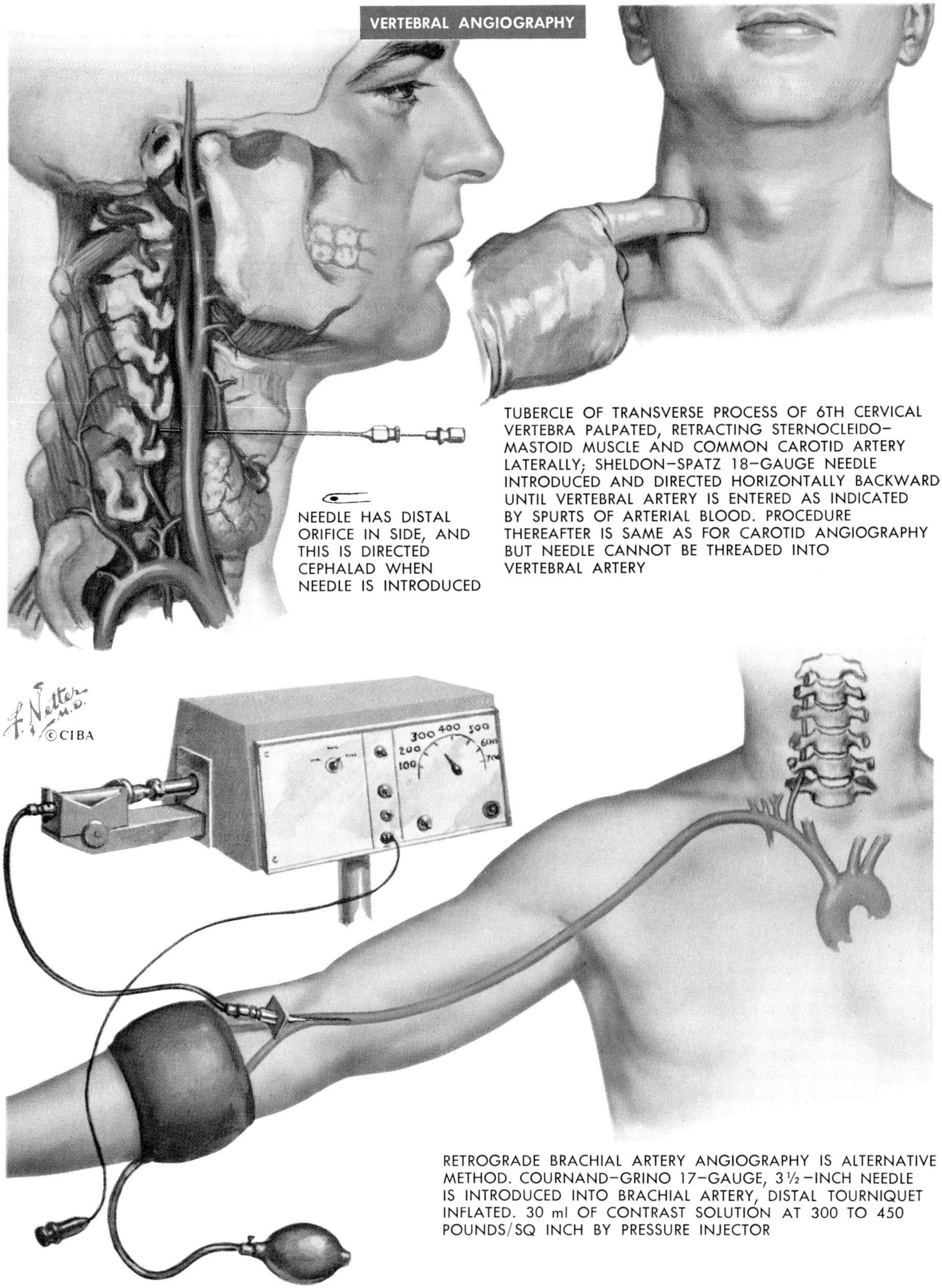
VERTEBRAL ANGIOGRAPHY
TUBERCLE OF TRANSVERSE PROCESS OF 6TH CERVICAL VERTEBRA PALPATED, RETRACTING STERNOCLEIDO-MASTOID MUSCLE AND COMMON CAROTID ARTERY LATERALLY; SHELDON-SPATZ 18-GAUGE NEEDLE INTRODUCED AND DIRECTED HORIZONTALLY BACKWARD UNTIL VERTEBRAL ARTERY IS ENTERED AS INDICATED BY SPURTS OF ARTERIAL BLOOD. PROCEDURE THEREAFTER IS SAME AS FOR CAROTID ANGIOGRAPHY BUT NEEDLE CANNOT BE THREADED INTO VERTEBRAL ARTERY
NEEDLE HAS DISTAL ORIFICE IN SIDE, AND THIS IS DIRECTED CEPHALAD WHEN NEEDLE IS INTRODUCED
F. Netter M.D.
©CIBA
300 400 500
200 600
100 700
RETROGRADE BRACHIAL ARTERY ANGIOGRAPHY IS ALTERNATIVE METHOD. COURNAND-GRINO 17-GAUGE, 3½-INCH NEEDLE IS INTRODUCED INTO BRACHIAL ARTERY, DISTAL TOURNIQUET INFLATED. 30 ml OF CONTRAST SOLUTION AT 300 TO 450 POUNDS/SQ INCH BY PRESSURE INJECTOR

PLATE V

VERTEBRAL ANGIOGRAPHY FOR VISUALIZATION OF POSTERIOR CEREBRAL ARTERY have deferred until now a discussion of those procedures which must always be considered as being ancillary to clinical observation.

X-Ray Examination

When time permits, one would like to have a number of views of the head and neck, x-ray of chest, abdomen, and any extremities suspected of containing fractures. However, in emergency, one should be provided with a minimum of five pictures—an AP and lateral view of the skull, an AP and lateral view of the cervical spine (be sure the shoulders are pulled down as far as possible to visualize C-6 and C-7), and an AP view of the chest.

A fracture line crossing a middle meningeal artery or one of the venous sinuses will alert the physician to the likelihood of life-threatening intracranial hemorrhage. A fracture line reaching the foramen magnum suggests brain stem injury. However, a negative x-ray should never form the basis for complacency, because serious and even fatal brain injury can exist in the absence of any x-ray abnormality.

Spinal Fluid

Examination of the spinal fluid with determination of pressure may be carried out in a patient with head injury. Yet, *in acute stages it rarely provides any useful information.* Moreover, it is potentially dangerous. If an evaluation of spinal fluid and pressure becomes necessary, several precautions should be observed:

1. Use a small bore (22 gauge) needle and never do a Queckenstedt test. This maneuver is designed to determine the presence of blockage along the route of spinal fluid. It involves compressing the jugular veins to see whether the increase in intracranial pressure thus produced will be reflected at the point of spinal tap. In acute head injury, any such artificial increase in pressure may force the cerebellar tonsils into the foramen magnum

with sudden death. An exception to the rule against the Queckenstedt test may be made where there is serious spinal injury with minimal involvement of the head.

2. As a general rule, take off no more fluid than that contained in the manometer. This will be ample for cell count, and removal of a greater amount of fluid will merely invite fatality.

The "curled-up" position in which spinal tap is usually carried out will, of itself, artificially raise cerebrospinal fluid pressure. Therefore, once the needle is in place, the patient should be straightened out by extending his limbs and back. This will usually result in 30 to 40 mm lower pressure than in the curled-up position. The normal spinal fluid pressure varies between 70 and 200. The critical point beyond which it will be impossible to maintain cerebral blood flow is about 600 mm.

Special Tests

The greatest threat to life that is amenable to surgery is intracranial hemorrhage. As discussed in our previous monograph, bleeding may be epidural, where expansion is somewhat circumscribed by the close attachment of dura to skull. Bleeding may be subdural, between dura and arachnoid, where the escaping blood tends to spread broadly over the surface of the brain. This latter type of hemorrhage may be acute with a rapidly fatal outcome unless operated. Or when bleeding is less profuse, a subacute or chronic hematoma may form, with symptoms that come and go and may even be so indefinite as to suggest a long-continuing psychoneurosis. A third type of hemorrhage is intracerebral. Unlike a subdural clot, this type does not tend to significant expansion, but the clot should be removed along with any pulpified brain.

In an acute situation, one must make exploratory burr holes without delay. However, when time permits and doubt exists, echo-encephalography, cerebral angiography, and brain scanning will be of great help in determining the presence and location of a hematoma.

The *echo-encephalogram* is a device to determine whether there has been any shift of midline structures which, in head injury, may indicate a space-occupying hematoma. A pulsed beam of high-frequency sound which is emitted by the transmitter will echo back to be recorded on an oscillographic screen whenever a change in density is encountered (Plate IV). When the transmitter is held against the temple, high spikes are recorded on the left and extreme right of the screen by reflections from the skull and temporal muscles. Midline structures produce a smaller blip. Where there is a displacement of midline structures, by an epidural hemorrhage for example, the central blip will be deflected toward the opposite side. This displacement can then be checked by placing the transmitter against the opposite temple and noting the location of the central blip.

This procedure can be carried out in a couple of minutes without disturbing the patient in any way. It is thus an excellent screening technique for the detection of any pressure-producing lesion, whether it be contusion with swelling or an intracranial hematoma, that will displace the midline structures of the brain.

Angiography: This, the most reliable method for the diagnosis and localization of an intracranial hemorrhage, depends upon visualizing a displacement of cerebral vessels which have been filled with a radiopaque substance.

An epidural hemorrhage in its most frequent location — the temporoparietal region — will often deflect the middle meningeal artery toward the midline. Because of the tenacity with which the dura adheres to the skull, this type of hemorrhage produces a lentil-shaped, inward bulge of the vessels. An epidural hemorrhage on the orbital surface of the frontal lobes will elevate the frontal polar branch of the anterior cerebral artery.

A subdural hematoma, since it tends to spread widely over the surface of the brain, displaces the vessels away from the skull more evenly. Also, if it has been possible to inject both internal and external carotid vessels, the meningeal artery, derived from the external carotid, will be found separated from the middle cerebral artery, a branch of the internal carotid.

Where a hemorrhage, either epidural or subdural, is located in the frontal region, the anterior cerebral vessels are displaced toward the opposite side. Where a hemorrhage is far anterior, there will be a lateral bowing of the anterior cerebral vessels.

Angiography is also helpful in the diagnosis of hemorrhage into the brain tissue, for here too, vessels will be displaced by the accumulation of blood.

Technique: Injection of the contrast medium into the carotid artery is followed by six synchronous AP and lateral x-ray exposures at intervals of 1½ seconds.

A number of techniques of injection have been used and recommended. The method we have found most successful is illustrated in Plates VI and VII.

Vertebral Angiography: Blood supply to the occipital lobes is derived from the posterior cerebral arteries, which are usually supplied from the vertebral arteries via the basilar. Therefore, to visualize the vessels in this area of the brain, it is usually necessary to inject one of the vertebral arteries. This can be accomplished by direct injection of the vertebral artery in the neck or by retrograde injection via the brachial artery in the antecubital space (Plate V). This is accomplished by placing an inflatable cuff on the forearm distal to the artery and injecting the opaque material with a pressure injector utilizing 30 ml of contrast material with a pressure of 300 to 450 psi.

Brain Scanning: In patients not requiring immediate surgery, photoscans follow-

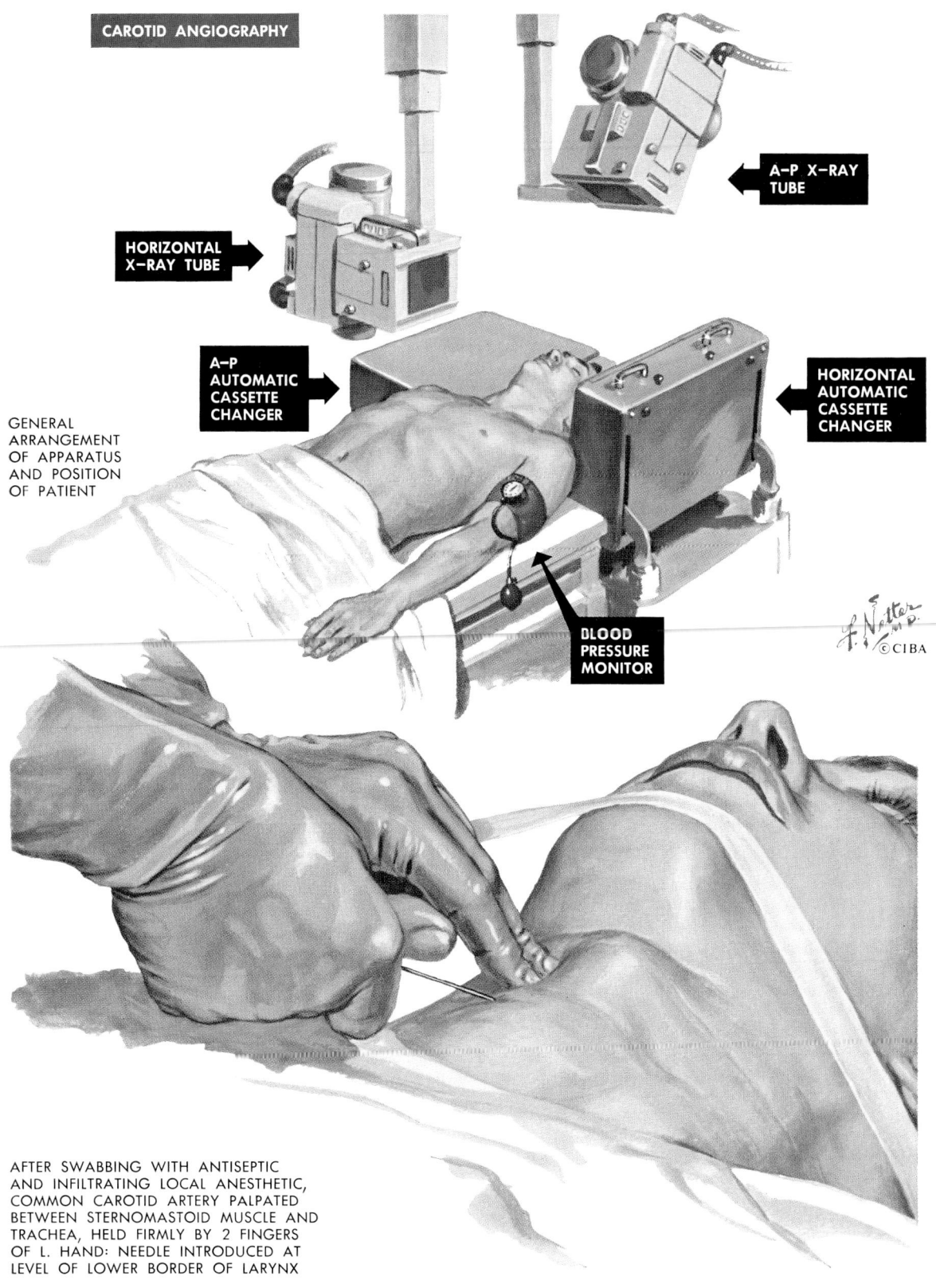

CAROTID ANGIOGRAPHY

A-P X-RAY TUBE

HORIZONTAL X-RAY TUBE

A-P AUTOMATIC CASSETTE CHANGER

HORIZONTAL AUTOMATIC CASSETTE CHANGER

GENERAL ARRANGEMENT OF APPARATUS AND POSITION OF PATIENT

BLOOD PRESSURE MONITOR

AFTER SWABBING WITH ANTISEPTIC AND INFILTRATING LOCAL ANESTHETIC, COMMON CAROTID ARTERY PALPATED BETWEEN STERNOMASTOID MUSCLE AND TRACHEA, HELD FIRMLY BY 2 FINGERS OF L. HAND: NEEDLE INTRODUCED AT LEVEL OF LOWER BORDER OF LARYNX

PLATE VI

TECHNIQUE OF CAROTID ANGIOGRAPHY

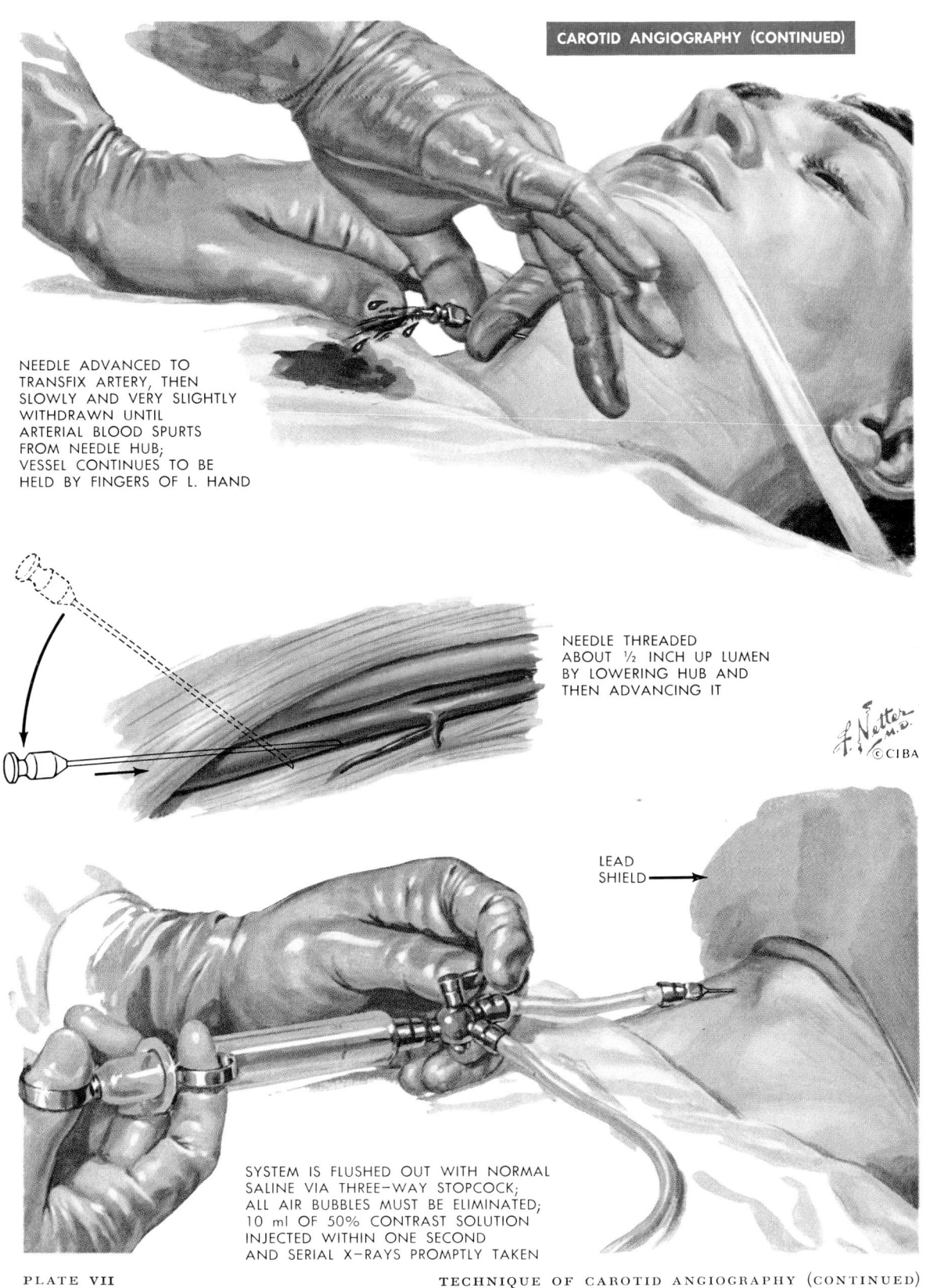

NEEDLE ADVANCED TO
TRANSFIX ARTERY, THEN
SLOWLY AND VERY SLIGHTLY
WITHDRAWN UNTIL
ARTERIAL BLOOD SPURTS
FROM NEEDLE HUB;
VESSEL CONTINUES TO BE
HELD BY FINGERS OF L. HAND

NEEDLE THREADED
ABOUT ½ INCH UP LUMEN
BY LOWERING HUB AND
THEN ADVANCING IT

LEAD
SHIELD ➤

SYSTEM IS FLUSHED OUT WITH NORMAL
SALINE VIA THREE—WAY STOPCOCK;
ALL AIR BUBBLES MUST BE ELIMINATED;
10 ml OF 50% CONTRAST SOLUTION
INJECTED WITHIN ONE SECOND
AND SERIAL X—RAYS PROMPTLY TAKEN

RAPID NEUROLOGIC EVALUATION OF CRANIAL NERVE FUNCTION

NERVE	FREQUENCY	SITES OF INVOLVEMENT	TESTS	ABNORMAL FINDINGS
I OLFACTORY	Uncommon	Fracture of cribriform plate or in ethmoid area	Apply simple odors such as peppermint to one nostril at a time	Anosmia
II OPTIC	Common	Direct trauma to orbit or globe, or fracture involving optic foramen	Light flashed in affected eye	Loss of both direct and consensual pupillary constriction
			Light flashed in normal eye	Direct and consensual pupillary constriction
	Common	Pressure on geniculocalcarine tract. Laceration or intracerebral clot in temporal, parietal, or occipital lobes (rarely from subdural clot)	Bring hand suddenly toward eye from the side	Absence of the blink reflex indicates a visual field defect (always homonymous)
III OCULOMOTOR	Very frequent	Pressure of herniating uncus on nerve just before it enters cavernous sinus or fracture involving cavernous sinus		Dilated pupil, ptosis, eye turns down and out
			Light flashed in affected eye	Direct pupil reflex absent. Consensual reflex present
			Light flashed in normal eye	Direct pupil reflex present. Consensual reflex absent
IV TROCHLEAR	Infrequent	Course of nerve around brain stem or fracture of orbit	Isolated involvement requires special equipment	Eye fails to move down and out
V TRIGEMINAL	Uncommon	Direct injury to terminal branches, particularly 2nd division in roof of maxillary sinus	Sensation: 1st division: Above eye and cornea 2nd division: Upper lip 3rd division: Lower lip and chin	Loss of sensation of pain and touch. Paresthesias
			Motor Function: "Bite down" or "Chew"	Palpated masseter and temporalis fail to contract
VI ABDUCENS	Quite frequent	Base of brain as nerve enters clivus. Fracture involving cavernous sinus or orbit	"Look to the right — Look to the left"	Affected eye fails to move laterally. Diplopia on lateral gaze

		Peripheral: Laceration or contusion in parotid region		Eye remains open. Angle of mouth droops. Forehead fails to wrinkle
VII FACIAL	Frequent	Peripheral: Fracture of temporal bone		As above plus associated involvement of acoustic nerve (see below) and chorda tympani (dry cornea and loss of taste on ipsilateral ⅔ of tongue)
	Frequent	Supranuclear: Intracerebral clot	"Wrinkle your forehead"	Forehead wrinkles because of bilateral innervation of frontalis. Otherwise paralysis of facial muscles as above
VIII ACOUSTIC	Common	Fractures of petrous portion of temporal bone. Seventh nerve also often involved	In children and uncooperative patients, slap hands close to ear	Startle reflex
			Weber Test: Tuning fork middle of forehead	Sound not heard by involved ear
IX GLOSSO-PHARYNGEAL	Rare	Brain stem or deep laceration of neck	Motor power of stylopharyngeus — impractical to test	Loss of taste posterior one-third of tongue
			Cotton applicator to soft palate	Loss of sensation on affected side of soft palate
X VAGUS	Rare	Brain stem or deep laceration of neck	Inspection of soft palate. Laryngoscopy	Sagging of soft palate; deviation of uvula to normal side. Hoarseness from paralysis of vocal cord
XI SPINAL ACCESSORY	Rare	Laceration of neck	Hand on side of chin: "Push your chin against my hand"	Palpated sternocleidomastoid fails to contract
			"Shrug your shoulders"	Palpated upper fibers of trapezius fail to contract
			"Stretch out your hands toward me"	Affected arm seems longer (scapula not "anchored")
XII HYPOGLOSSAL	Rare	Neck laceration usually associated with major vessel damage	"Stick your tongue out"	Tongue protrudes toward affected side. Dysarthria

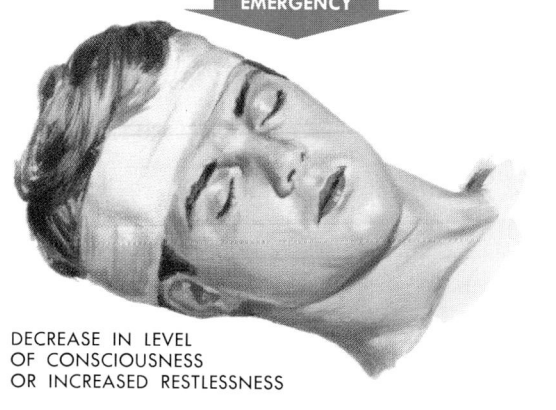

DECREASE IN LEVEL
OF CONSCIOUSNESS
OR INCREASED RESTLESSNESS

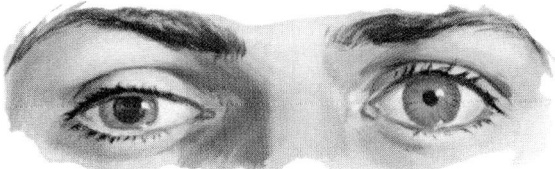

DEVELOPMENT OF UNILATERAL PUPIL DILATATION
AND/OR OCULAR PALSY

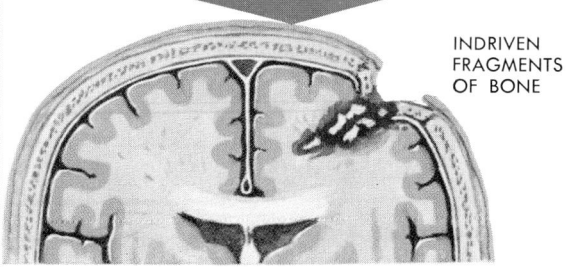

INDRIVEN
FRAGMENTS
OF BONE

"PING–PONG BALL"
DEPRESSION OF
SKULL IN AN
INFANT

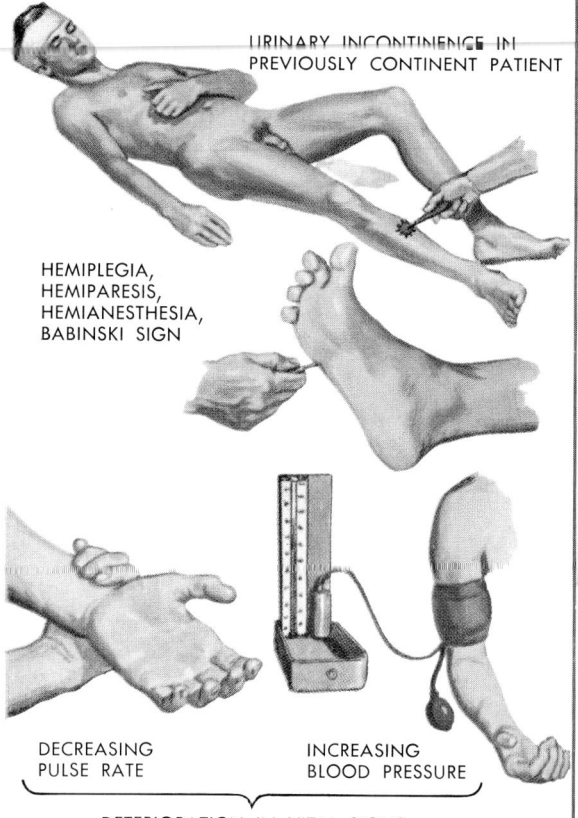

URINARY INCONTINENCE IN
PREVIOUSLY CONTINENT PATIENT

HEMIPLEGIA,
HEMIPARESIS,
HEMIANESTHESIA,
BABINSKI SIGN

DECREASING
PULSE RATE

INCREASING
BLOOD PRESSURE

DETERIORATION IN VITAL SIGNS

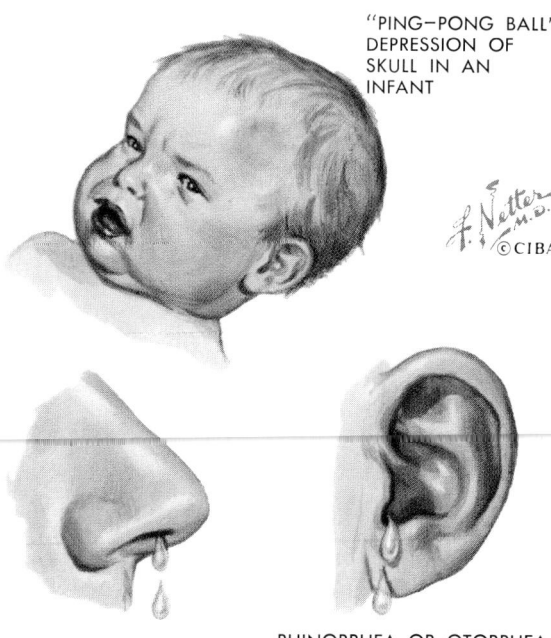

RHINORRHEA OR OTORRHEA;
PERSISTENT OR RECURRENT

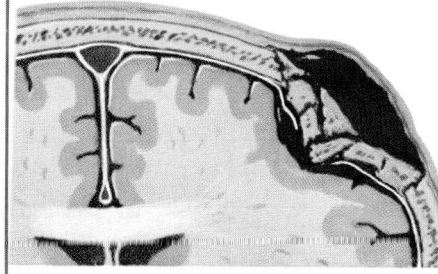

FRACTURE
DEPRESSED
MORE THAN
½ THICKNESS
OF SKULL

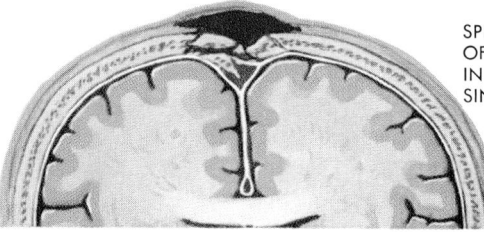

SPICULE
OF BONE
IN VENOUS
SINUS

PLATE VIII   SIGNS SUGGESTING NEED FOR OPERATION

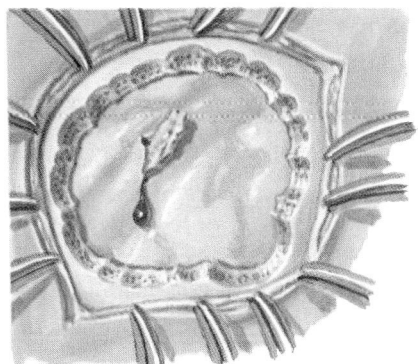

SPICULE OF BONE IN SUPERIOR
SAGITTAL SINUS

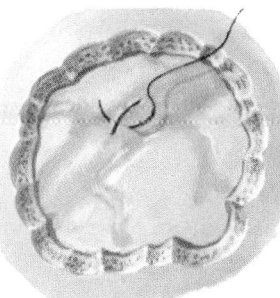

DIRECT SUTURE OF SMALL
TEAR IN SINUS WITH
6-0 SILK EYE SUTURES

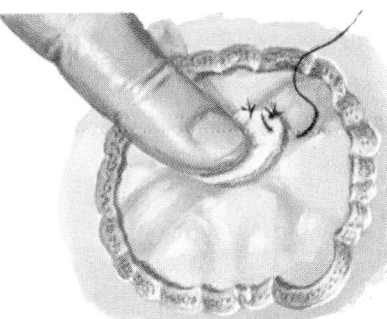

REPAIR OF LARGER SINUS TEAR BY
OVERSEWING GELFOAM OR MUSCLE;
MUSCLE MAY BE ACTUALLY INSERTED
IN SINUS WHICH RECANALIZES

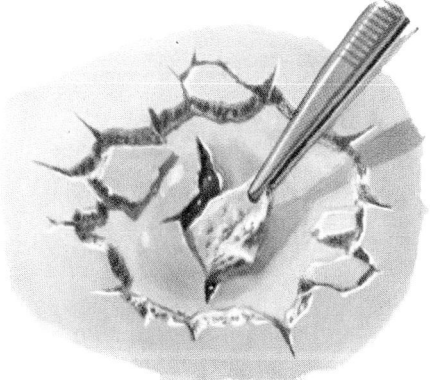

COMPOUND DEPRESSED SKULL FRACTURE;
ELEVATION AND REMOVAL OF FRAGMENTS

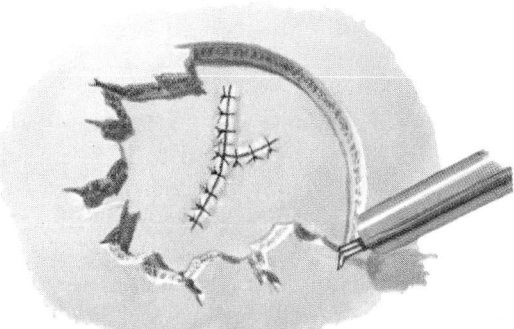

MARGINS OF FRACTURE SMOOTHED AND
ROUNDED BY TURBOBIT; DURA SUTURED

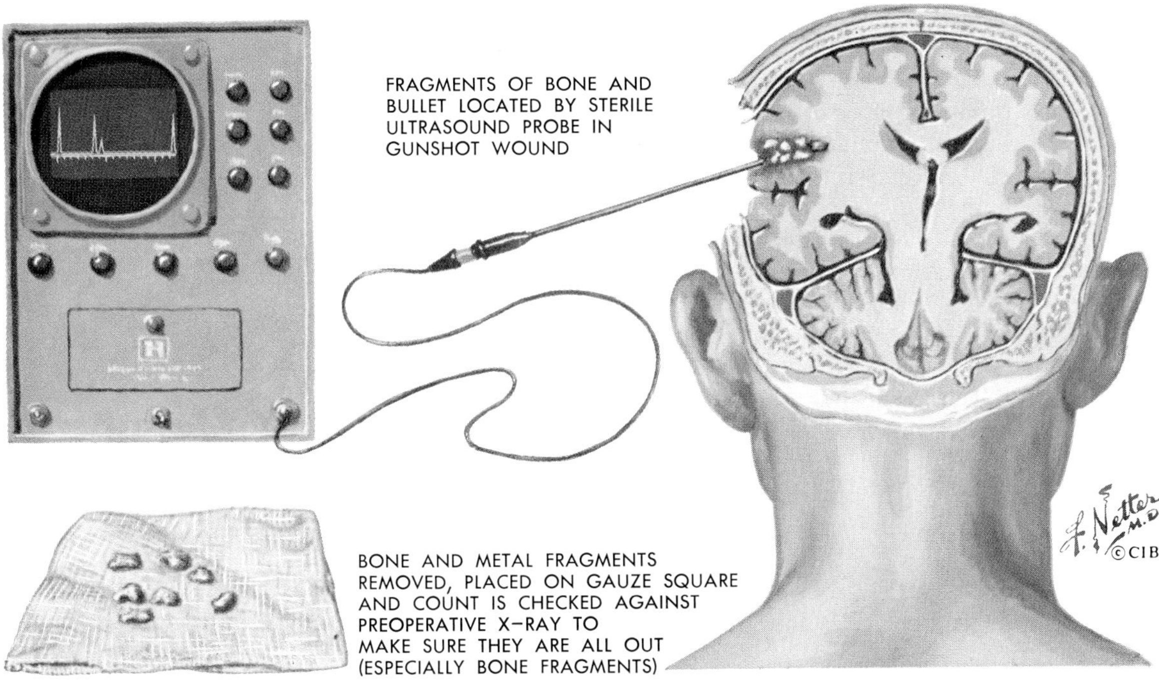

FRAGMENTS OF BONE AND
BULLET LOCATED BY STERILE
ULTRASOUND PROBE IN
GUNSHOT WOUND

BONE AND METAL FRAGMENTS
REMOVED, PLACED ON GAUZE SQUARE
AND COUNT IS CHECKED AGAINST
PREOPERATIVE X-RAY TO
MAKE SURE THEY ARE ALL OUT
(ESPECIALLY BONE FRAGMENTS)

PLATE IX

ADDITIONAL INDICATIONS FOR EARLY OPERATION: SINUS TEARS,
COMPOUND DEPRESSED FRACTURES, AND PENETRATING WOUNDS

ing the injection of radioactive isotopes have given accurate results in the diagnosis and localization of subdural and intracerebral hematomas.

An *electroencephalogram* is rarely helpful clinically in an acute case. In a subacute subdural hematoma, brain waves may show unilateral depression of electrical activity or, occasionally, slow waves underlying the hematoma. Localization of the hematoma is not completely dependable, however, because not infrequently the brain wave abnormalities will be greater on the opposite side.

DISPOSITION OF PATIENTS

Patients who, after thorough evaluation, are deemed to have minimal head injury may be discharged with instructions that they be aroused at two-hour intervals for several nights following the head injury. This will assure early recognition of those cases having intracranial hemorrhage after minor injury.

Those patients having more severe head injuries should be transferred to a hospital where an experienced staff is available, equipped to handle all of the possible complications and sequelae.

To assure the seriously injured patient the best chance of safe arrival, he should be accompanied by a trained attendant equipped with suction apparatus, an intubation tube, and a mechanical respirator so that pressure respiration can be given in the event of respiratory difficulty.

CARE OF THE UNCONSCIOUS PATIENT

The seriously head-injured patient may remain unconscious for days, weeks, or even months. During the period of unconsciousness, normally protective mechanisms like the cough reflex may be absent. In such patients, the degree of ultimate rehabilitation, and even life itself, must depend on meticulous attention to many details of nursing care and medical supervision.

Need for Frequent Reevaluation

Patients with head injury who are apparently stabilized may still deteriorate rapidly over a period of only a few hours. Therefore, they should be examined medically several times a day as a minimum and should have continuous nursing care. Pulse, respiration, and blood pressure should be taken at intervals of 15 minutes for the first 4 hours and every half hour thereafter. Temperature should be taken every 2 hours.

A physician should be notified immediately if there is any deterioration in the patient's state of consciousness, if the pulse goes below 60 or above 120, or if the blood pressure goes below 100 or above 160 systolic. Of all the indications for medical reevaluation, the state of consciousness is the most important. *If one waits for an alteration in vital signs, one may have already waited too long.*

INTRAVENOUS THERAPY

Patients immobilized over long periods have a marked tendency to develop thrombophlebitis, the incidence of which is 20 times greater in the lower extremities than in the upper extremities. Therefore, one should always use an upper extremity for intravenous fluids. Also, if possible, one should avoid the antecubital space which will necessitate fixation of the arm on a board. If the intravenous catheter is inserted in a vein of the forearm or wrist, immobilization becomes unnecessary.

Fluid and Electrolyte Requirements

Both overhydration (water intoxication) and dehydration can produce symptoms indistinguishable from those of head injury. If both of these are to be avoided, one must keep an accurate record of intake and output. Also, it is helpful to recall the usual effect of head injury on water and electrolytes.

Following cerebral trauma, a positive balance of both sodium and water persists for two to four days. Thus, despite the reduced urine volume, incident to the water retention, one should not administer fluids in larger quantity than that necessary to meet daily needs. To do so would be to invite water intoxication with signs and symptoms that might easily be confused with those of head injury: unconsciousness, delirium, coma with convulsions, and increased intracranial pressure. These symptoms, due to cellular overhydration, may be produced by a positive water balance of 3 to 4 liters per day. (They may be relieved by hypertonic saline or more slowly by water restriction.)

Retention of water is somewhat greater than that of sodium, so there is a moderate hyponatremia, the sodium concentration of the blood rarely going below 130 mEq/L. Since sodium stores are already high, this is *not* an indication to administer extra salt.

Dehydration, once recommended in the hope of reducing cerebral edema, will reduce blood volume, stimulate aldosterone secretion, and increase salt retention, thus increasing the hypernatremia induced by dehydration — a vicious cycle.

For maintenance after shock has been controlled, fluid intake for the first three or four days should be limited to 1,500 ml (plus any extrarenal losses). Since extra salt is unnecessary and even contraindicated, only 500 ml is given as normal salt solution (containing 5 percent dextrose). The remaining 1,000 ml is given as 5 percent dextrose in water.

After the first 3 or 4 days, when the urinary output begins to increase, intake of both salt and water is liberalized. 1,000 ml of 5 percent dextrose in normal saline is augmented by 1,500 ml of 5 percent dextrose in water to make a total of 2,500 ml of water with 4.5 Gm of salt daily.

It must be emphasized that the intake just mentioned is in addition to extrarenal losses, which include cerebrospinal rhinorrhea or otorrhea and loss by perspiration, which is particularly important in children, and when there is fever.

Also, one must be aware of the additional fluid loss that is brought about by feeding a high protein diet during the catabolic phase (see below). During this phase, protein cannot be utilized; therefore, it must be excreted along with an appropriate amount of water.

It is most important to anticipate the tremendous outpouring of urine that will follow the intravenous injection of urea or mannitol given to reduce cerebral edema (see page 31). Especially in infants, the great augmentation of urine flow can lead to hypovolemia and circulatory collapse unless the fluid loss is promptly replaced.

Perhaps the most common cause of difficulty with fluid balance is failure to keep an *accurate* record of intake and output. The phrase "taking fluids well" is meaningless and may be dangerously misleading.

Nitrogen Balance

Head injury is always followed by a variable period of negative nitrogen balance during which period catabolism exceeds anabolism. The average nitrogen loss, which has no correlation with the severity of injury, amounts to about 8 to 10 Gm per day. This indicates a loss of about 300 Gm of muscle mass daily, is not influenced by caloric intake, and very little affected by increasing the protein intake.

Blood

The importance of blood in the treatment of shock is universally recognized. Sometimes overlooked, however, is the importance of a satisfactory hematocrit in later stages of head injury. Not least in this latter respect, is the oxygen-carrying power of the blood, which is directly pro-

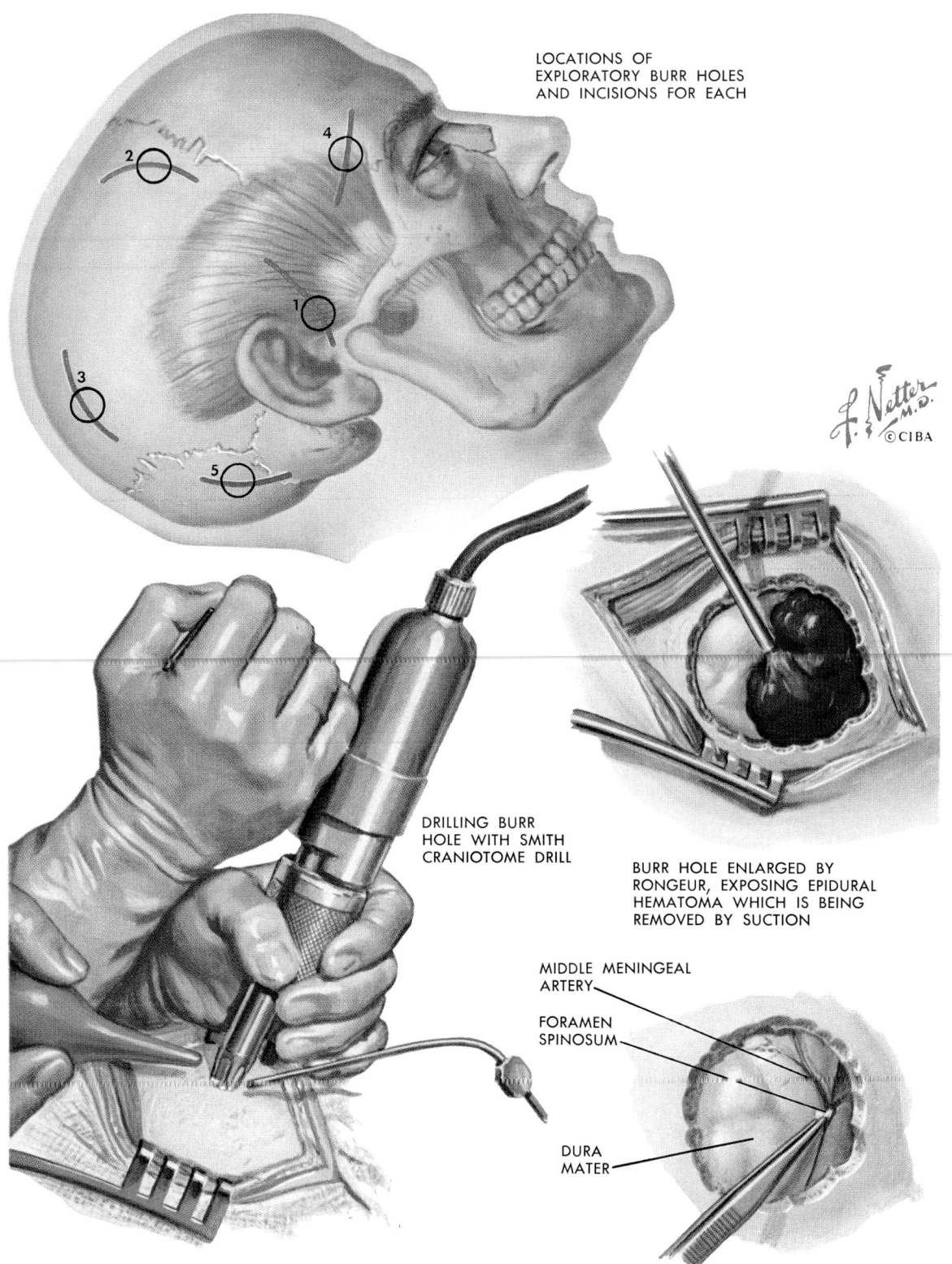

LOCATIONS OF
EXPLORATORY BURR HOLES
AND INCISIONS FOR EACH

DRILLING BURR
HOLE WITH SMITH
CRANIOTOME DRILL

BURR HOLE ENLARGED BY
RONGEUR, EXPOSING EPIDURAL
HEMATOMA WHICH IS BEING
REMOVED BY SUCTION

MIDDLE MENINGEAL
ARTERY

FORAMEN
SPINOSUM

DURA
MATER

PACKING FORAMEN SPINOSUM

PLATE X EXPLORATORY BURR HOLES AND REMOVAL OF MIDDLE FOSSA HEMATOMA

portional to the amount of hemoglobin contained. Indeed, when the hemoglobin is reduced to 10 grams percent, a 95 percent oxygen saturation would be equivalent only to a 63 percent oxygen saturation if the hemoglobin were a normal 15 grams percent!

GASTRIC FEEDING

Feeding by nasal tube can be started as soon as bowel sounds return — usually in about 48 hours. Once the tube is in place, the stomach should be aspirated. This should be repeated before each feeding in order to make sure there is no gastric retention.

Gastric feeding is started with 10 percent dextrose and water, given in a quantity of 50 ml every hour or 100 ml every 2 hours. This supplementation of intravenous fluids minus any fluid that has been aspirated from the stomach must, of course, be taken into account in estimating intake and output.

On the second day of nasal feeding, skim milk is added and given at the same rate and frequency. The following day, blenderized baby food may be given and a protein-containing supplement added.

The aim is to give about 3,000 calories per day. During the first 4 or 5 days, about 100 Gm of protein is given. After the catabolic phase has passed, the protein intake can be increased to 400 Gm per day in a patient of average adult weight.

In addition, an anabolic steroid given orally or parenterally to combat the negative nitrogen balance, and multiple vitamins, including several hundred mg of ascorbic acid, should be administered daily starting on the fifth day.

To avoid the possibility of pressure ulceration of the nasal mucosa covering turbinates and septum, the nasal tube should be brought laterally downward from the nose and maintained in that position by adhesive tape.

NURSING CARE

1. *Position of the Patient:* While unconscious and deprived of his cough reflex, the patient must never be allowed to lie continuously on his back, for there is no surer way to invite the onset of a fatal respiratory complication. Therefore, except in those cases of less severe head injury, where return of consciousness and recovery of the cough reflex are soon to be expected, a patient with a combination of severe head injury and a fractured femur should have intramedullary nailing of the bone or be placed in a 1½ hip plaster spica which will permit rolling from side to side.

The patient in coma should spend one-third of his time on each side, one-third of his time on his back — night and day. While on his side, he will be more comfortable with a pillow between his knees, one under his head, and one behind his back. To avoid contractures, all joints should be moved through their entire range of motion daily.

2. Where a *tracheostomy tube* has been inserted, the inner cannula should be removed and cleansed every four hours. Intratracheal suction should be used as necessary for aspiration of excess secretions or blood. Whenever there is the slightest question about respiratory insufficiency, intermittent positive-pressure breathing should be carried out for 5 minutes every one-half hour or 10 minutes every hour.

Whether or not oxygen should be added for its vasoconstrictive effect or CO_2 added for its vasodilatation and respiratory stimulation is controversial. Room air contains these gases in a physiological mixture, and it is certainly true that supplemental administration of oxygen cannot be considered an adequate substitute for the alveolar filling that is encouraged by the use of positive-pressure respiration. To counteract the drying effect of room air in the bronchi and bronchioles, the air should be moisturized with a humidifier.

Body Temperature: The elevation of temperature that accompanies head injury can usually be controlled quite well by keeping the patient nude except for a bikini, employing a fan to maintain a movement of air, and alcohol rubs with massage of the muscles to bring blood to the surface where it may be cooled. If the temperature is over 100° rectally, aspirin 0.6 Gm can be given by rectum every 3 hours as required, but will have little effect unless accompanied by the measures just described.

Hypothermia, with maintenance of body temperature between 28.5° and 30° C (83° and 86° F), is best employed early (within the first 8 hours) and in young patients with severe injuries.

However, hypothermia may mask the signs of infection, such as pneumonia or meningitis, as well as those of an advancing surgical lesion. Therefore, it is best employed in those cases in which such complications have been reasonably ruled out, or after craniotomy.

Restlessness may be a sign of fracture, full bladder, fecal impaction, or increasing intracranial pressure. Therefore, it is an indication for careful reappraisal. It is *not* an indication for restraint. To tie a patient down may save the nurse but lose the patient!

From the standpoint of medication, chlorpromazine 25 mg can be given at intervals of 2 hours as needed. Paraldehyde 6 ml can be given by rectum or deeply into the gluteal muscle. If there is pain, 32 mg codeine may be given, but *not* morphine. This latter drug constricts the pupils, thus tending to mask a most important neurologic sign. It also deepens coma, and it depresses respiration — three excellent reasons for interdicting its use.

Bowels should be evacuated every other day. This can usually be accomplished by use of a suppository or mild laxative. Fecal impaction must be avoided. There-fore, if necessary, a small enema containing a hypertonic solution of sodium phosphate may be used.

The *mouth* should be kept clean, the teeth brushed twice daily.

The *indwelling catheter*, which is so necessary to provide a dry bed and avoid bladder distention, invites urinary infection. Therefore, while the catheter is in place, we would recommend an antibacterial agent containing a sulfa having high solubility, alternated at intervals of two weeks with a nitrofuran.

The *eyes* demand attention, particularly where there is facial weakness. Whenever the eyes tend to remain open, the cornea will become dried and ulcerated. This may be prevented by instilling a few drops of an ophthalmic solution every 2 hours, with or without an antibiotic. If the eyes are likely to remain open longer than a day or so, the lids can be temporarily sutured together.

In the absence of normal moisture, *contact lenses* may adhere to the cornea causing ulceration. Therefore, they should be removed.

INDICATIONS FOR OPERATION

Early (but not emergency) operation is indicated by: 1. A fracture depressed more than one-half the thickness of the skull. 2. A Ping-Pong ball depression in an infant. 3. Persistent or recurrent rhinorrhea or otorrhea. 4. Indriven fragments of bone. 5. A spicule of bone lodged in a major sinus (Plates VIII and IX).

Emergency operation must be considered with any of the following conditions: 1. Decrease in the level of consciousness. 2. Unilateral dilatation of the pupil. 3. Hemiplegia or hemiparesis. 4. Hemianesthesia. 5. Deterioration in vital signs, particularly decreasing pulse rate with increasing blood pressure (Plate VIII).

If signs of neurological decompensation are developing gradually, there is usually time for angiography, carried out in the hope of revealing and localizing an intracerebral, subdural, or epidural hematoma. But if there is rapid progression, it may be necessary to operate immediately. If an angiogram cannot be taken or is unrevealing, one must depend on surgical exploration to disclose the pathology.

SURGICAL EXPLORATION

In those cases where deepening of unconsciousness or changes in vital signs previously discussed under "Neurologic Evaluation" indicate that the patient's condition is deteriorating too rapidly to allow time for angiography or even echoencephalography, the only course open is immediate surgical exploration.

Localizing signs can never be completely relied upon. Therefore, one cannot consider an exploration as being complete until either the responsible hematoma has been discovered or *at least* three burr holes have been made on each side. In some cases, it may be necessary also to trephine in the subfrontal and occipital regions before terminating the exploration.

In preparation for bilateral trephination, the patient is placed on a Light-Vealy headrest, which permits exposure of both sides without change of position.

The lines of incision and location of prospective burr holes are marked on the scalp, which is then prepared with an antiseptic solution such as Betadine and covered with a transparent plastic drape to maintain sterility.

When symptoms suggest a temporal pressure cone, the first incision is made just above the zygomatic arch, and within a finger's breadth of the ear to avoid branches of the facial nerve. The incision curves anteriorly upward so that it can be continued to meet the second incision if a flap must be turned (Plate X).

The temporalis muscle is incised in the long axis of the muscle fibers which are then retracted laterally, exposing the squamous portion of the temporal bone. A trephine opening is then made with a burr that will not injure the underlying dura. This opening, which we will call No. 1 for purposes of identification, exposes the floor of the middle fossa. It will reveal the presence of an epidural hemorrhage beneath the temporal lobe, if one is present. If not, the dura is opened in search of a subdural hemorrhage.

The next step is enlargement of the burr hole by rongeur to obtain exposure for inspection of the temporal lobe, exploration beneath the temporal lobe, or to pack the foramen spinosum for the arrest of middle meningeal hemorrhage.

If this initial opening fails to reveal the cause of increased pressure or does not permit removal of enough clotted blood, a second trephine opening is made directly toward the vertex and 5 cm from the midline. This skin incision is curved as shown in Plate X so that it can be extended if a flap is to be turned. A burr hole is made.

A third burr hole is then made 8 cm above the inion and 3 cm from the midline.

When these three openings have failed to reveal a hemorrhage, similar burr holes should be made in the already prepared contralateral side. Also, when symptoms, location of fractures, or external evidence of trauma suggest it, trephine exploration is carried out in the occipital region or beneath the frontal lobe. *We have never been sorry to have made additional burr holes; often sorry we did not!*

Exploration in the frontal region is carried out through a burr hole made just above the supraorbital margin of the frontal bone. This opening, which we will identify as burr hole 4, provides access to the orbital surface of the frontal bone just beneath the frontal lobe.

Exploration of the posterior fossa is made through a trephine opening which we will call 5. It is made 3 centimeters below and 3 centimeters lateral to the inion.

It has been shown experimentally that a single burr hole, or even multiple burr holes, will not reduce intracranial pressure. Instead, the tense underlying brain will simply bulge into the opening, creating necrotizing pressure at the edges. Therefore, when increased intracranial pressure persists and the multiple burr holes previously described have failed to reveal a correctable lesion, one may make a large opening (in severe cases bilaterally) to allow room for expansion of the compressed edematous brain. In those cases where epidural and subdural hemorrhage have been ruled out and intravenous urea or mannitol has failed to control elevated intracranial pressure, surgical decompression can be a lifesaving procedure.

Technique

The temporal burr hole above the zygomatic arch, which has been previously described, is enlarged by rongeur until an area approximately 8 cm by 8 cm has been removed. The dura is incised in a stellate fashion, the lines of incision having first been coagulated to decrease the possibility of bleeding.

The wound is then irrigated with Bacitracin solution 50,000 units/100 ml after which the muscle is sutured and the galea closed with 3-0 inverted mattress sutures. The skin is closed with .005 stainless steel wire.

In extreme cases requiring even greater decompression, the anterior 5 cm of the temporal lobe *on the nondominant side* may be removed. This is particularly desirable in those cases where contusion has caused maceration of brain tissue in this area. Indeed, pulpified necrotic brain had best be removed wherever found.

After surgical decompression has been performed, spinal tap to reduce the increased pressure by one-half can be carried out daily or every other day without fear of herniation of the hippocampus. Also, it may be necessary to give intravenous urea, mannitol, or adrenal corticoids to help control the edema. It has been our practice to use intravenous urea during the first 48 hours. Corticoids are given for edema, starting before the patient leaves the table and continuing thereafter for 5 to 7 days as needed. After recovery, the defect in the temporal bone may be plated.

REMOVAL OF AN EPIDURAL HEMATOMA

The most frequent cause of epidural hemorrhage is rupture of the middle meningeal artery *in the middle fossa.* This is usually, but not invariably, caused by a fracture line that crosses the course of the vessel.

Where this type of hematoma is present, as determined by angiography or located by surgical exploration through burr hole No. 1 previously described, the opening is enlarged to about 8 cm in diameter, as in a subtemporal decompression.

Through this opening the hematoma can be removed and the bleeding controlled by ligation or by packing the foramen spinosum from which the middle meningeal artery emerges.

An epidural hemorrhage can also occur *in the parietal region,* usually from rupture of a diploic vein. In this location, the clot is almost impossible to remove completely by irrigation. Therefore, to reduce operative time and eliminate uncertainty about complete removal, it is usually best to turn a flap. This can be accomplished quickly and easily by use of a turbobit craniotome,* which is powered by compressed CO_2, will not cut soft tissue, and will make it possible to complete the skull opening within a minute or two.

First, the skin incisions already de-

---

*Available from Midas Rex Pneumatic Tools, 2929 Race Street, Fort Worth, Texas 76111.

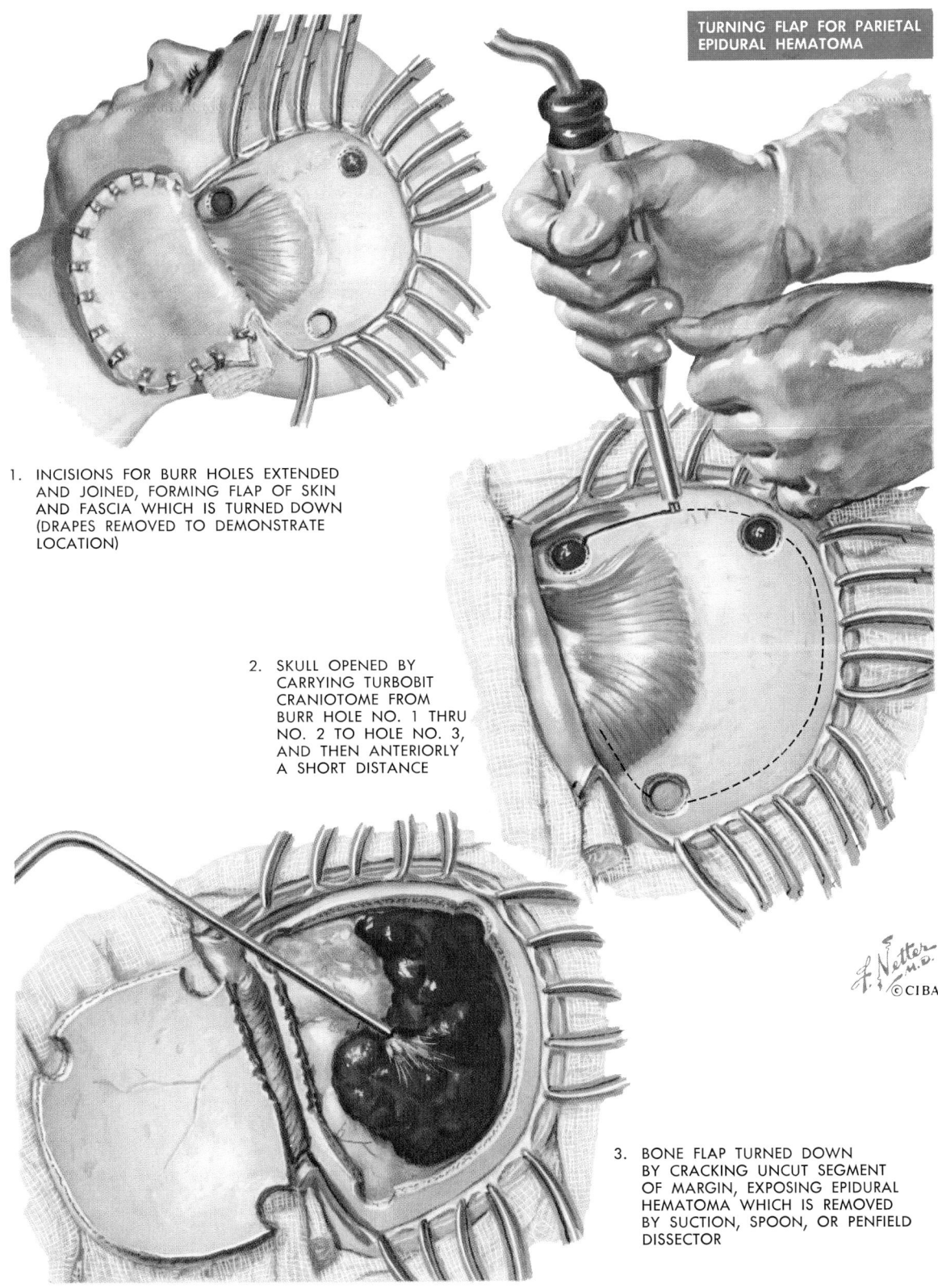

1. INCISIONS FOR BURR HOLES EXTENDED
   AND JOINED, FORMING FLAP OF SKIN
   AND FASCIA WHICH IS TURNED DOWN
   (DRAPES REMOVED TO DEMONSTRATE
   LOCATION)

2. SKULL OPENED BY
   CARRYING TURBOBIT
   CRANIOTOME FROM
   BURR HOLE NO. 1 THRU
   NO. 2 TO HOLE NO. 3,
   AND THEN ANTERIORLY
   A SHORT DISTANCE

3. BONE FLAP TURNED DOWN
   BY CRACKING UNCUT SEGMENT
   OF MARGIN, EXPOSING EPIDURAL
   HEMATOMA WHICH IS REMOVED
   BY SUCTION, SPOON, OR PENFIELD
   DISSECTOR

PLATE XI   OPERATION FOR PARIETAL EPIDURAL HEMATOMA

scribed as being made over the location of the three burr holes are extended as shown in Plate XI. Then the skull is opened by guiding the craniotome from burr hole 1 through burr hole 2 to burr hole 3, and then a short distance anteriorly. The flap of bone is then bent downward to break along a line as shown in Plate XI.

Beneath the frontal lobes, hemorrhage is caused by rupture of one of the anterior ethmoidal arteries. Since these vessels are relatively small, symptoms tend to develop rather slowly. When a hematoma has been demonstrated by angiogram or by burr hole No. 4, a frontal flap is turned. This is accomplished as follows: Starting at hole No. 4, which has been made just above the supraorbital margin of the frontal bone, the turbobit is carried transversely toward the midline just above the frontal sinuses. (Where these sinuses are unusually large and cannot be avoided, they may be entered without fear of infection if the contained mucous membrane is removed.) The turbobit is then turned upward just short of the midline to a point above the hairline, from whence it curves laterally and then downward to terminate just in front of the ear (Plate XII). The flap is then bent downward as shown in Plate XII, exposing the frontal lobe unilaterally and providing exposure for removal of the hematoma and control of the bleeding vessel if necessary.

In the posterior fossa, an epidural hemorrhage is to be suspected when there is external evidence of trauma in that area, particularly with a linear fracture of the occipital bone and if papilledema is present. With these symptoms, burr hole No. 5 is made 3 cm below and 3 cm lateral to the inion. With hemorrhage in the posterior fossa, another exploratory burr hole may be made 2 cm *above* and 2 cm lateral to the inion to rule out an associated epidural clot above the tentorium (Plate XII).

Over the sagittal sinus, an epidural hem-orrhage is usually caused by a spicule of bone penetrating the sinus. Surgical treatment of this condition consists of removing the spicule of bone and repairing the sinus. (Following penetration of a venous sinus by bone, the continuity of the sinus must always be preserved if possible. However, in the anterior one-half of the sagittal sinus, ligation can be carried out with relative impunity, although the risk of neurologic damage increases as you approach the vertex.)

At operation, bone is removed to provide proximal and distal exposure and control of the sinus before the penetrating spicule is dislodged. If possible, the sinus tear is repaired by simple suture. If loss of tissue has occurred, the opening must be closed with transplanted fascia. In order to control venous bleeding, it may also be necessary to utilize tamponade with gelfoam or muscle (Plate IX).

REMOVAL OF SUBDURAL HEMATOMA

In contrast to the localized bulging of an epidural clot, a subdural hematoma tends to spread over the surface of the brain. A very recent hemorrhage appears as a reddish liquid, consisting of blood and spinal fluid. After 24 hours, the blood begins to clot, becoming thicker and jelly-like. This thickened consistency usually makes complete removal by irrigation through burr holes impossible. Therefore, one must turn a flap.

After 5 to 7 days, the clot begins to break down and change to the color and consistency of crankcase oil. Still later, as pigment is absorbed, the liquid becomes lighter and more xanthochromic.

After a while, the clot begins to organize, forming an outer membrane which is tough, thick, and avascular and an inner membrane, which is thin and filamentous. The thick portion of the membrane is derived from the dura; the thin part is derived from the arachnoid. After organization has occurred, it is necessary to remove at least 90 percent of the membrane.

MEDICAL MEASURES TO CONTROL INCREASED INTRACRANIAL PRESSURE

The brain, like other tissues subjected to trauma, becomes edematous. Being enclosed in a rigid cavity, the swelling so produced increases intracranial pressure. This may reach a point (about 600 mm) where cerebral circulation can no longer be maintained.

Stressing the importance of control of elevated pressure is the fact that death has occurred in cases where the only postmortem finding was edema.

One is tempted to think first of spinal tap as being the simplest and most direct way to reduce intracranial pressure. However, as already pointed out, this is potentially dangerous, particularly in an *acute* rise in intracranial pressure. Moreover, it is questionable whether in acute stages one would be able to remove sufficient cerebrospinal fluid to make a significant or prolonged reduction in the pressure.

Dehydration was once recommended with the same aim in view, but as previously mentioned, the results of dehydration may be more injurious than helpful. Indeed, it is probably as illogical to attempt to relieve cerebral edema by dehydration as it would be to treat the swelling of a sprained ankle by dehydration.

Short of subtemporal decompression, the most rapid and dependable method of reducing intracranial pressure is intravenous urea. Dosage of 1 to 1½ Gm per kilogram at intervals of 12 to 24 hours will cause the brain to shrink rapidly, the effect becoming maximal in 30 to 90 minutes and disappearing after about 6 hours. This osmotic diuresis produces a great outpouring of urine (2,000 to 4,000 ml). Unless this fluid loss is replaced, the patient will become acutely dehydrated, even to the point of hypovolemic shock.

Mannitol (2.5 to 3 Gm/kg) given intravenously will have much the same effect. However, maximal shrinkage will not occur until 2 to 4 hours after injection.

Though extremely effective in reducing intracranial pressure, osmotic diuretics such as urea and mannitol should be used with caution until *after* intracranial hemorrhage has been ruled out by angiography, echo-encephalography, or surgical exploration.

Another method of reducing cerebral edema is the administration of adrenal corticoids. For this purpose we have used dexamethasone phosphate 10 mg intravenously, followed by 4 mg given 4 times a day for three to five days, then gradually decreased. This type of therapy reduces intracranial pressure less rapidly, but its effect is more prolonged.

COMPLICATIONS MIMICKING HEAD INJURY

Two complications, *dehydration* and *water intoxication,* which may produce symptoms mimicking those of an expanding intracranial hematoma may be avoided by careful measurement of intake and output and administering fluid either by vein or nasal tube as we have suggested. Other complications, which may produce similar confusion, include respiratory acidosis, cerebral fat embolism, and carotid artery thrombosis.

Respiratory Acidosis

Any impairment of pulmonary ventilation, whether from involvement of the respiratory center or concomitant chest injury, will result in a reduction of pO_2 and an increase of pCO_2 from its normal level of about 40 mm Hg. As the blood CO_2 rises, the dissolved gas rapidly penetrates neurons to produce a cellular acidosis. This will produce early symptoms including confusion, headache, restlessness, disorientation, and occasionally hyperactivity to the point of mania. Physical signs include tremor, incoordination, papilledema, retinal hemorrhages, occasionally cranial nerve signs, and frequently decreased or absent tendon reflexes. An acute elevation of pCO_2 to 70 or 80 mm Hg will produce coma. In more slowly developing respiratory acidosis pCO_2 may go to 100 mm Hg before coma develops.

Cerebral Fat Embolism

The mechanism of this embolic phenomenon is obscure since symptoms will not be produced by injection of fat into the bloodstream. However, following injury, particularly when one of the long bones is involved, fat droplets may be found in sputum, spinal fluid, and urine. Petechiae appear on the chest, axillary folds, under the eyelids, and on the sclera. Hemorrhages and exudates may be found in the eyegrounds. Incidence does not seem to correlate with severity of head injury. Usually, embolism occurs 24 to 72 hours after injury, although "free intervals" as short as 30 minutes and as long as 9 days have been reported.

The first symptom is usually restlessness. However, much more serious symptoms can occur, which may be cardiac (increase in pulse rate, fall in blood pressure, rise in venous pressure) and respiratory (increased respiratory rate, cough, stertorous breathing, cyanosis, rales). X-ray may reveal a butterfly pattern of miliary deposits bilaterally about the hilum.

Cerebral symptoms may consist of loss of sphincter control, generalized disorientation, deepening coma, tonic and clonic seizures, aphasia, and hemiplegia.

Treatment is symptomatic and supportive. Sodium heparin, 10 to 50 mg every six to eight hours, for its chylolytic effect and Dextran-40, 500 ml every 12 hours, have been recommended. Incidence is probably reduced by early fixation of fractures. Where doubt exists, one should not hesitate to perform carotid angiography or

to make exploratory burr holes to rule out an expanding intracranial hemorrhage.

Thrombosis of the Carotid or Vertebral Artery

The frequent association of neck injuries with those involving the head, which have been previously mentioned, may on occasion lead to carotid artery thrombosis. This may be caused primarily by intimal damage secondary to blunt trauma. Cerebral vasoconstriction, with slowing of the circulation, may be a contributing factor.

Speed of onset of symptoms and their severity will depend on several factors: (1) extent of the thrombosis; (2) presence of arteriosclerosis; (3) competency of collateral circulation through the circle of Willis; (4) degree of vasospasm; (5) severity of associated craniocerebral injury; (6) competency of the airway.

Differential diagnosis will depend on arteriography.

Treatment: Because of the importance of adequate oxygenation, tracheotomy and positive-pressure breathing should be applied. The only definitive treatment is vascular surgery.

Pneumonia

This is a frequent cause of death in the comatose, head-injured patient. It is almost certain to develop if the patient is tied down on his back because of restlessness or immobilized in suspension traction for a fractured femur.

The best prophylactic measures are movement of the patient from side to-back-to-side so that he spends only one-third of the time on his back, with intermittent positive-pressure breathing to prevent atelectasis and good nursing care to prevent aspiration.

Symptoms are apt to be masked by

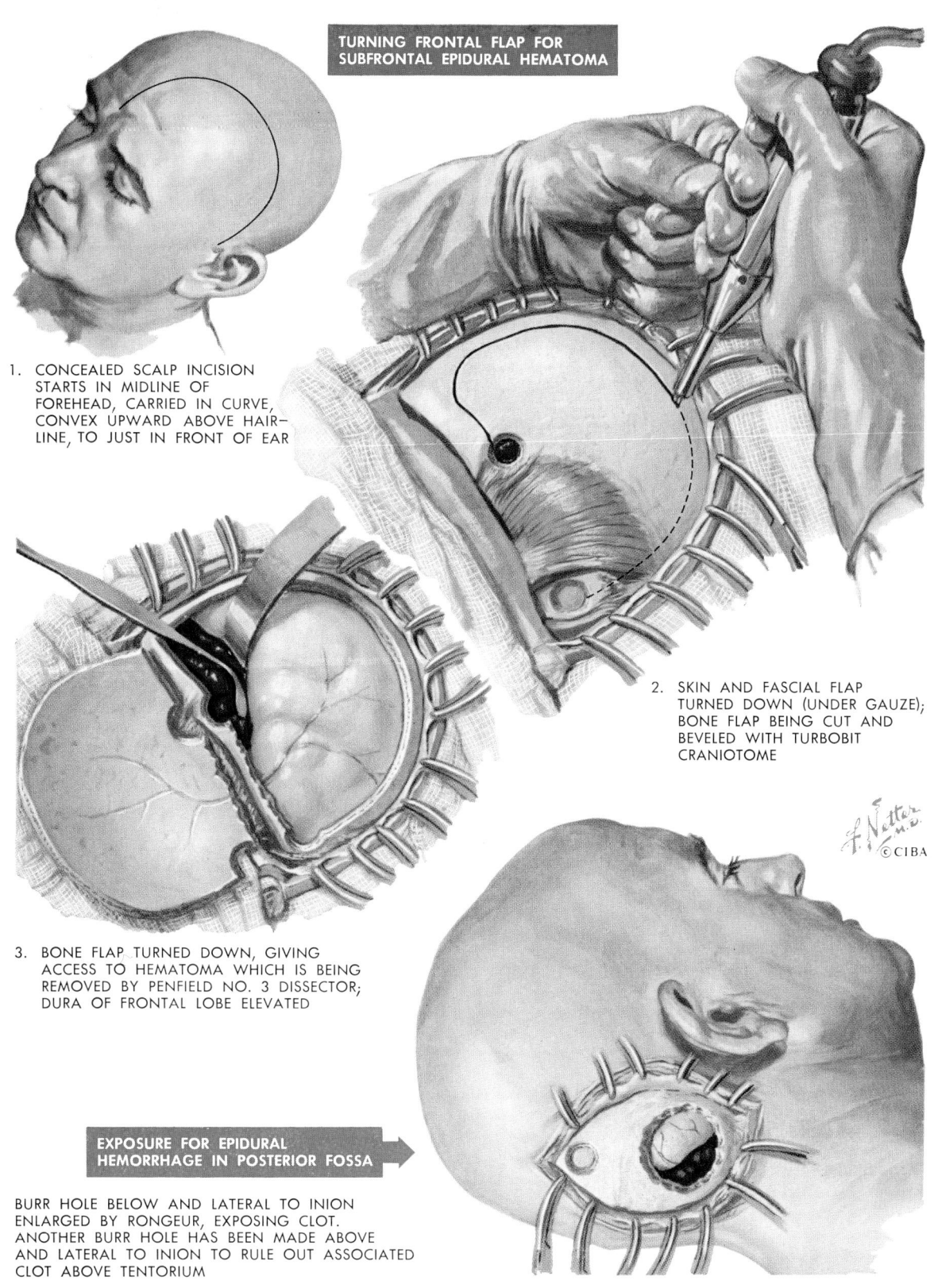

TURNING FRONTAL FLAP FOR SUBFRONTAL EPIDURAL HEMATOMA

1. CONCEALED SCALP INCISION STARTS IN MIDLINE OF FOREHEAD, CARRIED IN CURVE, CONVEX UPWARD ABOVE HAIR–LINE, TO JUST IN FRONT OF EAR

2. SKIN AND FASCIAL FLAP TURNED DOWN (UNDER GAUZE); BONE FLAP BEING CUT AND BEVELED WITH TURBOBIT CRANIOTOME

3. BONE FLAP TURNED DOWN, GIVING ACCESS TO HEMATOMA WHICH IS BEING REMOVED BY PENFIELD NO. 3 DISSECTOR; DURA OF FRONTAL LOBE ELEVATED

EXPOSURE FOR EPIDURAL HEMORRHAGE IN POSTERIOR FOSSA

BURR HOLE BELOW AND LATERAL TO INION ENLARGED BY RONGEUR, EXPOSING CLOT. ANOTHER BURR HOLE HAS BEEN MADE ABOVE AND LATERAL TO INION TO RULE OUT ASSOCIATED CLOT ABOVE TENTORIUM

PLATE XII

OPERATIVE TREATMENT OF SUBFRONTAL AND POSTERIOR FOSSA EPIDURAL HEMATOMA

hypothermia. Daily physical examination and frequently repeated x-ray will help to prevent this complication being overlooked.

Acute Gastrointestinal Ulceration

The association of severe stress and acute gastrointestinal ulceration was first reported by Curling in 1842 in a patient with burns, and first reported in association with cerebral lesions in 1932 by Harvey Cushing. While relatively rare and of unknown pathogenesis, an occasional post-traumatic patient will suddenly develop tachycardia and go into hypovolemic shock as a result of gastrointestinal hemorrhage from ulcerations. These may be multiple and involve the gastrointestinal tract from stomach to sigmoid. Treatment is, of course, transfusion and gastrointestinal surgery. Occasionally, hemorrhage has been so profuse that patients have expired while blood was being transfused into both arms simultaneously.

Rupture of the Aorta

Another cause of sudden death in a patient who seems to be progressing satisfactorily is rupture of the aorta. This is to be suspected in patients who have had an associated chest injury.

The most common site is just distal to the left subclavian artery, where the aorta loses some of its support. Here the intima and media suffer a linear laceration and, if one waits until the adventitia gives way, the only result can be sudden death.

Signs suggesting beginning rupture and indicating surgical intervention to prevent a lethal blow-out include one or more of the following: 1. Widening of the superior mediastinum by percussion and x-ray. 2. A harsh systolic murmur heard throughout the pericardium being loudest to the left of the sternum in the second interspace. 3. High blood pressure with a bounding pulse in the upper extremities with weak pulse and lower pressure in the lower extremities. 4. Unexplained anemia (leakage into mediastinum or pleura).

Acute Fulminating Pulmonary Edema

This complication, occasionally seen following acute head injuries, usually occurs 1 to 24 hours after the injury, may be rapidly fatal, and is usually due to a primary or secondary hypothalamic lesion.

SUMMARY

1. The patient with a head injury has often suffered multiple injuries and therefore requires careful head-to-foot examination with first attention given those conditions that are most life-threatening. If neurons are to survive, a clear airway with adequate ventilation and the treatment of shock demand top priority.

2. *Not* a substitute for careful, complete physical examination and expert clinical judgment are the various diagnostic tests and procedures. Of these, echo-encephalography and angiography provide the most accurate information on the presence and location of an intracranial hemorrhage.

3. An unconscious patient must have continuous nursing care and frequent medical reevaluation for early detection of indications for surgical intervention.

4. Surgical exploration should not be considered unrevealing unless at least six trephine openings have been made.

5. One must be aware of those complications which may simulate the effects of head injury and of those which may suddenly cause the death of a patient who is apparently progressing satisfactorily.

6. The patient who is provided with meticulous care while unconscious, prompt surgical intervention when indicated, and adequate control of intracranial pressure, will have an increased chance of survival and (perhaps more important) better cerebration after recovery.

SECTION B

C I B A

RHEUMATOID ARTHRITIS
John J. Calabro, M.D., F.A.C.P.

RHEUMATOID ARTHRITIS

BY JOHN J. CALABRO, M.D., F.A.C.P.

J. HAROLD WALTON, M.D., *Editor*

FRANK H. NETTER, M.D., *Illustrator*

CIBA PHARMACEUTICAL COMPANY

SUMMIT, NEW JERSEY 07901

RHEUMATOID ARTHRITIS

A Potentially Crippling Disease That May Attack At Any Age

JOHN J. CALABRO, M.D., F.A.C.P.
Professor of Medicine, Tufts University
School of Medicine, Boston, Massachusetts
Physician-in-Chief, Department of Medicine
Director of Rheumatology, Saint Vincent Hospital
Worcester, Massachusetts 01610

Due to my retirement, this issue marks the end of a very stimulating experience, that of editing CLINICAL SYMPOSIA since its inception, 23 years ago. Most appreciated has been the loyalty of our readers, many of whom have assured me that they have saved every issue from the very beginning. Most rewarding has been the contact with our authors, so generous with their knowledge and their time. To both loyal readers and outstanding authors, my heartfelt thanks!

J. HAROLD WALTON, M.D., *Editor*

Rheumatoid arthritis, once considered a disease of the joints, is now recognized as a chronic systemic disorder in which signs of articular and periarticular inflammation predominate. This predominance of joint involvement over systemic manifestations is present in practically every case of adult rheumatoid arthritis and most cases that begin in childhood.

However, as will be described later, in about 20 percent of cases of rheumatoid arthritis beginning in childhood, severe systemic symptoms predominate. Arthritic involvement in these cases may be limited to arthralgia.

It will be our purpose to review briefly the various types of rheumatoid arthritis with particular emphasis on the childhood forms, since these present the greatest difficulty in diagnosis.

ADULT RHEUMATOID ARTHRITIS

Rheumatoid arthritis most often occurs between 25 and 45 years of age. It is primarily a disease of women, whom the disease affects three times as often as it does men.

The cause of rheumatoid arthritis remains unknown, despite world-wide research into etiologic factors as varied as bacterial and viral infections, metabolic and endocrine abnormalities, hypersensi-

tivity, autoimmunity, and even psychic disturbances. The most recent investigations suggest that one or more etiologic agents trigger a self-perpetuating, chronic inflammation of the synovial membrane within the joints.

Pathology (Plate I)

Initially, the synovial membrane becomes thickened by edema and cellular infiltration. The earliest invading cells are polymorphonuclear leukocytes, later replaced by lymphocytes and plasma cells that are distributed both diffusely and in nodular aggregates. The lining cells become elongated and hyperplastic, while synovial villi display marked hypertrophy. The synovial membrane is further thickened by infiltrating granulation tissue (pannus) that extends over the surface of the articular cartilage. Areas of cartilage, and subsequently even subchondral bone, are eroded by lysosomal enzymes derived from cells of the invading pannus. In some instances, adhesions between opposing layers of pannus lead to fibrous ankylosis and later bony ankylosis of the joint.

The bones in the vicinity of the diseased joints become osteoporotic. Periarticular tissues, notably tendons and muscles, become edematous and infiltrated with cells. Contractures of the joint capsule and surrounding ligaments or muscles may result from fibrosis, particularly after prolonged immobilization.

Signs and Symptoms

In most patients, prodromal symptoms of fatigue, weakness, weight loss, or numbness and tingling of the hands and feet precede joint symptoms by several weeks or months. Often these symptoms have been preceded by unusual physical strain or emotional stress.

In 20 percent of adult patients, arthritis begins suddenly. In the majority, however, the onset is insidious with vague aches and stiffness, often poorly localized to the joints. Pain, warmth, swelling, limitation of motion, and early morning stiffness gradually occur in a few joints or in only a single joint. Then, before these joint symptoms completely subside, other joints become involved. Transient muscular aches may also be present.

Over 90 percent of adult patients have a polyarticular onset. Their arthritis affects the small joints of the hands and feet, as well as the large joints, especially the knees. Rheumatoid arthritis tends to be symmetrical, affecting the same joints on each side, usually to the same degree.

Hand Involvement (Plates II and III)

Early involvement of the hands produces a characteristic appearance, consisting of fusiform enlargement of the proximal interphalangeal joints and swelling of the metacarpophalangeal and wrist joints. But the distal interphalangeal joints are not involved as they are in osteoarthritis. The hands are often cold and clammy. Later, they appear shrunken, because of atrophy of interosseous muscles. The grip is weak, and the patient cannot make a tight fist. Progressive disease of the metacarpophalangeal joints often leads to volar subluxation and ulnar deviation of the phalanges.

Foot Involvement (Plate IV)

Although much has been written concerning the characteristic initial changes of the hands of rheumatoid arthritis patients, almost no attention has been focused on early involvement of the feet, which occurs in about 85 percent of cases. The metatarsophalangeal joints are usually the first to become tender and swollen. Because of the stretching of the ligaments that hold the forefoot together, the metatarsals gradually begin to spread. The metatarsal heads then become unusually prominent in the sole of the foot, and unusually thick calluses develop. Rheumatoid inflammation of the forefoot causes contractures of contiguous tendons that promote the development of hammer toes and hallux valgus.

Pain at the back of the heel is due to rheumatoid achillotendinitis or retrocalcaneal bursitis. Pain at the bottom of the heel is from inflammation of the plantar fascia. Progressive x-ray examinations will reveal the following stages: a rarefaction of the subjacent bone, followed by erosions, then remineralization or healing, and tiny blunt spurs or roughening of the involved calcaneal surfaces.

Course and Prognosis

Remissions and exacerbations of arthritis are the hallmarks of this disease. Remission, characterized by sustained absence of all joint inflammation, is observed in about 20 percent of all adult patients. In a small percentage of patients, however, the disease progresses relentlessly to joint destruction and crippling.

Systemic Manifestations

While it is recognized that rheumatoid arthritis is a chronic disorder in which signs of articular and periarticular inflammation predominate, certain systemic manifestations also occur. The typical patient looks chronically ill. Malaise, anorexia, weight loss, early afternoon fatigue, and slight fever (to 100°F or 37.8°C) are frequent early manifestations. The spleen is palpable in 5 to 10 percent of patients

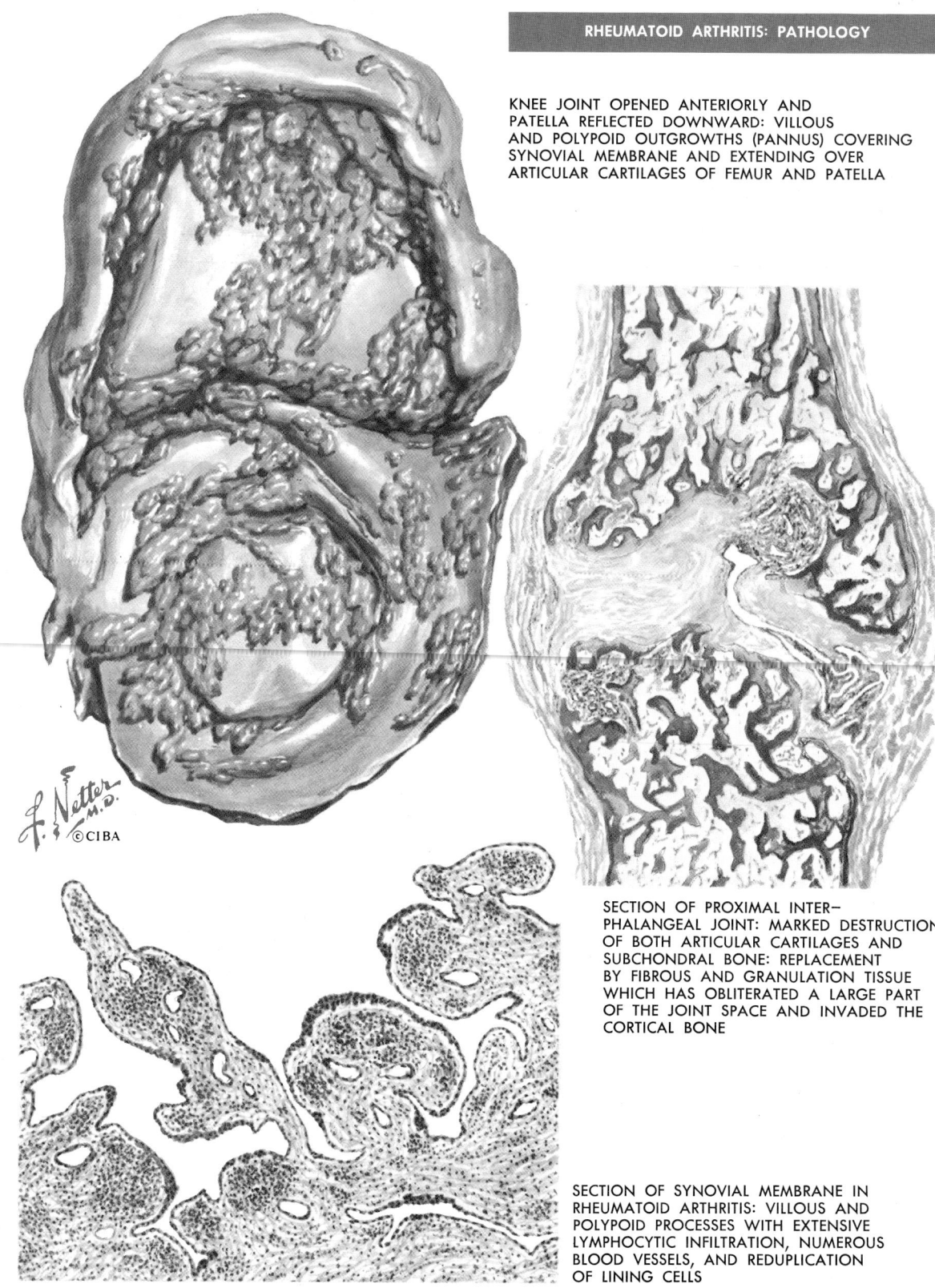

KNEE JOINT OPENED ANTERIORLY AND
PATELLA REFLECTED DOWNWARD: VILLOUS
AND POLYPOID OUTGROWTHS (PANNUS) COVERING
SYNOVIAL MEMBRANE AND EXTENDING OVER
ARTICULAR CARTILAGES OF FEMUR AND PATELLA

SECTION OF PROXIMAL INTER—
PHALANGEAL JOINT: MARKED DESTRUCTION
OF BOTH ARTICULAR CARTILAGES AND
SUBCHONDRAL BONE: REPLACEMENT
BY FIBROUS AND GRANULATION TISSUE
WHICH HAS OBLITERATED A LARGE PART
OF THE JOINT SPACE AND INVADED THE
CORTICAL BONE

SECTION OF SYNOVIAL MEMBRANE IN
RHEUMATOID ARTHRITIS: VILLOUS AND
POLYPOID PROCESSES WITH EXTENSIVE
LYMPHOCYTIC INFILTRATION, NUMEROUS
BLOOD VESSELS, AND REDUPLICATION
OF LINING CELLS

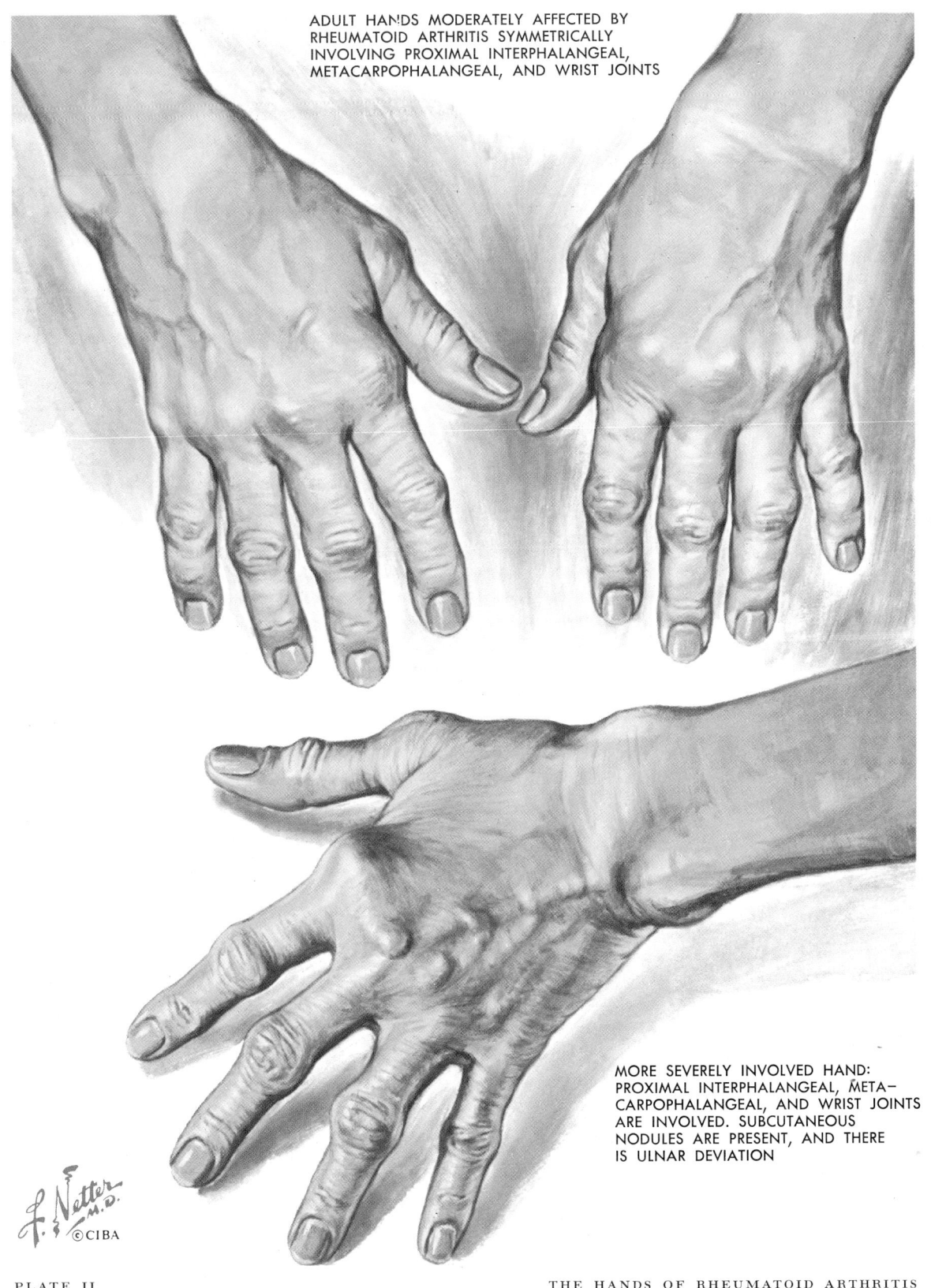

ADULT HANDS MODERATELY AFFECTED BY RHEUMATOID ARTHRITIS SYMMETRICALLY INVOLVING PROXIMAL INTERPHALANGEAL, METACARPOPHALANGEAL, AND WRIST JOINTS

MORE SEVERELY INVOLVED HAND: PROXIMAL INTERPHALANGEAL, META-CARPOPHALANGEAL, AND WRIST JOINTS ARE INVOLVED. SUBCUTANEOUS NODULES ARE PRESENT, AND THERE IS ULNAR DEVIATION

PLATE II

THE HANDS OF RHEUMATOID ARTHRITIS

and is often associated with focal or generalized lymphadenopathy.

Other systemic manifestations include Raynaud's phenomenon, episcleritis, pericarditis, or pleuritis. Vasculitis may induce peripheral neuropathies or ulcers of the skin of the legs, particularly over the malleoli (Plate IV). Unlike systemic lupus erythematosus (SLE), renal involvement is rare in rheumatoid arthritis. When it occurs, it is usually due to secondary amyloidosis.

Subcutaneous Nodules (Plate III)

These appear in up to 20 percent of adult patients and generally indicate a severe form of disease. Nodules usually lie free in the subcutaneous tissue and are located over bony prominences or at sites, such as the elbow or back of the heel that are subject to repeated pressure. On rare occasions, nodules appear in the eye (scleromalacia), lung (Caplan's syndrome), or even on the valves of the heart.

Histologic examination reveals that the rheumatoid nodule has three distinct zones: a central area of necrosis; a palisade of elongated, connective tissue cells that are arranged radially in a corona about the necrotic zone; and an enveloping granulation tissue with chronic inflammatory cells.

Laboratory Findings

During active disease, the majority of patients have a mild, normocytic, hypochromic anemia, and a moderate leukocytosis (12,000 to 15,000) with a slight shift to the left. C-reactive protein and an accelerated erythrocyte sedimentation rate are also present.

Urinalysis reveals no abnormalities in a patient with uncomplicated disease. (The presence of red cells and casts in the sediment raises the strong possibility of SLE.) The occurrence of massive albuminuria seen in a patient with long-standing disease suggests underlying amyloidosis.

Hyperglobulinemia with elevations of the gamma and alpha$_2$ globulins and hypoalbuminemia are frequently present when rheumatoid arthritis is active. None of these protein electrophoretic abnormalities are diagnostic. However, when a protein "spike" appears in the globulin region, it should suggest a diagnosis of multiple myeloma or macroglobulinemia, while marked hyperglobulinemia may be a clue to sarcoidosis or lupoid hepatitis.

Rheumatoid Factor: A positive test for this complex macroglobulin is obtained in 50 to 85 percent of adults with rheumatoid arthritis. This factor will agglutinate a number of different particles, including tanned sheep erythrocytes and latex particles that have been previously coated with gamma globulin. Titers reflect the severity of the disease, being low in mild, but high in advanced disease. High titers are also present in patients with vasculitis, Felty's syndrome (splenomegaly and neutropenia), and Sjögren's syndrome (keratoconjunctivitis sicca and dryness of the mouth.)

Rheumatoid factor is found in less than 5 percent of the general population, but in up to 30 percent of people past the age of 70. This macroglobulin is present in about 15 percent of patients with certain other rheumatic disorders.

Synovial Fluid Analysis: In a patient with persistent swelling of one or only a few joints, synovial fluid analysis should be done primarily to rule out infectious arthritis (see table, page 18). One should also search for crystals to eliminate a diagnosis of gout or pseudogout (chondrocalcinosis). Since acute infectious arthritis may be superimposed on underlying joint disease, arthrocentesis should also be done in a patient with well-established rheumatoid arthritis in whom a single joint exhibits greater swelling than do others.

Differential Diagnosis

SLE, osteoarthritis, and gout must all be ruled out as part of the differential diagnosis of rheumatoid arthritis.

Systemic Lupus Erythematosus (SLE)

Most of these patients have pain and swelling of the same joints affected by rheumatoid arthritis. Mild deformities may develop in SLE, but contractures, ankylosis, or erosions on x-ray examination are unusual, except for aseptic necrosis of the femoral head. Features supporting a diagnosis of SLE include the characteristic "butterfly rash" over the malar eminences, thrombocytopenia, hemolytic anemia, and renal involvement.

LE cells are found in about 10 percent of patients with rheumatoid arthritis, but do not correlate with the severity of the disease. Therefore, their presence should not alter therapy.

In certain patients, it may be difficult to decide between rheumatoid arthritis and SLE. In such patients, the absence of antinuclear antibodies virtually precludes a diagnosis of SLE. While antinuclear antibodies are present in low titers in up to 30 percent of patients with rheumatoid arthritis, high titers are found primarily in SLE.

Osteoarthritis (Plates V and VI)

Unlike rheumatoid arthritis, which is a systemic disease primarily involving the joint synovium, osteoarthritis is a localized degenerative disorder of articular cartilage.

The normally smooth, translucent cartilage loses its elasticity, becoming frayed and opaque. Later, clefts and pits appear, followed by erosions. Where the articular cartilage is thinned, subchondral bone proliferates, especially at the joint margins, forming bony spurs or ridges called osteophytes. These are composed of spongy bone covered with cartilage.

Joint cartilage degenerates as part of a physical or metabolic process at different rates in different individuals. The disease may occur in patients under the age of 50, although it is predominantly found in later life.

Weight-bearing and finger joints are generally involved. Joint pain is usually mild, except in hip involvement, which may be exceedingly painful. Characteristically, pain is intensified by overuse of a joint, but is relieved by rest. Gelling, or stiffness that follows rest, is less noticeable and of shorter duration than in rheumatoid arthritis. Affected joints are usually swollen, and an unusual amount of crepitus, creaking, and grating can often be demonstrated. Except in the hip, permanent loss of motion and ankylosis are unusual.

An important diagnostic consideration is the appearance of the hand in osteoarthritis (Plate VI). Unlike rheumatoid arthritis, the metacarpophalangeal and carpal joints are spared in osteoarthritis. Involvement occurs primarily at the distal (terminal) interphalangeal joints. These are the familiar Heberden's nodes that are found primarily in women shortly after the menopause. Occasionally, osteophytes occur at the proximal interphalangeal joints. These are the Bouchard's nodes, which never appear alone, but always together with Heberden's nodes. Pain at the base of the thumb is due to involvement of the carpometacarpal joint.

In rare instances, Heberden's nodes develop acutely with swelling, tenderness, and pain. However, they usually begin insidiously and painlessly. Nodes are found on the dorsolateral aspects of the involved finger joint. They feel hard on palpation and may or may not be tender.

When the disease is advanced, the fingers will show slight flexion or lateral deviation of the terminal phalanx. X-ray study will reveal enlargement of the bone ends with spurs laterally and at the attachment of extensor tendons. The joint space is narrowed because of distortion of the cartilage surfaces and occasionally by erosions of the bone (erosive osteoarthritis).

Unlike in rheumatoid arthritis, the erythrocyte sedimentation rate and other laboratory indices of systemic disease are

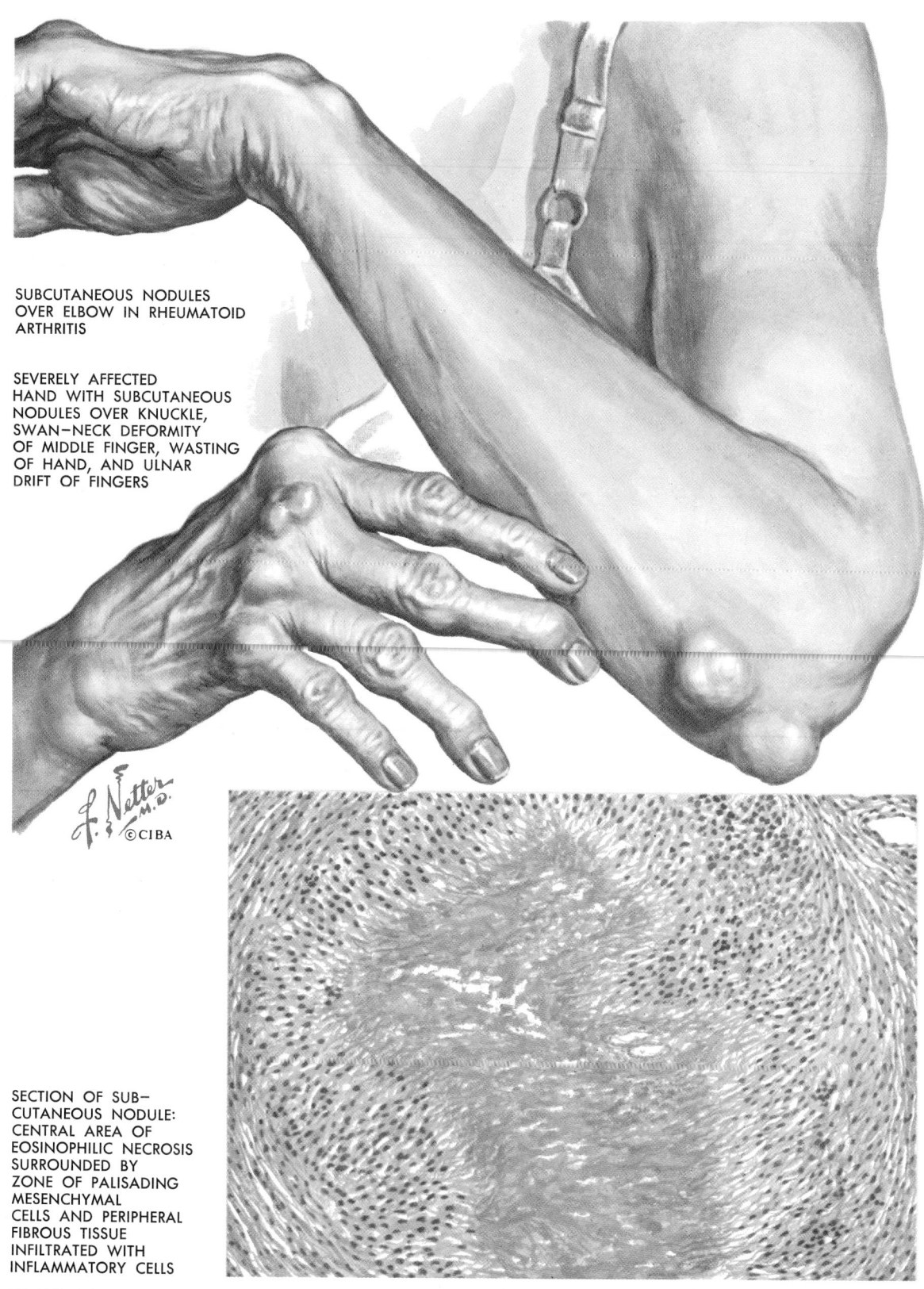

SUBCUTANEOUS NODULES
OVER ELBOW IN RHEUMATOID
ARTHRITIS

SEVERELY AFFECTED
HAND WITH SUBCUTANEOUS
NODULES OVER KNUCKLE,
SWAN–NECK DEFORMITY
OF MIDDLE FINGER, WASTING
OF HAND, AND ULNAR
DRIFT OF FINGERS

SECTION OF SUB–
CUTANEOUS NODULE:
CENTRAL AREA OF
EOSINOPHILIC NECROSIS
SURROUNDED BY
ZONE OF PALISADING
MESENCHYMAL
CELLS AND PERIPHERAL
FIBROUS TISSUE
INFILTRATED WITH
INFLAMMATORY CELLS

PLATE III

SEVERELY AFFECTED HAND AND SUBCUTANEOUS NODULES
OF RHEUMATOID ARTHRITIS

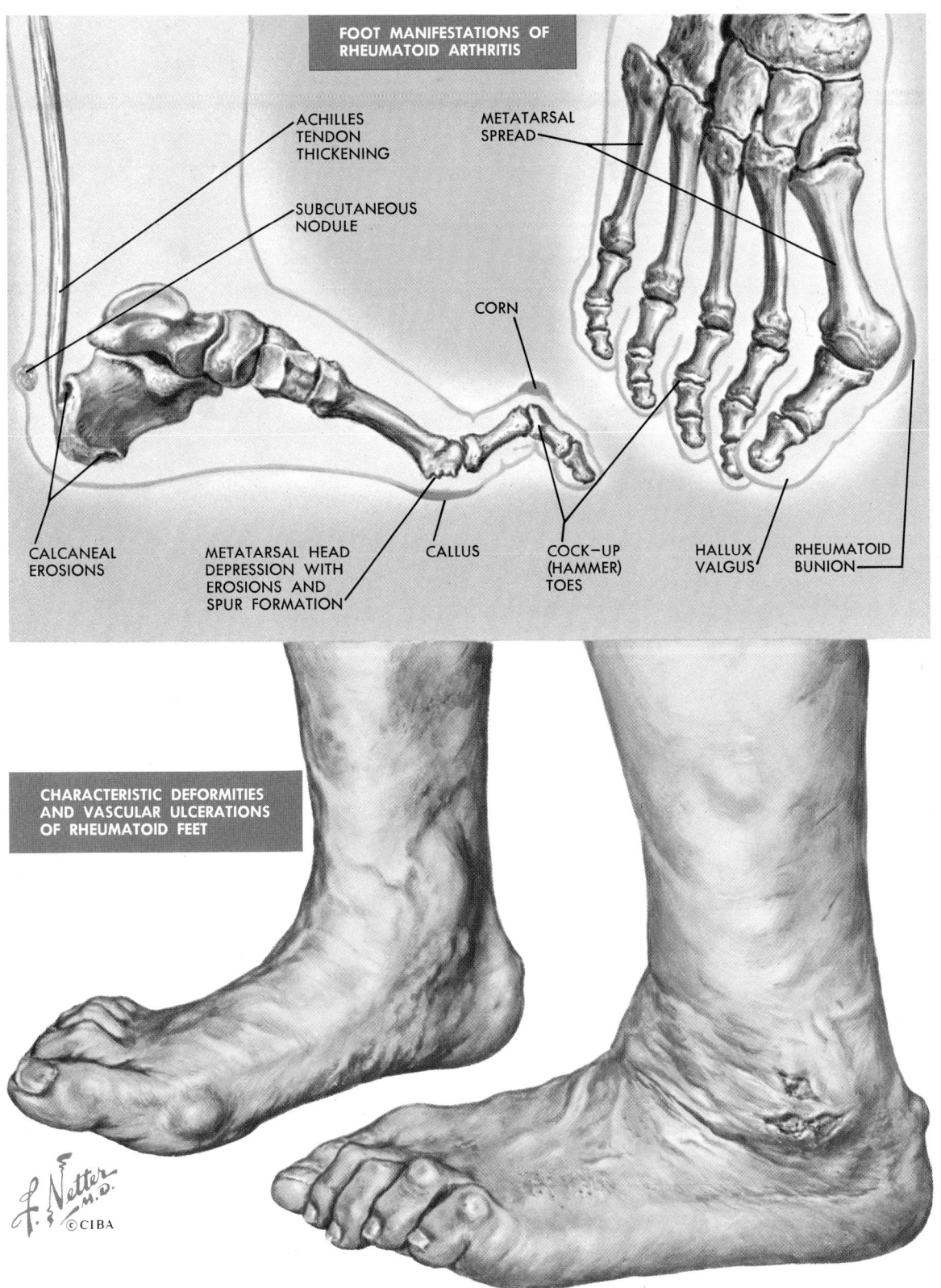

FOOT MANIFESTATIONS OF RHEUMATOID ARTHRITIS

ACHILLES TENDON THICKENING

SUBCUTANEOUS NODULE

METATARSAL SPREAD

CORN

CALCANEAL EROSIONS

METATARSAL HEAD DEPRESSION WITH EROSIONS AND SPUR FORMATION

CALLUS

COCK–UP (HAMMER) TOES

HALLUX VALGUS

RHEUMATOID BUNION

CHARACTERISTIC DEFORMITIES AND VASCULAR ULCERATIONS OF RHEUMATOID FEET

F. Netter M.D.
©CIBA

PLATE IV

THE FEET IN RHEUMATOID ARTHRITIS

normal in osteoarthritis. As it is in traumatic arthritis, the synovial fluid from an osteoarthritic joint is characteristically noninflammatory (see table, page 18).

Gouty Arthritis

Both gout and rheumatoid arthritis may begin with acute arthritis of a single joint. But involvement of a big toe, the instep, or a heel suggests gout, since these areas are rarely the only joints affected by rheumatoid arthritis. Other indications of gout are an elevated serum uric acid, a prompt response to therapy with colchicine, and the finding of urate crystals in the synovial fluid.

Chronic tophaceous arthritis, which occurs in one third of patients with gout, can closely simulate the advanced deformities of rheumatoid arthritis (Plate VI). In these patients, joint involvement is asymmetric, and draining tophi may be present. There are typical punched-out areas on x-ray examination, serum uric acid values are high, and urate crystals can be demonstrated in tophaceous material.

JUVENILE RHEUMATOID ARTHRITIS (JRA)

Despite many similarities, juvenile rheumatoid arthritis has certain features that are quite distinct from adult disease. Among these are the more frequent occurrences in children of high fever, a characteristic rash, splenomegaly, lymphadenopathy, chronic iridocyclitis, single-joint involvement, failure to grow, a striking leukocytosis, and the infrequency in the child of subcutaneous nodules and rheumatoid factor.

Whereas the adult form of rheumatoid arthritis is relatively easy to differentiate from other forms of arthritis, the juvenile variety often imposes tremendous diagnostic difficulties.

When mild, the disease may remain undetected and therefore untreated. When severe, it may mimic other childhood diseases. Adding to the difficulty of recognition, juvenile rheumatoid arthritis (JRA) has three distinct and quite dissimilar modes of onset, with each type requiring its own precise differential diagnosis.

JRA is the leading musculoskeletal disorder causing crippling in childhood. It is the major cause of childhood blindness due to its associated chronic iridocyclitis. Moreover, it is the underlying condition that most often predisposes to amyloidosis in children.

Therefore, an understanding of this disease is of greatest importance to every physician, and it will be our purpose to review briefly the important diagnostic problems that may be encountered in each of the three different modes of onset.

POLYARTICULAR ONSET

About one half of all cases of JRA begin with the simultaneous involvement of four or more joints, usually the knees, ankles, feet, hands, and wrists. Affected joints are usually warm and swollen, but not necessarily painful. They may or may not be tender and red. However, motion is almost always restricted.

When onset is abrupt and the arthritis is generalized, with typically symmetrical involvement of the hands and feet, diagnosis is easy. In children under 5, a fusiform swelling between the joints of the fingers often replaces the more typical swelling at the joints (Plate VII). Frequently, however, careful differentiation must be made from other rheumatic disorders of childhood, particularly rheumatic fever, serum sickness, and drug reaction, as will be discussed later. This is especially true when the arthritis is confined to large joints, and involvement is asymmetric and migratory.

Often, the patient will not complain of pain in an involved joint, but he will wince on movement, limp on walking, and "guard" the joints by adopting a fixed position of unnatural flexion (Plate XI).

One rather unique characteristic of JRA is involvement of the apophyseal joints between the facets of the cervical vertebrae. This causes limitation of motion of the cervical spine, and typically the head is held projecting rather stiffly forward (Plate VIII). In addition, vertebral bodies fail to develop normally, which contributes to a shortened stature. Often there is associated lack of mandibular development due to early closure of ossification centers. This produces a markedly receding chin, which is permanent (Plate VIII).

Cervical apophyseal involvement also may occur in adult rheumatoid arthritis, and is also seen in ankylosing spondylitis. In this latter condition, the dorsal and lumbar vertebrae are also involved, as are the costovertebral joints with fixation of the rib cage; whereas in JRA, only the cervical apophyseal and the sacroiliac joints are affected. The latter involvement, which may be demonstrated on x-ray as a narrowing, usually with erosion, is asymptomatic.

Systemic Manifestations

Patients usually look sick. They are listless, anorectic, and tend to lose weight. In contrast to the acute febrile type of onset (to be described later), the fever is low grade (under 102°F or 39°C). Usually it has the daily peaks of the quotidian fever that are typical of JRA. Occasionally, however, the temperature chart will show a double quotidian fever with 2 peaks daily (Plate VIII). Usually there is tachycardia out of proportion to the fever.

Rash, generalized lymphadenopathy, and splenomegaly occur frequently with this type of onset. However, subcutaneous nodules are rare.

Laboratory Tests

These are variable and nonspecific. White counts are often elevated, but rarely exceed 20,000. Occasionally, the white count is normal or a slight leukopenia is noted. An elevation of the erythrocyte sedimentation rate roughly parallels the intensity of the arthritis.

Rheumatoid factor may be detected in the serum of patients by either the sheep-cell agglutination or latex fixation test. The occurrence of rheumatoid factor in children is related to the age of onset, being found in only 10 percent of children in whom the disease started before age 12, but as high as 80 percent when it commenced later. Frequency bears no relationship to any particular type of onset.

X-ray findings may be helpful, but are not specific. They include juxta-articular demineralization, soft tissue radiodensities, and premature closure of epiphyses. Periosteal proliferation occasionally occurs, but disappears despite persistence of arthritis. All of these findings may be present by the fourth month. However, in children, the cartilage is exceptionally thick, being two or three times the thickness in adults. Also, it is more readily regenerated. Therefore, joint erosions are rarely seen until quite late.

Differential Diagnosis

The diseases that must be considered in the differential diagnosis of the polyarticular type of JRA include rheumatic fever, serum sickness, drug reaction, rubella, and hypogammaglobulinemia.

Rheumatic Fever

In its early stages, polyarticular JRA may be mistaken for rheumatic fever. In both diseases, polyarticular involvement may be asymmetric. Both may have low grade fever, rash, pericarditis, abdominal pain, and an elevated antistreptolysin-O titer.

The *fever pattern* in JRA is typically quotidian, with a daily peak returning to normal. That of rheumatic fever is typically of a sustained or remittent type that may fluctuate, but does not return to normal. In those few early cases of JRA that have a sustained or remittent fever, the temperature chart is of little assistance.

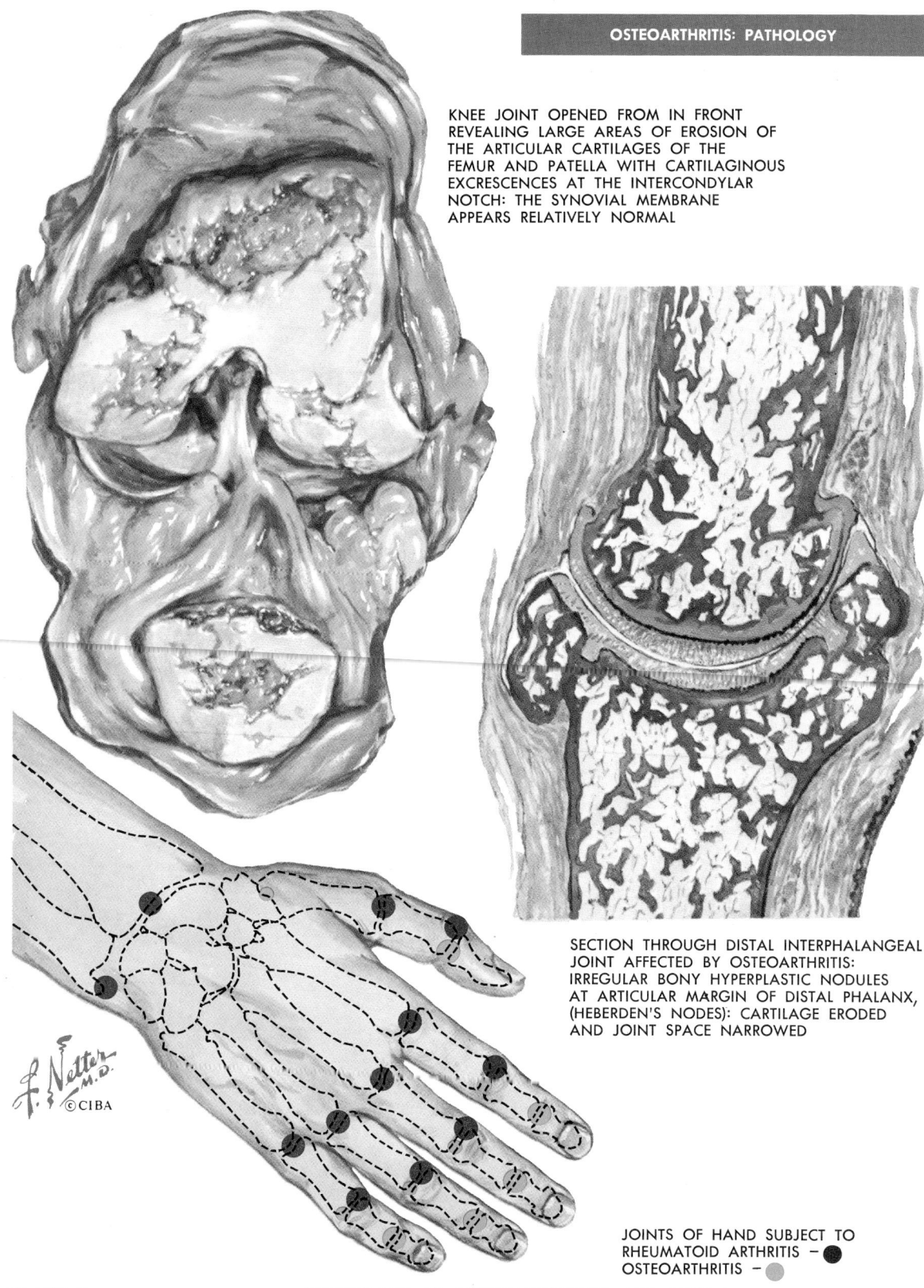

KNEE JOINT OPENED FROM IN FRONT
REVEALING LARGE AREAS OF EROSION OF
THE ARTICULAR CARTILAGES OF THE
FEMUR AND PATELLA WITH CARTILAGINOUS
EXCRESCENCES AT THE INTERCONDYLAR
NOTCH: THE SYNOVIAL MEMBRANE
APPEARS RELATIVELY NORMAL

SECTION THROUGH DISTAL INTERPHALANGEAL
JOINT AFFECTED BY OSTEOARTHRITIS:
IRREGULAR BONY HYPERPLASTIC NODULES
AT ARTICULAR MARGIN OF DISTAL PHALANX,
(HEBERDEN'S NODES): CARTILAGE ERODED
AND JOINT SPACE NARROWED

JOINTS OF HAND SUBJECT TO
RHEUMATOID ARTHRITIS – ●
OSTEOARTHRITIS – ●

PLATE V   PATHOLOGY OF OSTEOARTHRITIS AND JOINTS USUALLY INVOLVED

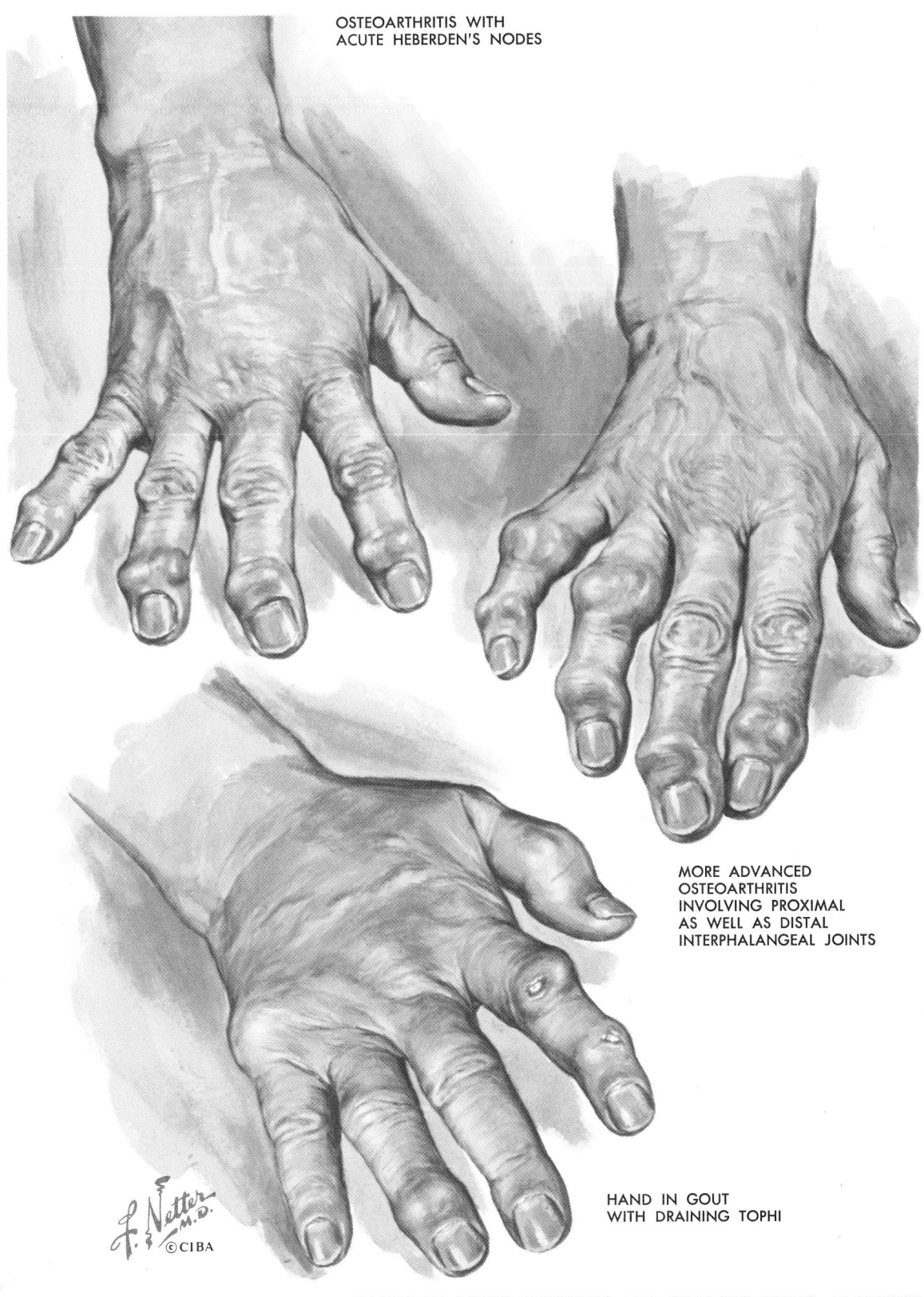

OSTEOARTHRITIS WITH
ACUTE HEBERDEN'S NODES

MORE ADVANCED
OSTEOARTHRITIS
INVOLVING PROXIMAL
AS WELL AS DISTAL
INTERPHALANGEAL JOINTS

HAND IN GOUT
WITH DRAINING TOPHI

Heart murmurs suggest rheumatic fever. However, the myocarditis of JRA may produce transient functional murmurs. Thus, to be diagnostic of rheumatic fever, a heart murmur must be persistent. If it lasts for 2 or 3 months, it cannot be due to JRA.

Response to salicylates is almost always more dramatic in rheumatic fever, symptoms being controlled within 24 hours. In contrast, aspirin usually takes up to a week to control the fever and arthritis of JRA. However, in some cases these are suppressed within the first day. Thus, the effect of aspirin, while often suggestive, is not an infallible guide to diagnosis.

The duration of arthritis in rheumatic fever is usually only about two weeks, even if untreated. Thus, if the arthritis persists a month or more, one is almost certainly dealing with JRA.

The rash of JRA is distinctive in appearance, location, and duration. Although it is present in only about 25 percent of JRA having a polyarticular onset, when it is found, it is so different from the rash of rheumatic fever as to be practically diagnostic (see Plate XII).

The rash is composed of discrete macules or maculopapules that are faintly pink in color. This is in contrast to the erythema marginatum of rheumatic fever, which is composed of peripherally expanding, open rings, with sharp outer edges and pale centers.

In JRA, the rash is migratory and usually evanescent. It may appear only at the height of fever and then be gone. It tends to be found in areas of pressure or irritation.

If the rash has been seen by a parent, but is not present at the time of examination, it may be brought out in a susceptible area by scratching or rubbing (the Koebner phenomenon, see Plate XII). If it is found on the face, soles, or palms, it is *not* due to rheumatic fever. While the rash of rheumatic fever is gone within a week or two, that of JRA will tend to recur over a period of months or years.

Serum Sickness and Drug Reactions

These conditions may cause polyarthritis with fever. However, the rash is urticarial, and the fever is remittent or sustained, instead of the quotidian pattern found in JRA.

Rubella Synovitis

When severe, this condition may cause confusion. However, the synovial fluid contains a predominance of mononuclear cells instead of the polys found in JRA. Also, there will be a rising H-I (hemagglutination-inhibition) antibody titer in the sera. A benign synovitis has also appeared following rubella vaccination, where it may persist for as long as eight weeks.

Hypogammaglobulinemia

Infants having a congenital deficiency of gamma globulin are highly susceptible to infection. One third of these patients also develop joint or diffuse connective tissue disorders, the synovitis of which may mimic JRA.

Usually the arthritic manifestations are asymmetric and transient. However, arthritis may persist for years with only minimal effusion and slight tenderness. The sedimentation rate is normal, and x-ray fails to reveal any abnormalities. Definite differentiation is made by gamma globulin determination, because in JRA this may be elevated instead of depressed.

Course and Prognosis

The course of polyarthritis is usually intermittent, characterized by exacerbations and remissions that may continue for many years. Remissions are common, being observed in 60 percent of patients that have been followed for 10 years. Sometimes, a remission will seem complete, only to be followed by a severe exacerbation, as long as 30 years later. Thus, once the diagnosis is made, the patient can never be discharged as "cured."

Occasionally, the course is unremitting

and progressively downhill, with marked joint deformities, and an enhanced susceptibility to secondary amyloidosis and vasculitis. The latter complication is marked by peripheral neuropathies and ulcerations of the extremities. In these chronically ill patients, amyloidosis should be suspected when hepatosplenomegaly persists or when proteinuria or hematuria is found in the urine and is not related to gold therapy.

MONARTICULAR JRA

In about 30 percent of cases of JRA, the onset is monarticular. Unlike the polyarticular variety, previously discussed, where the hands and feet were frequently involved, here it is the larger joints. Most frequently affected is the knee, followed by the hip, the elbow, and the ankle.

There are several other sharp distinctions between the poly- and the monarticular forms of onset. In the former, epiphyseal closure may lead to permanent decrease in growth of neighboring bones (limbs, mandible, and vertebral bodies). In the monarticular variety of onset, adjacent bones may grow more rapidly (Plate IX). This accelerated growth may result in a leg an inch or two longer than its mate; a foot several inches longer and wider than the contralateral one. Fortunately, this difference is temporary. With control of the arthritis, the opposite member catches up, so that eventually the sizes on the two sides are approximately equal.

The onset of monarticular involvement is usually insidious, and symptoms are mild. Except for the hip, which may be quite painful, other joints will have only a minimal degree of swelling, stiffness, and pain. Objectively, the only evidence of involvement of a knee may be a slight bulging alongside the infrapatellar tendon of the flexed knee (Plate IX). Quite often the only abnormality to be found is an antalgic (pain-relieving) limp.

A few patients, usually those under 5, appear listless and irritable, have low grade fever, and fail to gain weight. Otherwise, patients look well. Only occasionally will there be lymphadenopathy, splenomegaly, or rash. Myocarditis and pericarditis are rare.

Thus, the entire picture suggests an exceedingly mild, perhaps innocuous disease process. Yet, it is this form of JRA that has the highest incidence of the sight-threatening complication, iridocyclitis.

Chronic Iridocyclitis: The anterior portion of the uveal tract of the eye, consisting of the iris and ciliary body, becomes chronically inflamed in about 20 percent of cases of monarticular JRA. As a result, clumps of white cells and protein appear in the aqueous and vitreous humors and may adhere to the cornea as discrete white precipitates (Plate X). Later, gray adhesions (synechiae) develop between the iris and lens so that the pupil becomes irregular and reacts sluggishly. Blockage of the canals of Schlemm may lead to secondary glaucoma.

Calcium salts, deposited on the cornea, beginning at the nasal and temporal edges, will gradually restrict the visual field as they progress toward the center. Coincidentally, the posterior cortex of the lens becomes involved with gradual loss of vision from cataract formation.

Acute iridocyclitis (frequently associated with ankylosing spondylitis and Reiter's syndrome, but not with JRA) is quickly apparent because of redness and pain. The chronic form, however, remains silent and hidden. There are no symptoms until vision is decreased. The earliest manifestations, clumps of cells and protein, can only be visualized by slit-lamp examination (Plate X).

Since chronic iridocyclitis may develop as long as 10 years after the onset of arthritis, and even during a period of remission, slit-lamp examination should be carried out at intervals of every 3 months in all patients having monarticular JRA.

Treatment, which should be supervised

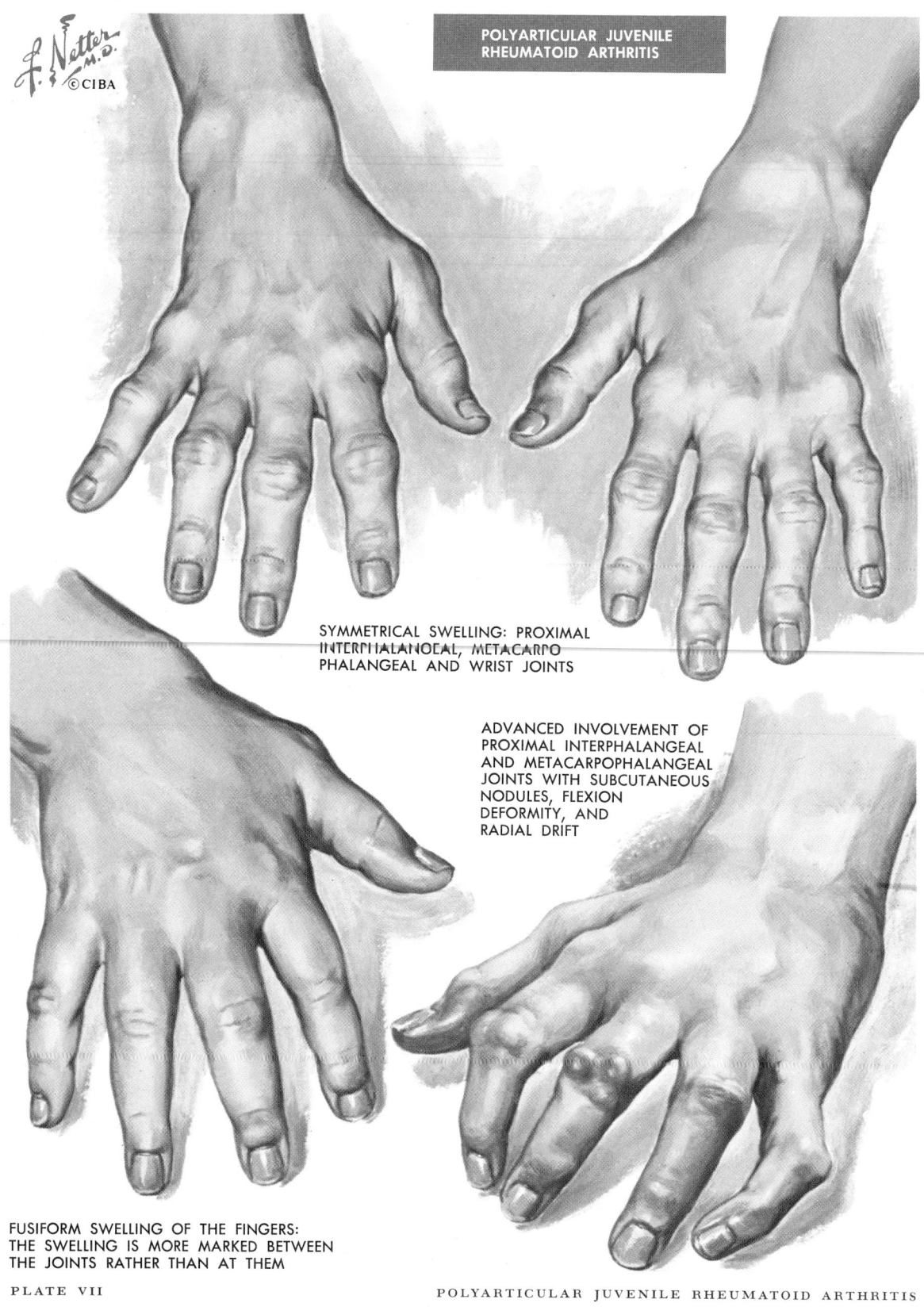

SYMMETRICAL SWELLING: PROXIMAL
INTERPHALANGEAL, METACARPO
PHALANGEAL AND WRIST JOINTS

ADVANCED INVOLVEMENT OF
PROXIMAL INTERPHALANGEAL
AND METACARPOPHALANGEAL
JOINTS WITH SUBCUTANEOUS
NODULES, FLEXION
DEFORMITY, AND
RADIAL DRIFT

FUSIFORM SWELLING OF THE FINGERS:
THE SWELLING IS MORE MARKED BETWEEN
THE JOINTS RATHER THAN AT THEM

PLATE VII

POLYARTICULAR JUVENILE RHEUMATOID ARTHRITIS

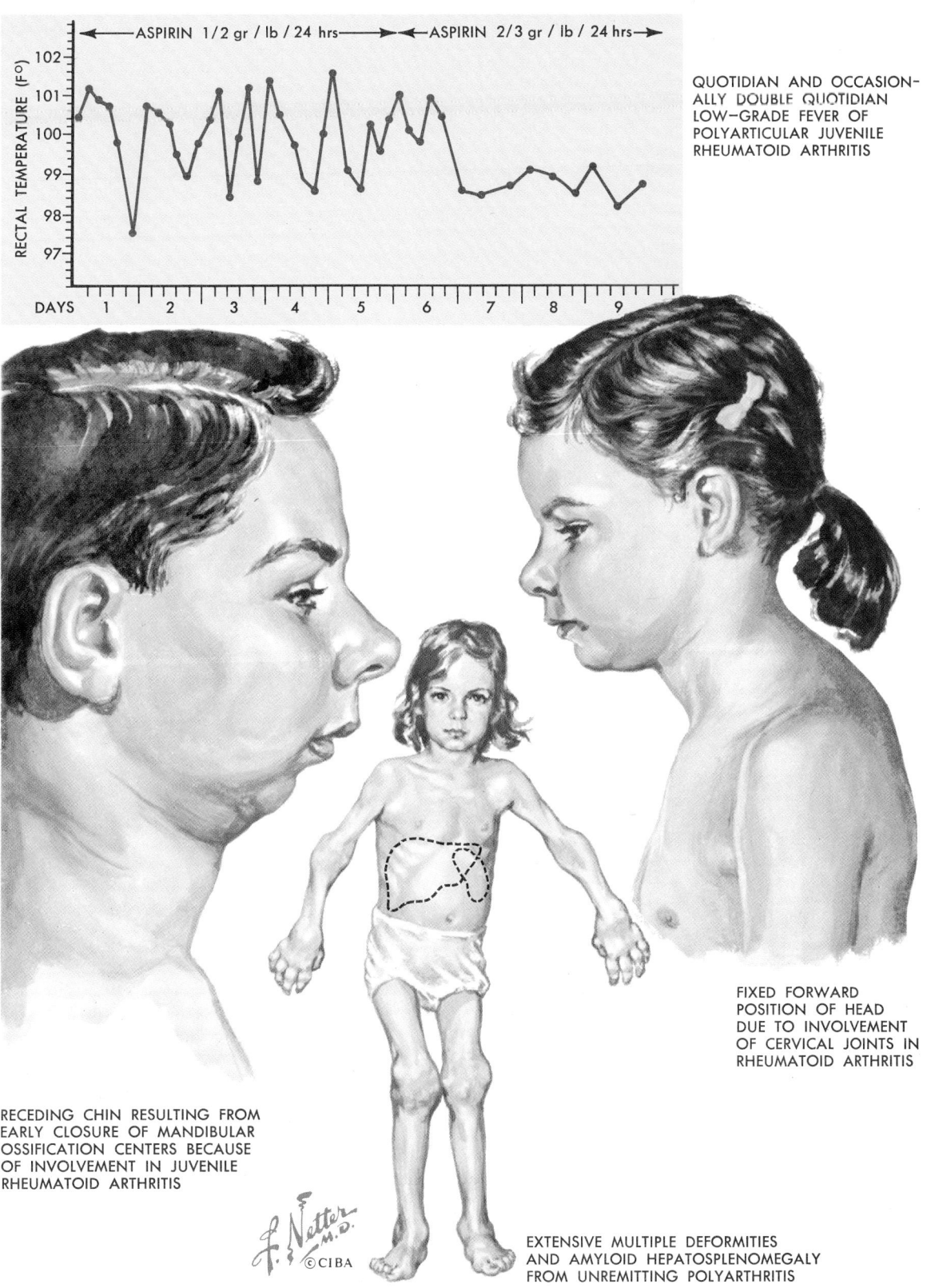

ASPIRIN 1/2 gr / lb / 24 hrs → ←ASPIRIN 2/3 gr / lb / 24 hrs →

RECTAL TEMPERATURE (F°)

DAYS 1 2 3 4 5 6 7 8 9

QUOTIDIAN AND OCCASIONALLY DOUBLE QUOTIDIAN LOW-GRADE FEVER OF POLYARTICULAR JUVENILE RHEUMATOID ARTHRITIS

FIXED FORWARD POSITION OF HEAD DUE TO INVOLVEMENT OF CERVICAL JOINTS IN RHEUMATOID ARTHRITIS

RECEDING CHIN RESULTING FROM EARLY CLOSURE OF MANDIBULAR OSSIFICATION CENTERS BECAUSE OF INVOLVEMENT IN JUVENILE RHEUMATOID ARTHRITIS

EXTENSIVE MULTIPLE DEFORMITIES AND AMYLOID HEPATOSPLENOMEGALY FROM UNREMITTING POLYARTHRITIS

PLATE VIII

POLYARTICULAR JUVENILE RHEUMATOID ARTHRITIS
TYPICAL FEVER, POSITION OF HEAD, AND SEQUELAE

CAUSE	GROSS APPEARANCE	MUCIN CLOT	WHITE-CELL COUNT	PERCENT OF NEUTROPHILES	GLUCOSE DIFFERENCE*
TRAUMATIC	Clear or hemorrhagic	Good	<5,000	<50	<10 mg/100 ml
RHEUMATOID	Clear to opalescent	Good to poor	15,000 to 25,000	50-90	10-25 mg/100 ml
INFECTIOUS	Cloudy or turbid	Poor	50,000 to 100,000	>90	>50 mg/100 ml

*Reduction of glucose level in synovial fluid as compared with simultaneously drawn blood.

by an ophthalmologist, includes the topical use of steroids and mydriatics.

Differential Diagnosis

Hematocrit, sedimentation rate, and the white-cell count are frequently normal. X-ray findings include osteoporosis, accelerated epiphyseal maturation, and periosteal proliferation.

Synovial Fluid Examination: This is the most important and rewarding study in the diagnosis of monarticular arthritis (see table above).

When aspirating joint fluid, the syringe should be coated with sterile heparin to prevent clotting prior to analysis. Also, one should be sure to use isotonic saline, instead of glacial acetic acid, to dilute the joint fluid for a white-cell count. Otherwise, the fluid may coagulate and cause a spuriously low cell count.

Synovial fluid analysis first includes the gross appearance of the fluid, since this may provide the earliest clue. Next, the character of the synovial fluid mucin is measured by adding a few drops of fluid to a small beaker containing about 20 ml of 5 percent acetic acid. After allowing a minute for the clot to form, the beaker is shaken. *A good clot* forms a firm ropy mass, which does not fragment on shaking. *A poor clot* fragments, quickly forming flakes and shreds, producing cloudiness in the surrounding solution.

Microscopic examination of a drop of fresh uncentrifuged synovial fluid, under low and high power, may reveal bacteria. All of these techniques are simple and may be done in any routine office or clinic laboratory.

Traumatic Arthritis

A history of trauma may be obtained in about 20 percent of cases of monarticular JRA. The significance of this is uncertain, but to differentiate the joint that remains "traumatic" from the one which becomes rheumatoid, one need only do arthrocentesis. The differences may be visualized in the table, where it will be noticed that the cell count and preponderance of polys is much higher in JRA, as is the reduction in sugar content. The mucin clot may be good in JRA, as it is in traumatic arthritis, or it may be poor.

Infectious Arthritis

Since infection may ruin a joint in a matter of 7 to 10 days, this differentiation must have highest priority. As shown in the table at the top of the page, the synovial fluid in infectious arthritis is cloudy or turbid with a tremendously high white count and a great preponderance of polys. The mucin clot is poor, and the sugar content is greatly reduced. Microorganisms can usually be demonstrated in uncentrifuged smears of synovial fluid. Cultures may or may not be positive.

Where tuberculous arthritis is suspected, synovial biopsy should be carried out in a search for caseating granulomas and giant cells. In JRA, the synovium is hypertrophied, with increased vascularity and round cell infiltration; but there are no giant cells.

Other Monarticular Disorders

Osteochondritis, epiphysitis, or meniscus tear may be differentiated by their distinctive clinical and x-ray findings. In a condition known as "transient synovitis of the hip," pain is minimal. This is a benign and self-limited disorder, primarily of young boys. The erythrocyte sedimentation rate is normal, as are other laboratory and x-ray studies.

Course and Prognosis

In about 75 percent of cases of monarticular JRA, a few other joints (less than four) will become involved. The disease is then called oligoarticular or pauciarticular. In about 25 percent, the pattern will change to the polyarthritic form. Both the oligo- and polyarthritic courses will be marked by remissions and exacerbations.

Even during remission, chronic iridocyclitis continues as a constant threat, since it may persist or recur long after arthritis has become inactive. Because chronic iridocyclitis is usually asymptomatic and thus escapes early detection, half of the children with this complication have gone blind. Therefore, periodic slit-lamp examinations should be carried out until patients reach adulthood, when attacks of iridocyclitis tend to become acute, and routine screening for silent iridocyclitis no longer has the same urgency.

ACUTE FEBRILE JRA

This mode of onset, which accounts for about 20 percent of Juvenile Rheumatoid Arthritis, usually offers the greatest diagnostic challenge. The articular findings may be minimal, limited only to arthralgia; and in any case, they tend to be overshadowed by the severity of systemic manifestations.

Often one can only infer the existence of joint involvement by the patient's "guarding" of tender joints by sitting or lying in a knee-flexed position to protect a knee or hip, without any complaint of pain.

Systemic Manifestations

These children are irritable, listless, eat poorly, and are losing weight. They are feverish and may present generalized lymphadenopathy, splenomegaly, myocarditis, pericarditis, pneumonitis, pleuritis, and rash, separately or in any combination. The fever pattern and rash are of greatest diagnostic value. Myocarditis is the most dangerous.

Fever: The pattern is typically quotidian or double quotidian, with a daily peak or peaks, usually above 102°F (39°C) and often going to hyperpyrexia (greater than 105°F or 40.5°C). It will then fall to normal or subnormal levels and is thereby characterized by wide diurnal swings on each succeeding day. Indeed, the diurnal fluctuations may be as much as 8° or 9°F (Plate XI).

This fever pattern, which can only be brought out by suitable charting, is most important diagnostically, because it helps to differentiate JRA from those conditions characterized by remittent or sustained fevers (which fail to reach normal in their diurnal swings) and relapsing or periodic fevers (where febrile periods are interrupted by days or months of normalcy). Thus, every patient suspected of JRA should have rectal temperature recorded every four hours around the clock. After a month or two, the quotidian fever of JRA may give way to relapsing, periodic, or remittent fever. Thus, the importance of charting from the beginning. The fever may precede joint involvement by days, months, or even years.

Rash: The characteristics of the JRA rash

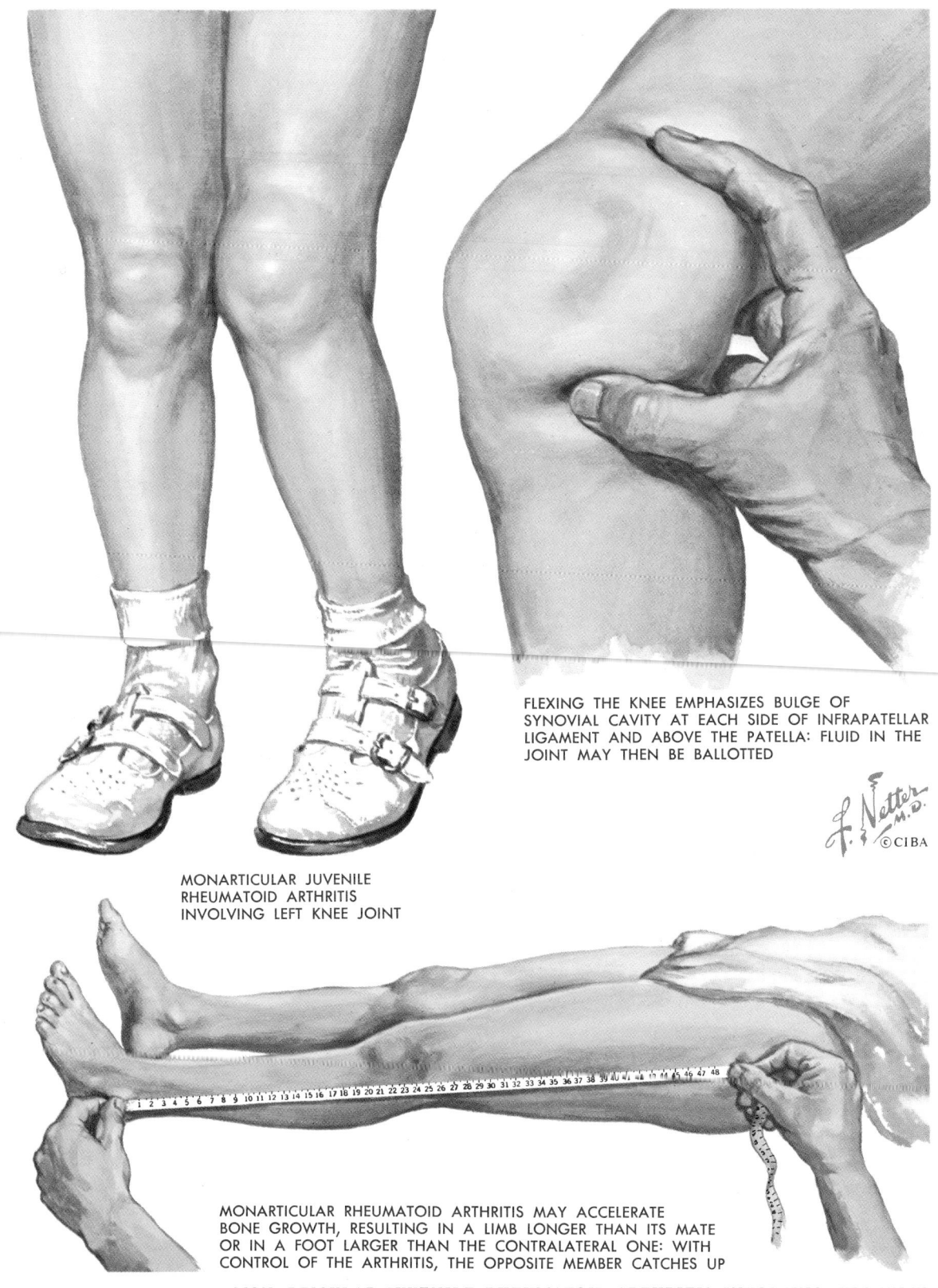

FLEXING THE KNEE EMPHASIZES BULGE OF
SYNOVIAL CAVITY AT EACH SIDE OF INFRAPATELLAR
LIGAMENT AND ABOVE THE PATELLA: FLUID IN THE
JOINT MAY THEN BE BALLOTTED

MONARTICULAR JUVENILE
RHEUMATOID ARTHRITIS
INVOLVING LEFT KNEE JOINT

MONARTICULAR RHEUMATOID ARTHRITIS MAY ACCELERATE
BONE GROWTH, RESULTING IN A LIMB LONGER THAN ITS MATE
OR IN A FOOT LARGER THAN THE CONTRALATERAL ONE: WITH
CONTROL OF THE ARTHRITIS, THE OPPOSITE MEMBER CATCHES UP

OCULAR PATHOLOGY OF JUVENILE RHEUMATOID ARTHRITIS

CORNEA
CONJUNCTIVA
CANAL OF SCHLEMM
ANTERIOR CHAMBER
IRIS
CILIARY BODY
POSTERIOR CHAMBER
LENS
SCLERA
CHOROID
RETINA
VITREOUS
OPTIC NERVE
BAND KERATOPATHY
DEPOSITS OF WHITE CELLS AND PROTEIN IN ANTERIOR CHAMBER
SYNECHIAE
POSTERIOR OPACITY OF LENS (CATARACT)
F. Netter M.D.
©CIBA

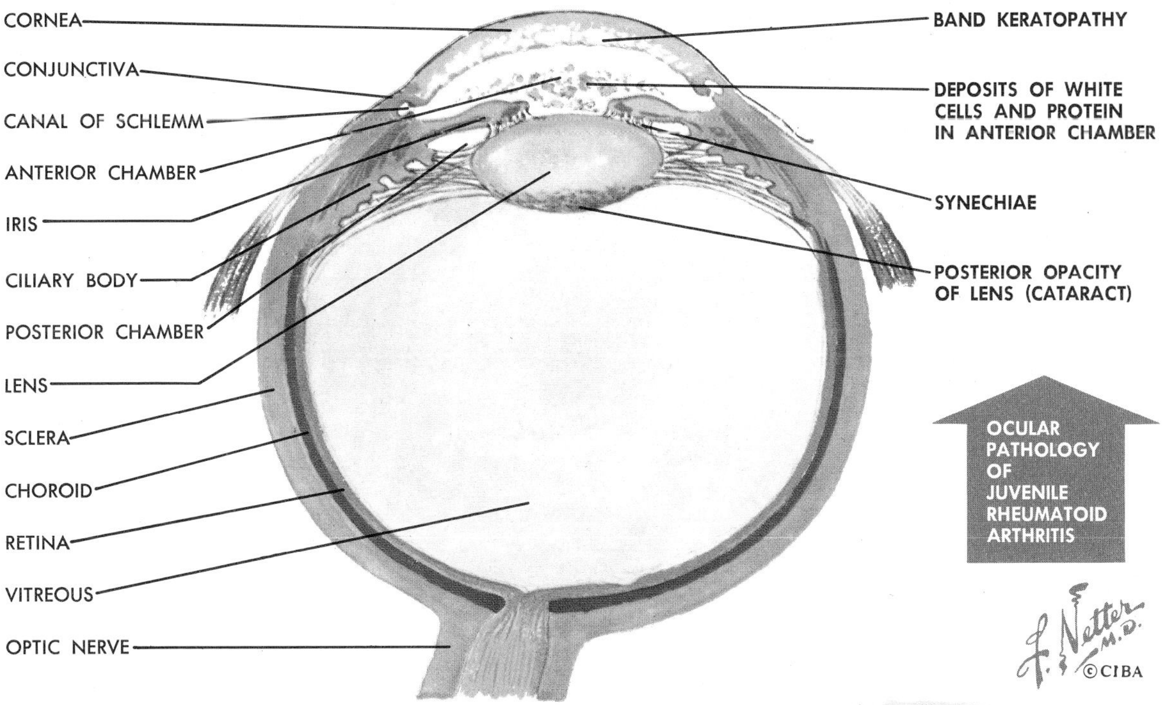

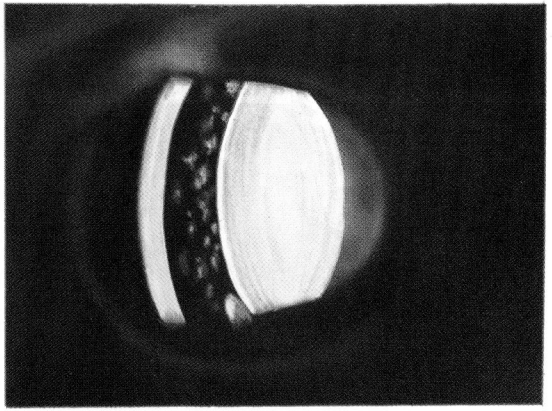

DEPOSITS IN ANTERIOR CHAMBER
VIEWED BY SLIT–LAMP ILLUMINATION

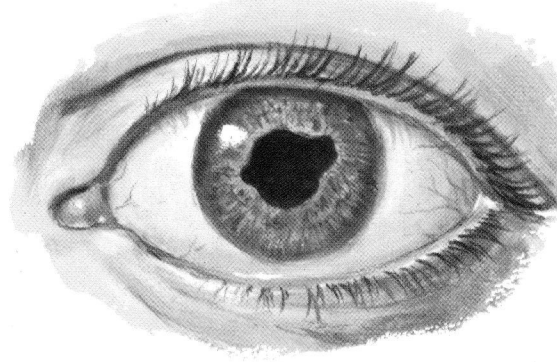

IRREGULAR PUPIL DUE TO SYNECHIAE

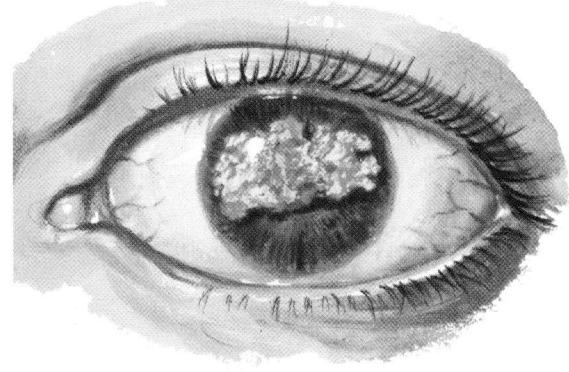

BAND KERATOPATHY

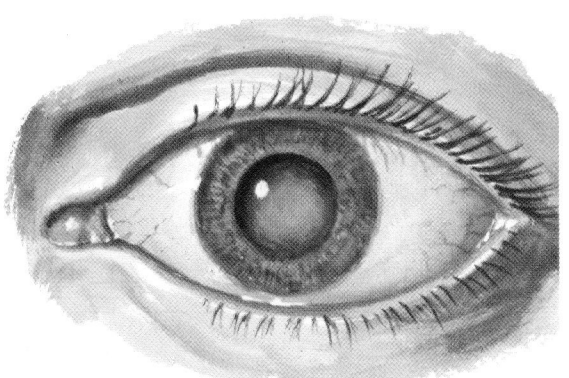

CATARACT

PLATE X

CHRONIC IRIDOCYCLITIS OF JRA
PARTICULARLY FOUND IN MONARTICULAR ONSET

have already been described (page 14). It is more frequently present in the JRA of acute febrile onset than in any other variety, appearing in 90 percent of cases.

However, it is usually evanescent, so that one must be alert to its possible appearance; diligent in search of its existence. The rash appears primarily in the late afternoon or early evening, often in conjunction with fever spikes. As previously mentioned, it can be brought out in susceptible areas by scratching or rubbing (Plate XII). This Koebner phenomenon is not to be confused with the pale, raised wheals of dermatographia.

The rash may be present for only a few hours during the day or the week, but it may still be found after the fever has been suppressed by medication, even over a period of years. (The mean duration of recurring rash is one year.) Like the typical fever, the characteristic rash may be found months or even years before obvious swelling of joints.

Splenomegaly is present in about 50 percent of cases of acute febrile JRA. It is often associated with hepatomegaly and generalized lymphadenopathy.

Lymphadenopathy may be so prominent as to suggest acute leukemia or lymphoma. Indeed, axillary glands may become so enlarged as to cause bulging of the axillary folds (Plates XI and XII). Enlargement of mesenteric nodes may cause abdominal pain and vomiting to such an extent as to suggest an acute surgical abdomen, leading to needless surgical exploration.

Pericarditis: This is the most frequent form of cardiac involvement. It is usually benign and will be detected only by serial electrocardiograms, x-ray for cardiac enlargement, and frequent auscultation for an evanescent friction rub. Symptoms may consist only of unexplained dyspnea or disproportionate tachycardia.

However, some cases can be severe, with sharp stabbing pain across the front of the chest, which is aggravated by respiration or change in posture.

The course of rheumatoid pericarditis is variable, lasting from one to fifteen weeks or for an average of eight weeks. It does not lead to tamponade, but can recur even years after the initial episode.

Myocarditis: This is the most serious complication of acute febrile JRA. Often overshadowed by a coexisting pericarditis, the myocardial muscle may be insidiously infiltrated with mononuclear cells. Thus weakened, heart failure with cardiac dilatation may ensue rapidly and even lead to a fatal outcome.

The treatment is the *prompt* administration of adrenocorticosteroids.

Differential Diagnosis

As with other forms of JRA, there is no single clinical finding or laboratory test that will make the diagnosis. Rather, it must be based on an evaluation of the combination of fever, rash, and arthralgia, along with other systemic features that have been described.

So far as the laboratory is concerned, the most important finding is a striking neutrophilic leukocytosis. The white-cell count is usually between 15,000 and 25,000, but may be as high as 50,000. Sedimentation rate is usually elevated, but does not correlate with the height of the fever. A moderate normocytic, normochromic anemia is commonly present.

The serum electrophoretic pattern is often normal. However, albumin may be low, the alpha$_2$ and gamma globulins high. Febrile proteinuria is the only abnormality of the urine.

In the absence of arthritis, the early diagnosis of acute febrile JRA depends on repeated examinations to detect the presence of an evanescent rash accompanying the characteristic fever pattern, or on the observation of minimal signs of asymptomatic joint involvement, such as painless swelling or limitation of motion.

Despite the presence of such clues, even more difficult tasks must be assumed: (1)

The ruling out of infection, and (2) Elimination of other causes of fever, rash, and joint pain. Among the latter diseases that must be ruled out are systemic lupus erythematosus, polyarteritis, hypersensitivity angiitis, Schönlein-Henoch (anaphylactoid) purpura, and leukemia.

Systemic Lupus Erythematosus (SLE)

This disease does not usually affect a child younger than five. Several other considerations may prove helpful in differentiating SLE from JRA. Moderate leukocytosis (rarely exceeding 20,000 cells) or leukopenia will be seen, but not the marked leukocytosis of JRA.

The early skin lesions of childhood SLE may resemble the characteristic JRA rash, particularly when localized to the arms and face. However, the rash of SLE is not evanescent, does not recur at the time of fever spikes, and unlike the rash of JRA, cannot be brought out by scratching or rubbing (Koebner phenomenon).

The presence of oral lesions, renal abnormalities, and LE cells will help confirm the diagnosis of SLE. The absence of antinuclear antibodies virtually excludes SLE. This test should be performed in a reliable laboratory. Actually, antinuclear antibodies may be detected in both JRA and SLE. However in JRA, the titers are low. In SLE, they are high.

Polyarteritis, Hypersensitivity Angiitis, Schönlein-Henoch Purpura

A macular erythema of the trunk and face is often observed in the early stages of these disorders. However, it is frequently associated with purpuric or ecchymotic patches that do not occur in JRA. Also, unlike in JRA, renal manifestations are common in each of these vascular disorders.

Childhood Leukemia

Leukemia may masquerade as JRA for many months or even a year or two. This occurs because both disorders may have similar signs and symptoms; such as high fever, marked leukocytosis, lymphadenopathy, splenomegaly, and joint pain, which may be alleviated by antirheumatic drugs. Severe anemia or the presence of purpura should suggest the possibility of leukemia; peripheral blood and bone marrow studies help to confirm the diagnosis.

Etiocholanolone Fever, Familial Mediterranean Fever, or "Periodic Fever"

In those cases of JRA having a periodic fever pattern, these disorders must be ruled out as a possible cause. The simplest way to differentiate them from JRA is by noting the absence of marked leukocytosis and the evanescent rash; both of which are typical only of acute febrile JRA.

Course and Prognosis

About one-half the patients with an acute febrile onset of JRA will continue with this form of the disease. This will be a cyclic course, with one to ten recurrences each year, marked by acute recurrence of fever and the other systemic features previously described. As patients approach adulthood, attacks subside slowly, leaving no deformities.

About one half of cases develop a polyarthritic course, which may continue with remissions and exacerbations into adult life.

CHANGES IN DIAGNOSIS

Perhaps because of the close, but as yet poorly defined, relationship between the various rheumatic diseases, diagnosis must sometimes be revised, even after months or years.

For example, an occasional patient, believed to have JRA, will subsequently be found to have the arthritis characteristic of psoriasis, ulcerative colitis, or regional enteritis, since these underlying disorders may appear after the arthritis.

Sometimes, ankylosing spondylitis develops after years of a chronic polyarthri-

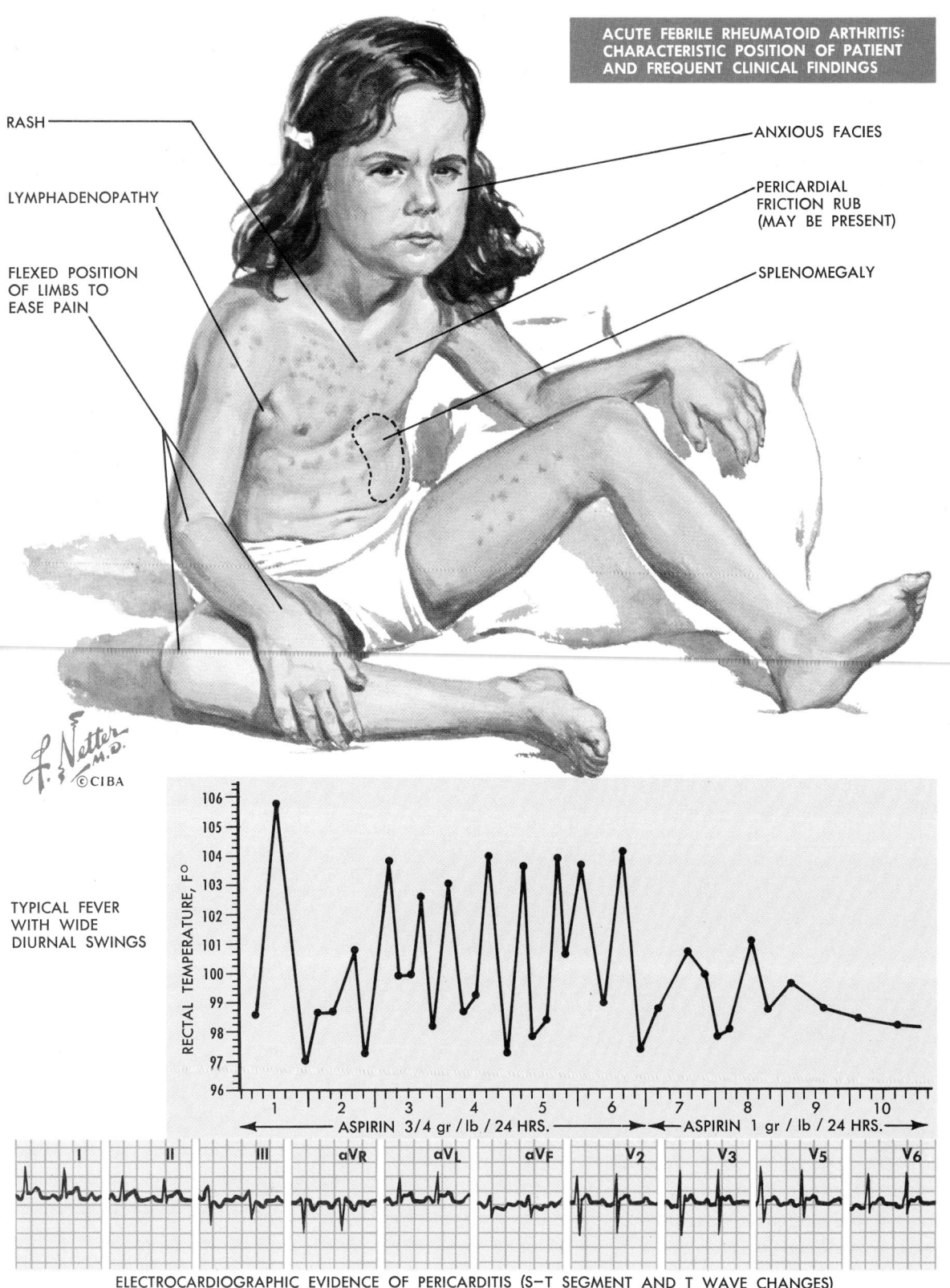

ACUTE FEBRILE RHEUMATOID ARTHRITIS: CHARACTERISTIC POSITION OF PATIENT AND FREQUENT CLINICAL FINDINGS

RASH

LYMPHADENOPATHY

FLEXED POSITION OF LIMBS TO EASE PAIN

ANXIOUS FACIES

PERICARDIAL FRICTION RUB (MAY BE PRESENT)

SPLENOMEGALY

TYPICAL FEVER WITH WIDE DIURNAL SWINGS

RECTAL TEMPERATURE, F°

←—— ASPIRIN 3/4 gr / lb / 24 HRS. ——→ ←— ASPIRIN 1 gr / lb / 24 HRS. —→

I   II   III   aVR   aVL   aVF   V2   V3   V5   V6

ELECTROCARDIOGRAPHIC EVIDENCE OF PERICARDITIS (S–T SEGMENT AND T WAVE CHANGES)

PLATE XI

ACUTE FEBRILE JRA: COMMON PHYSICAL FINDINGS, FEVER PATTERN, AND ECG OF PERICARDITIS

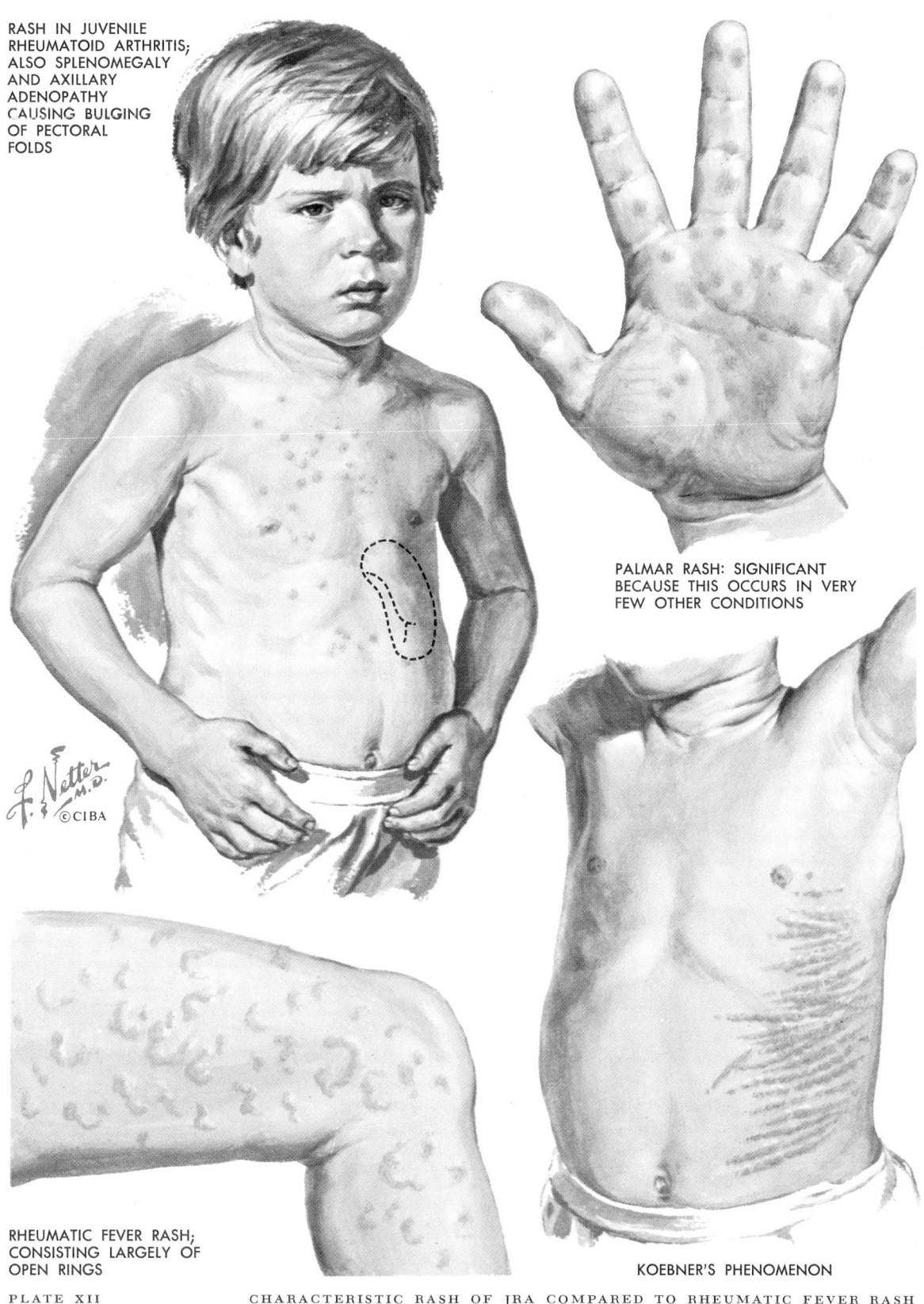

RASH IN JUVENILE RHEUMATOID ARTHRITIS; ALSO SPLENOMEGALY AND AXILLARY ADENOPATHY CAUSING BULGING OF PECTORAL FOLDS

PALMAR RASH: SIGNIFICANT BECAUSE THIS OCCURS IN VERY FEW OTHER CONDITIONS

RHEUMATIC FEVER RASH; CONSISTING LARGELY OF OPEN RINGS

KOEBNER'S PHENOMENON

PLATE XII

CHARACTERISTIC RASH OF JRA COMPARED TO RHEUMATIC FEVER RASH

tis. These patients are usually young boys with peripheral arthritis that is primarily confined to the joints of the lower extremities. An early clue to the development of juvenile ankylosing spondylitis is the presence of asymptomatic costovertebral joint involvement. This is not a feature of JRA. It may be detected by noting that chest expansion is limited to less than 3 cm, rather than the normal of 5 to 6 cm.

MANAGEMENT

Treatment may be difficult because the long course of disease for the individual patient is so unpredictable and may change at any time. Consequently, management must include an active treatment program and regular follow-up care.

Treatment Philosophy

From the first, the physician must be aware of his limitations. He can only initiate and supervise therapy. The actual treatment will be done at home, and results will depend on establishing a good working collaboration. Therefore, the most important task of the physician comes at the very beginning of treatment. He must educate and motivate the patient or the parents. Often, the physician must help to overcome unreasonable expectations of an immediate or decisive "cure." False hopes and fantasies should be examined and discussed openly so they can be replaced by active participation in a long-range treatment plan carried out primarily in the home. The most important part of home care is physical therapy, which can be made possible by use of drugs that reduce joint inflammation.

Drug Therapy

Patients and parents must be made to understand that no drug exists that will cure the disease or prevent disability. The extreme usefulness and versatility of aspirin should be stressed, since too many patients regard this drug as merely a "home remedy" that is of little value except for minor aches and pains. Also, it must be stressed that even after active disease stops, a drug must be continued for weeks or months before it is gradually withdrawn.

Aspirin: Whether child or adult, and whatever the mode of onset, aspirin in individualized doses is the drug of choice. Active disease can be suppressed in the majority of patients by four to six daily doses that total 90 to 130 mg per kg (2/3 to 1 grain per lb). Patients with prominent systemic manifestations, such as the acute febrile onset of JRA, require the more frequent and higher dosage.

Side effects of aspirin include acute toxicity, which in infants and younger children may cause intense ketosis, acidosis, and paradoxically, hyperpyrexia. Older children, like adults, usually develop respiratory alkalosis. Since early signs of chronic salicylate intoxication are easily overlooked in children, parents should be taught to watch for the occurrence of lethargy and episodic hyperpnea, signs that are especially important in the child too young to complain of tinnitus. When they occur, aspirin should be stopped for 24 hours and then reinstituted at a slightly lower dosage.

Systemic Adrenocorticosteroids: Systemic use is indicated in children only when disease threatens "life" or "sight." Oral steroids are used in heart failure due to myocarditis, in vasculitis, or in protracted iridocyclitis. For short periods and in moderate dosages, steroids may also be given to patients who do not tolerate or fail to respond to aspirin. If prolonged steroid treatment is necessary, every effort must be made to maintain the lowest dosage possible (for the average adult, 5 mg of prednisone daily, or equivalent). This is because serious adverse reactions occur so quickly, and large amounts will benefit the patient no more than lower doses.

The risks of long-term steroid administration are many and include decreased resistance to infection, retarded growth or skeletal maturation in the child, vertebral collapse (osteoporosis), glaucoma, cataract, peptic ulceration, myopathy, psychosis, and hypertension.

A rare adverse reaction to corticoids is pseudotumor cerebri, a form of intracranial hypertension causing headache, nausea, vomiting, and papilledema. It occurs primarily in children on long-term steroid therapy and is due either to an abrupt decrease in maintenance dosage or to a change from one steroid compound to another. Should it occur, one must return to the previous maintenance dosage or resume treatment with the original drug.

Intra-articular Corticosteroids: While the hazards of oral steroids are significant, intrasynovial injections of long-acting preparations carry little risk and may be extremely helpful in patients with minimal joint involvement. Even in patients with generalized polyarthritis, when only one or two joints are so seriously affected that exercise and activity are compromised, intra-articular steroid injections often enable resumption of such activities. The use of prednisolone or other steroid preparations, combined with a salt such as tertiary butylacetate, will prolong the effect from four to six weeks. Employing sterile precautions and after local infiltration with 1 or 2 percent lidocaine at the site of maximum periarticular swelling, remove as much synovial fluid as possible. Then inject 5 to 20 mg of the steroid medication, the amount depending on the size of the joint. Remember to caution patients that increased pain and swelling may occur 12 to 24 hours after the injection, and that this steroid-induced flare-up will promptly subside within a day or two. Do not inject the same joint more often than every three or four months. More frequent injections encourage abuse of inflamed joints that may promote mechanical derangement.

Gold: Chrysotherapy may be useful in patients with generalized arthritis who respond poorly to aspirin. The major difficulties with gold are that one cannot predict which patients will respond, and it takes at least three months before showing any benefit. Aspirin should therefore be continued until the benefit of gold is apparent. *But only the physician knowledgeable of its use and potential toxicity should employ gold.*

Gold sodium thiosulfate or gold sodium thiomalate is injected intramuscularly at weekly intervals in a dosage of 1 mg/kg. Weekly therapy is continued for six months and stopped at this point if there has been no response. If the patient responds, the interval is then reduced to every two weeks for 4 injections, then every three weeks for 4 injections, and monthly thereafter.

Gold therapy is continued as long as it is beneficial and there are no adverse reactions. Complications are more frequent in children under six and in the early months of therapy. These include nephrotoxicity, various blood dyscrasias, skin rash, or a metallic taste that often precedes stomatitis. Renal and hematopoietic complications are potentially fatal, and it is therefore urgent to monitor the blood and urine of each patient and evaluate the results before each injection. Anemia, leukopenia, granulocytopenia, or thrombocytopenia, as well as proteinuria or hematuria, are warnings to stop gold, and to treat the toxicity with ACTH or steroid. An eosinophilia may precede toxicity, particularly skin rash, and is therefore a sign to skip one injection and resume treatment at a slightly lower dosage.

Antimalarials: Chloroquine and hydroxychloroquine are not recommended for routine use. In dosage of 200 to 500 mg daily, they may be of some value in adult patients with polyarthritis responding poorly to aspirin. However, these agents are especially dangerous in children because accidental ingestion of as little as 1 gm may rapidly produce cardiorespiratory arrest. Since no antidote

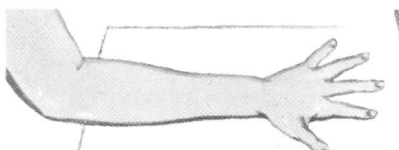

HAND AND FOREARM FLAT ON TABLE, PALM DOWN: SPREAD FINGERS APART AND BRING TOGETHER

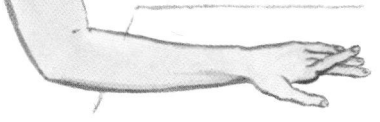

EACH FINGER IN TURN LIFTED OFF TABLE (DORSIFLEXED). THEN ALL FINGERS LIFTED TOGETHER

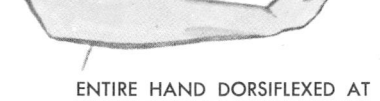

ENTIRE HAND DORSIFLEXED AT WRIST KEEPING FOREARM ON TABLE

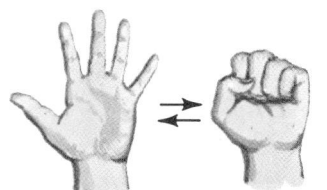

THE HAND IS SUCCESSIVELY OPENED AND CLENCHED, SPREADING FINGERS WIDELY AS IT IS OPENED

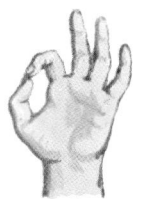

EACH FINGER IN TURN IS THEN TOUCHED TO THE THUMB, PINCHING FIRMLY

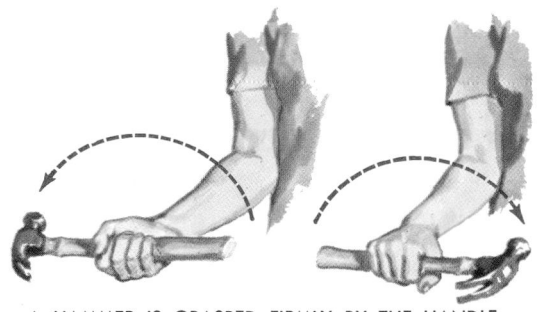

A HAMMER IS GRASPED FIRMLY BY THE HANDLE, THE ARM HELD SNUGLY TO THE SIDE: ROTATE THE FOREARM SO THAT HAMMER HEAD SWINGS FROM SIDE TO SIDE: DEGREE OF RESISTANCE CAN BE VARIED BY MOVING GRIP CLOSER TO OR FARTHER FROM HAMMER HEAD

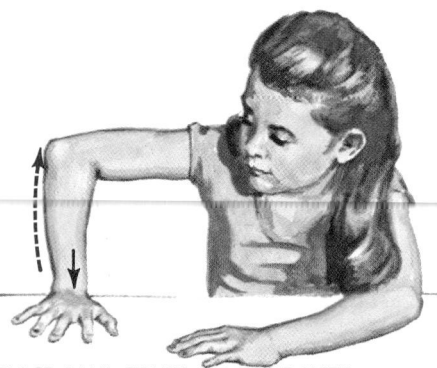

PLACE PALM FIRMLY ON TABLE WITH FOREARM HORIZONTAL: RAISE ELBOW HIGH AS POSSIBLE WHILE PRESSING DOWN ON TABLE

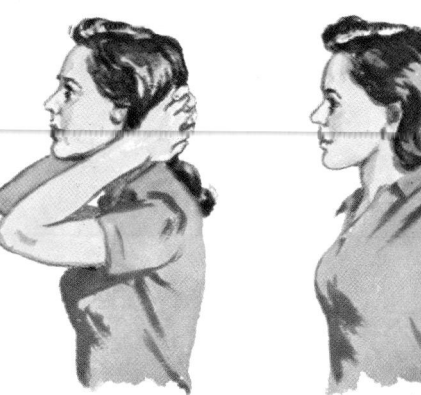

PLACE HANDS BEHIND HEAD; THEN DRAW ELBOWS BACKWARD AS FAR AS POSSIBLE, SIMULTANEOUSLY PULLING CHIN IN AND HEAD BACK

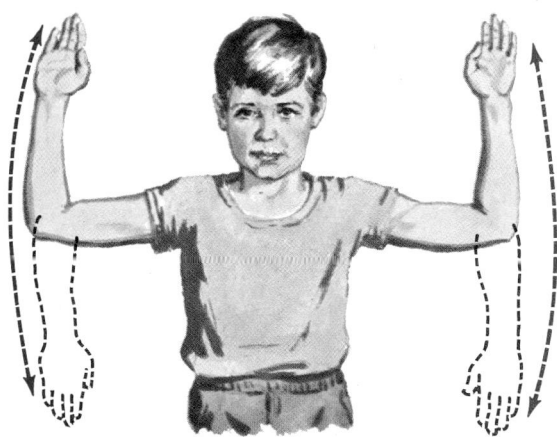

ARMS EXTENDED SIDEWARD WITH ELBOWS FLEXED TO 90°: SWING HANDS AND FOREARMS DOWNWARD AND THEN UPWARD AGAIN, THUS ROTATING THE SHOULDERS

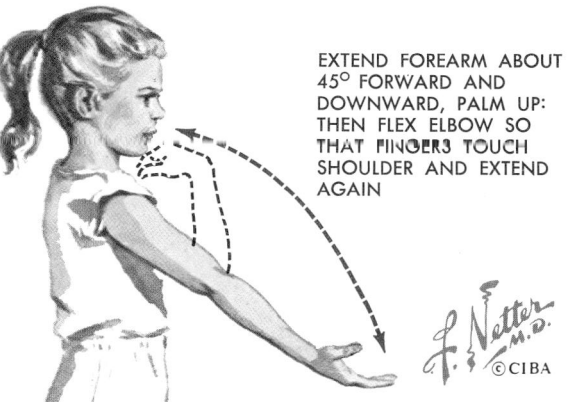

EXTEND FOREARM ABOUT 45° FORWARD AND DOWNWARD, PALM UP: THEN FLEX ELBOW SO THAT FINGERS TOUCH SHOULDER AND EXTEND AGAIN

PLATE XIII

EXERCISES FOR THE UPPER EXTREMITIES

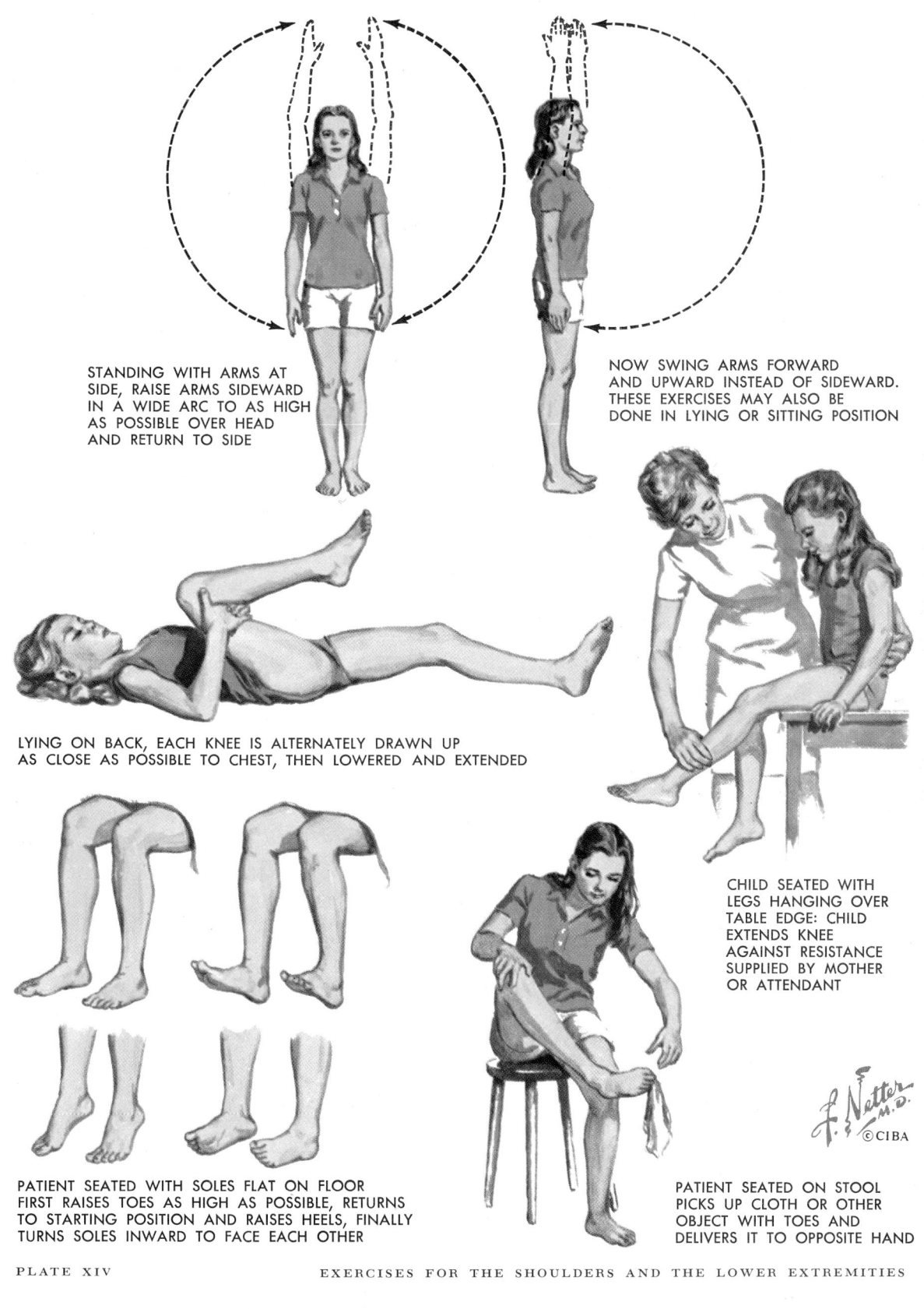

STANDING WITH ARMS AT SIDE, RAISE ARMS SIDEWARD IN A WIDE ARC TO AS HIGH AS POSSIBLE OVER HEAD AND RETURN TO SIDE

NOW SWING ARMS FORWARD AND UPWARD INSTEAD OF SIDEWARD. THESE EXERCISES MAY ALSO BE DONE IN LYING OR SITTING POSITION

LYING ON BACK, EACH KNEE IS ALTERNATELY DRAWN UP AS CLOSE AS POSSIBLE TO CHEST, THEN LOWERED AND EXTENDED

CHILD SEATED WITH LEGS HANGING OVER TABLE EDGE: CHILD EXTENDS KNEE AGAINST RESISTANCE SUPPLIED BY MOTHER OR ATTENDANT

PATIENT SEATED WITH SOLES FLAT ON FLOOR FIRST RAISES TOES AS HIGH AS POSSIBLE, RETURNS TO STARTING POSITION AND RAISES HEELS, FINALLY TURNS SOLES INWARD TO FACE EACH OTHER

PATIENT SEATED ON STOOL PICKS UP CLOTH OR OTHER OBJECT WITH TOES AND DELIVERS IT TO OPPOSITE HAND

PLATE XIV EXERCISES FOR THE SHOULDERS AND THE LOWER EXTREMITIES

exists, survival depends on prompt endotracheal intubation and repeated gastric lavage. Retinal toxicity continues as the major drawback of prolonged treatment, since visual deterioration may continue months after antimalarial therapy has been terminated.

Phenylbutazone, Oxyphenbutazone, and Indomethacin: These drugs are consistently effective in alleviating the articular symptoms of ankylosing spondylitis. In fact, if clear-cut relief of even severe discomfort is not obtained with one of these drugs, the diagnosis of ankylosing spondylitis should be questioned.

In rheumatoid arthritis, the long-term use of these agents is controversial, primarily because their effectiveness is variable and unpredictable. Occasionally, they are beneficial in the short-term treatment of acute flare-ups of arthritis, being added to the basic aspirin regimen for a few weeks and then withdrawn. For phenylbutazone and oxyphenbutazone, the average daily dosage is 300 to 400 mg, for indomethacin, it is 75 to 150 mg.

The serious adverse reactions of phenylbutazone and oxyphenbutazone include hepatitis, thrombocytopenia, and agranulocytosis. Toxicity occurs more frequently in younger children and may be fatal. Indomethacin is currently contraindicated in children. According to the manufacturer, the drug should not be used in children 14 years of age and under. Routine use of this drug in children could have serious medicolegal implications.

Rest and Splinting

Moderate use of rest, eight to ten hours of sleep and a nap during the day, facilitates resolution of synovial inflammation. Complete bed rest must be avoided, however, since this may cause flexion contractures, because patients will flex an inflamed joint to ease pain and spasm. Also, other complications of prolonged bed rest must be avoided. These include muscle atrophy (which may occur within the short span of two weeks), decubitus ulcer, renal calculus, osteoporosis, and fracture.

Lightweight bivalved splints, made of plaster of Paris but preferably of plastic, must be fitted to the individual patient. One use is to rest inflamed joints, another to correct deformities (Plate XV).

Resting splints are used on the hand, wrist, or knee. When a joint is acutely inflamed, generally for no more than 1 to 4 weeks, splints are worn throughout the day and night. They may be needed only part of the time as swelling and pain subside. Sandbags, traction, or other methods of keeping joints in proper alignment are alternatives to resting splints.

If a joint deformity has already been sustained (a flexion contracture of the knee, for example), serial splinting may be useful. A new bivalved splint is applied every 7 to 10 days as the range of motion improves. It may be removed to permit daily therapeutic exercise and then replaced.

Two types of casts should be avoided, the cylindrical plaster cast and the wedging circular cast. The former may in time cause fibrous ankylosis and marked muscular atrophy, while the latter may produce fracture by over-vigorous wedging.

Exercise and Activity

Prescribed exercise is an intrinsic part of the patient's daily care. However, the capacity to exercise depends on how effectively drugs have suppressed the arthritis. Ordinarily, this takes no more than a week or two. When drugs have not achieved their objectives quickly enough, warm tub baths or showers, or hot paraffin applications, also help to alleviate joint pain and stiffness.

Exercise is fundamental to the prevention and correction of deformity. Plan exercises that emphasize extension rather than flexion. The aim is to build up muscle groups that oppose the direction of potential deformities and strengthen extensor, rather than flexor, muscle groups. Sug-

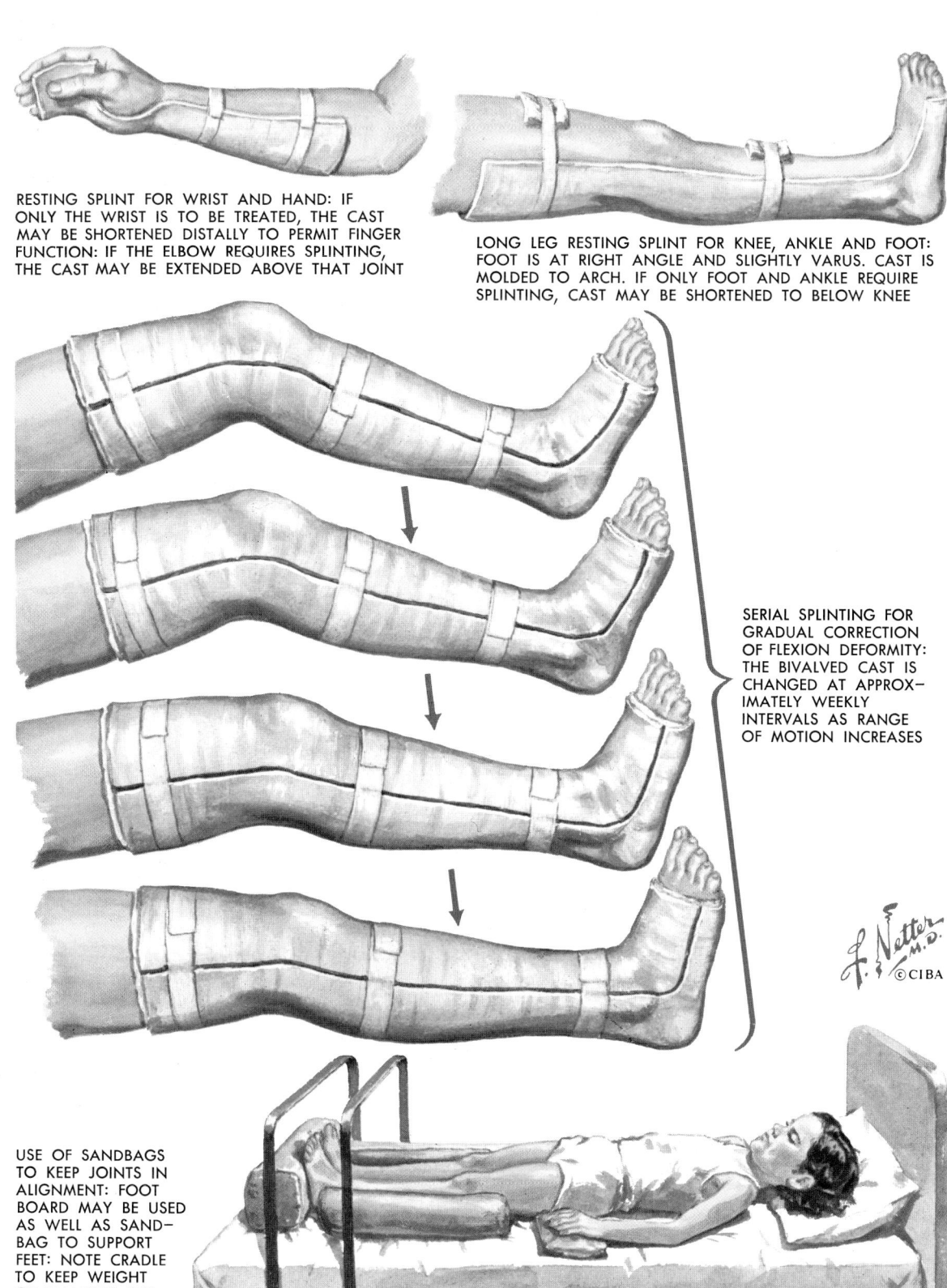

RESTING SPLINT FOR WRIST AND HAND: IF ONLY THE WRIST IS TO BE TREATED, THE CAST MAY BE SHORTENED DISTALLY TO PERMIT FINGER FUNCTION: IF THE ELBOW REQUIRES SPLINTING, THE CAST MAY BE EXTENDED ABOVE THAT JOINT

LONG LEG RESTING SPLINT FOR KNEE, ANKLE AND FOOT: FOOT IS AT RIGHT ANGLE AND SLIGHTLY VARUS. CAST IS MOLDED TO ARCH. IF ONLY FOOT AND ANKLE REQUIRE SPLINTING, CAST MAY BE SHORTENED TO BELOW KNEE

SERIAL SPLINTING FOR GRADUAL CORRECTION OF FLEXION DEFORMITY: THE BIVALVED CAST IS CHANGED AT APPROX— IMATELY WEEKLY INTERVALS AS RANGE OF MOTION INCREASES

USE OF SANDBAGS TO KEEP JOINTS IN ALIGNMENT: FOOT BOARD MAY BE USED AS WELL AS SAND— BAG TO SUPPORT FEET: NOTE CRADLE TO KEEP WEIGHT OF BLANKETS OFF FEET; ALSO BED BOARD

PLATE XV

SPLINTS TO REST INFLAMED JOINTS AND CORRECT DEFORMITIES

gested exercises are illustrated in Plates XIII and XIV.

Therapeutic exercises must be tailored to the patient and the degree of arthritis. A physiatrist or physical therapist must teach the patient or parents a program of regular daily exercises that can be performed in the home. When arthritis is acute, and especially if the joints are being splinted, exercise is performed gently and only when the patient is assisted by the therapist or a member of the family. As soon as possible, the patient should perform active extension-type exercises, changing next to active-resistive exercises when symptoms permit.

Daily activities, in addition to formal exercise, should be those that maintain strength and move joints through motions of extension. Recreation and sports can help to achieve these goals, but those which involve sharp impact to the joints (basketball, football, bowling) must be avoided. Swimming is an excellent sport, since it requires mainly extension-type movement with the added advantage of the positive buoyancy of water.

Keeping the adult at work, or keeping the child in school, also assures that mental activities are maintained. However, provision must be made to allow the patient more freedom than others. Patients need a sensible, well-balanced diet, but no special dietary measures are necessary.

Eye Care

The diagnosis and treatment of chronic iridocyclitis, a problem unique to children, are difficult and should be undertaken only by an ophthalmologist. Yet, the attending physician has the responsibility of early referral.

Because examination with an ophthalmoscope may not detect early iridocyclitis, periodic slit-lamp examinations should be carried out at six-month intervals in all patients with JRA. Monarticular-onset patients, the most susceptible group, require slit-lamp examinations every three months, even if the arthritis is in remission. Those who have had previous iridocyclitis should have this examination on a monthly basis.

Treatment of iridocyclitis consists of the topical application of steroids and mydriatics. In protracted cases, oral steroids may be needed since the hazard of steroid-induced glaucoma is greater following prolonged topical use. Surgery for cataract or glaucoma and chelating agents for band keratopathy may be helpful for even these serious ocular complications.

Surgery

The surgical therapy of rheumatoid arthritis, particularly early synovectomy, is an area of current, major interest. The object is to remove granulation tissue (pannus) early enough to prevent erosion of cartilage and bone. Most important is the correct timing of the procedure and the proper selection of patients. The usual criteria for selection of a joint for early synovectomy are persistence of swelling and absence of contracture, provided adequate medical measures have been tried for at least eight months. Patients six years or younger are poor risks, because of their inability to cooperate fully with important postoperative measures.

Established deformities can be successfully corrected by surgery, even in the presence of active disease. When arthroplasty is required, it is usually delayed until the patient is fully grown. Young patients may also need orthodontic care or plastic reconstruction of mandibular recession. Fortunately, most patients with rheumatoid arthritis will never require corrective surgery as part of their lifelong care.

SECTION C

CIBA

THORACIC-OUTLET SYNDROMES
Jere W. Lord, Jr., M.D., and Louis M. Rosati, M.D.

Illustrated by Frank H. Netter, M.D.

THORACIC-OUTLET SYNDROMES

BY JERE W. LORD, JR., M.D., AND
LOUIS M. ROSATI, M.D.

RICHARD H. ROBERTS, M.D., *Editor*
J. HAROLD WALTON, M.D., *Editor Emeritus*
FRANK H. NETTER, M.D., *Illustrator*

CIBA PHARMACEUTICAL COMPANY
SUMMIT, NEW JERSEY 07901

THORACIC-OUTLET SYNDROMES

JERE W. LORD, JR., M.D.
Professor of Clinical Surgery

LOUIS M. ROSATI, M.D.
Professor of Clinical Surgery

From the Department of Surgery, New York University School of Medicine, and Department of Surgery, Columbus Hospital, New York, New York

Thirteen years have elapsed since publication of the CLINICAL SYMPOSIA issue dealing with neurovascular-compression syndromes. Substantial progress in several areas has occurred, and we wish to update our earlier observations.

Currently, the most popular title for problems of the shoulder girdle causing compression of the neurovascular bundle is the term coined by Rob,[1] Thoracic-Outlet Syndromes.

Development of the transaxillary approach to resection of the first rib is of considerable importance in the operative correction of pressure on the subclavian artery and vein and elements of the brachial plexus by the clavicle and first rib and their fascial and muscular attachments.[2,3] Concurrently, we now reserve clavicular resection for primary abnormalities of the clavicle such as nonunion and faulty union either on a congenital or posttraumatic basis. For reconstruction of the subclavian artery rendered abnormal by trauma or atherosclerosis, total or near-total resection of the clavicle with removal of the periosteum and section of the scalenus anticus allows satisfactory and safe exposure.

Recognition of the carpal-tunnel syndrome as an entity, not only as an isolated phenomenon but also in its relation to the thoracic-outlet syndromes, has helped in the selection of correct surgical procedures.

Extensive use of improved diagnostic procedures, such as phlebography of the subclavian vein and arteriographic studies of the subclavian artery and its entire tree including the digital vessels by the transfemoral method of Seldinger, is a must in the careful evaluation of the potential surgical patient. Electrodiagnostic studies are accurate and identify the site of neural entrapment. We believe that these diagnostic advances coupled with further clinical experiences of the past 13 years enable those physicians concerned with patients suffering from thoracic-outlet syndromes to achieve a favorable operative result in better than 90 percent of patients.

The signs and symptoms encountered in the upper extremity may include pain, paresthesias, numbness, weakness, discoloration, swelling, ulceration, gangrene, and in some cases Raynaud's phenomenon.

These findings are common to all of the syndromes to be discussed. Moreover, they may also be produced by other conditions. Therefore, it is impossible to make a differential diagnosis from symptoms alone.

To assist the physician in arriving at a diagnosis and advising definitive treatment, we shall briefly review the anatomy of the region, enumerate the most frequent areas of pressure, and describe certain helpful (but not infallible) diagnostic maneuvers. Case histories illustrating the diagnostic difficulties and pitfalls, as well as the operative results, will be presented.

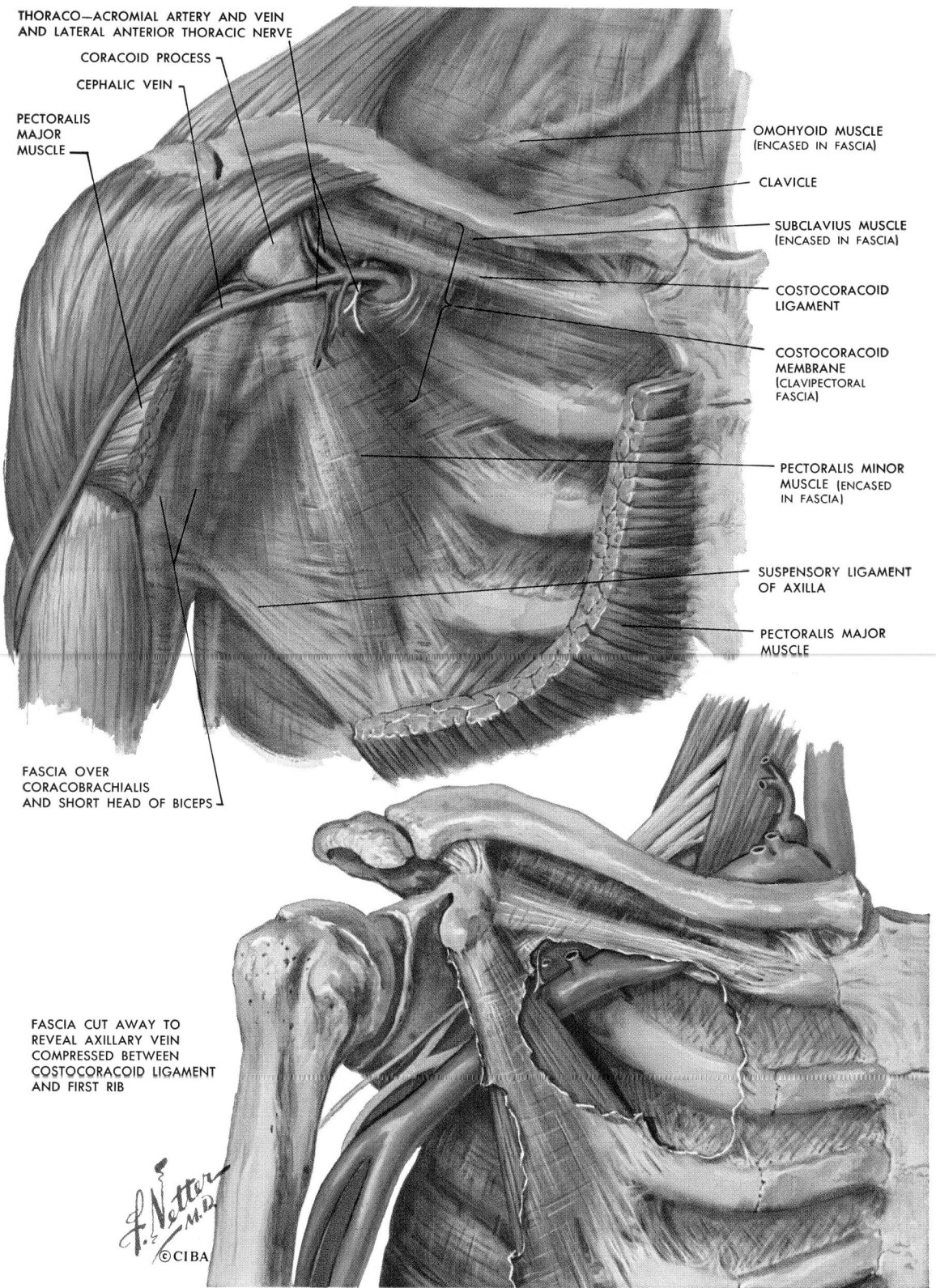

THORACO—ACROMIAL ARTERY AND VEIN
AND LATERAL ANTERIOR THORACIC NERVE

CORACOID PROCESS

CEPHALIC VEIN

PECTORALIS
MAJOR
MUSCLE

OMOHYOID MUSCLE
(ENCASED IN FASCIA)

CLAVICLE

SUBCLAVIUS MUSCLE
(ENCASED IN FASCIA)

COSTOCORACOID
LIGAMENT

COSTOCORACOID
MEMBRANE
(CLAVIPECTORAL
FASCIA)

PECTORALIS MINOR
MUSCLE (ENCASED
IN FASCIA)

SUSPENSORY LIGAMENT
OF AXILLA

PECTORALIS MAJOR
MUSCLE

FASCIA OVER
CORACOBRACHIALIS
AND SHORT HEAD OF BICEPS

FASCIA CUT AWAY TO
REVEAL AXILLARY VEIN
COMPRESSED BETWEEN
COSTOCORACOID LIGAMENT
AND FIRST RIB

©CIBA

PLATE I

FASCIAL SHEATHS OF THE CERVICOTHORACIC REGION

The subclavian artery leaves the thorax by arching over the first rib behind the scalenus anticus muscle and in front of the scalenus medius. It then passes under the subclavius muscle and clavicle and finally enters the axilla beneath the pectoralis minor muscle. Except that it passes anteriorly rather than posteriorly to the scalenus anticus muscle, the subclavian vein has an identical course. The brachial plexus follows the route of the subclavian artery, but it lies a little more posteriorly and laterally.

Fascial Coverings

From its origin at the root of the neck to the lowermost boundary of the axilla, the neurovascular supply of the upper limb is closely confined within rather rigid spaces by an overlying myofascial layer (Plate I). From above downward, this consists of:

(1) The *fascia of the omohyoid* (so-called muscular fascial division of the enveloping layer of the deep cervical fascia); (2) the *posterior belly of the omohyoid,* which is enclosed in this fascia; (3) below the omohyoid, this fascia splits to envelop the *subclavius muscle;* (4) it then joins again to form the *clavipectoral fascia,* whose thickened lateral portion forms the *costocoracoid membrane;* (5) this fascial layer is prolonged inferiorly and splits again to enclose the *pectoralis minor;* (6) finally, it rejoins again to form the *suspensory ligament of the axilla.*

In dissection or surgery, this continuous myofascial layer is a reliable guide to the vital neurovascular structures which lie beneath it.

Spaces of Potential Compression

The neurovascular bundle traverses the following spaces, in each of which some abnormal structural variation may decrease the function by pressing on the nerves and vessels:

1. Intervertebral foramina (brachial plexus roots only),
2. Interscalene triangle,
3. Cervico-axillary canal or costoclavicular space, and
4. The axilla with its unyielding anterior structures, including the pectoralis minor muscle near its insertion into the coracoid process, and the "scissorlike" encirclement of the axillary artery by the heads of the median nerve.

Fortunately, most individuals are so constructed that the artery, vein, and nerves we have mentioned have adequate space to perform their functions, regardless of changes in position or posture.

In addition to the anatomic relationships which provide potential areas of pressure leading to the production of neurovascular-compression syndromes, there are five contributing factors to consider: dynamic, static, congenital, traumatic, and arteriosclerotic.

Dynamic Factors

There is an unusually wide latitude of motion in the components of the shoulder joint. A moderate degree of motion takes place at the sternoclavicular articulation, this being one of the few universal joints in the body. The acromioclavicular articulation permits the inferior angle of the scapula to move laterally, approximately 45 degrees, during elevation of the arm. Finally, the articulation between the humerus and scapula permits the widest range of motion of any joint in the body. These movements, involving changes in relative position of regional structures, may result in compression or impingement upon either vessels and/or nerves. For example, when the arm is in full hyperabduction above the head, the axillary

5

artery is bent 180 degrees from its position when the arm is at the side. This motion pulls the vessel across the coracoid process and head of the humerus, as across a pulley.

Static Factors

Vigorous work or muscular exercise may result in an increase of muscular bulk, thereby reducing the space through which the artery, vein, and nerves must pass. On the other hand, a reduction in muscle mass and tone may cause middle-aged sagging of local structures. That the latter is the more important factor is indicated by the greater frequency of these syndromes in middle-adult life.

Congenital Factors

The presence of a cervical rib, a bifid clavicle, or a bony protuberance on the first rib may cause pressure on the vessels or nerves when the arm is in certain positions. Also there may be a fascial band behind the scalenus anticus or an abnormal insertion of the scalenus medius on the first rib.

Traumatic Factors

The most common traumatic causes of these syndromes are fractures of the clavicle and subacromial dislocation of the humeral head. Occasionally, a crushing injury of the upper thorax may unduly stretch parts of the brachial plexus and/or thrombose the artery or vein.

Arteriosclerotic Factors

The degree of activity and effort that is well tolerated by a healthy, flexible artery may cause thrombosis in a vessel that is narrowed and sclerotic. This situation has been observed in several individuals in their sixth and seventh decades of life, whose shoulder girdles were anatomically normal for their age, but whose arteries were hardened and relatively inflexible.

The symptomatology of the neurovascular symptoms is dependent upon the frequency, duration, and degree of compression of the subclavian or axillary vessels and the lower cords of the brachial plexus. However, the character of the symptoms is of no help in localizing the exact site or sites of pressure. Neither do the symptoms of themselves differentiate these syndromes from other conditions which will be mentioned later.

In general, the symptoms consist of pain in the fingers, hand, forearm, arm, and shoulder, along with paresthesias, which are usually perceived in the area of distribution of C_8 and T_1.[*]

Numbness, most frequently involving the fingers and less frequently affecting the hand and forearm, may also be noted. Ischemic symptoms secondary to intermittent compression of the subclavian artery include numbness, coldness, weakness, and discoloration. More profound degrees of ischemia may result in ulceration or gangrene. Symptoms are usually most marked in the fingers and hands, although there may be numbness and weakness in the forearm as well.

In most cases it is difficult to evaluate the importance of ischemia in the production of pain. Although direct compression of nerve fibers is probably the major cause of referred pain, ischemia may also contribute by producing a local peripheral neuritis, thus increasing the pain. Intermittent interruption of blood flow may be sufficient to cause a peripheral neuritis with lancinating pain lasting as long as

---

[*] C_8 supplies most of the posterior aspect of the arm from just below the posterior axillary crease down to and including the two middle fingers. Also included is the central part of the palm and a narrow area on the anterior aspect of the forearm. T_1 supplies the ulnar aspect of the forearm and hand as well as the little finger.

five or six months, even after pressure on the vessels has been relieved. The pain of neuritis is usually intermittent; whereas in thrombosis, the pain is constant. In some instances, typical Raynaud's phenomenon is apparently activated by one of these syndromes.

Less commonly, the presenting symptoms are those of venous obstruction or occlusion. Characteristically, this results in edema and cyanotic discoloration of the extremity. Dilatation of the superficial veins of the extremity and about the shoulder is a common accompaniment. A considerable number of terms have been applied to the syndrome of axillary and/or subclavian venous thrombosis, perhaps the most popular of which is "effort thrombosis."

SCALENUS-ANTICUS AND CERVICAL-RIB SYNDROMES

Diagnosis of the cervical-rib syndrome was first made by Willshire[4] in 1860 and by Gruber[5] in 1869. In 1905 Murphy[6] described changes in the neurovascular mechanism occurring as a result of pressure between a cervical rib and the scalenus anticus muscle. Naffziger and Grant,[7] and Ochsner, Gage, and DeBakey[8] in 1935 pointed out the fact that the scalenus anticus muscle, without a cervical rib, can be responsible for pressure on the neurovascular bundle, with consequent clinical symptoms.

Interscalene Triangle

As shown in the illustrations, a normally occurring space between the anterior portion of the scalene muscle mass called the scalenus anticus and a posterior portion called the scalenus medius permits passage of the brachial plexus and the subclavian artery from within outward. That this cleavage plane should occur with such clear-cut regularity, free of compression, is a tribute to human anatomic reliability and constancy.

However, as in all nature, *anatomic variations* may occur. For example, an accessory cervical rib or its fibrous extension may narrow the muscular interval between the scalene muscles, causing greater angulation of the subclavian artery and the lower components of the brachial plexus (Plate VII, upper left).

Also the scalene muscles vary considerably in regard to their insertions into the first rib and the arrangement of their fibers.[9,10] The subclavian artery may pass *through* instead of behind the anterior scalene muscle, or portions of the brachial plexus may pass *through* the scalenus medius.

In addition, muscle slips (scalenus minimus) may act as compressing agents on various portions of the neuroarterial axis.

Other pressure-producing anomalies in this area include the presence of anomalous arteries or an elongated transverse process of the seventh cervical vertebra.[11]

Numerous *embryologic, anatomic, and physiologic factors* predispose the nerves and vessels to pressure in this area. These may be summarized as follows:

1. In quadrupeds and the human embryo, the blood vessels and nerves to the upper extremities, along with the ribs, come off more or less at right angles to the spinal column when the latter is carried parallel to the ground.

As man assumes the upright position, however, the upper extremities pull downward toward the ground. Consequently, the lower cords of the brachial plexus and the subclavian vessels on leaving the spinal cord and the thoracic cage must bend rather sharply over the first rib. If a large cervical rib is present, there is additional pressure on these structures.

2. The thoracic cage in quadrupeds and human embryos is deeper from front to back; whereas, in adult man the cage is broader from side to side. This increased lateral diameter adds to the traction on

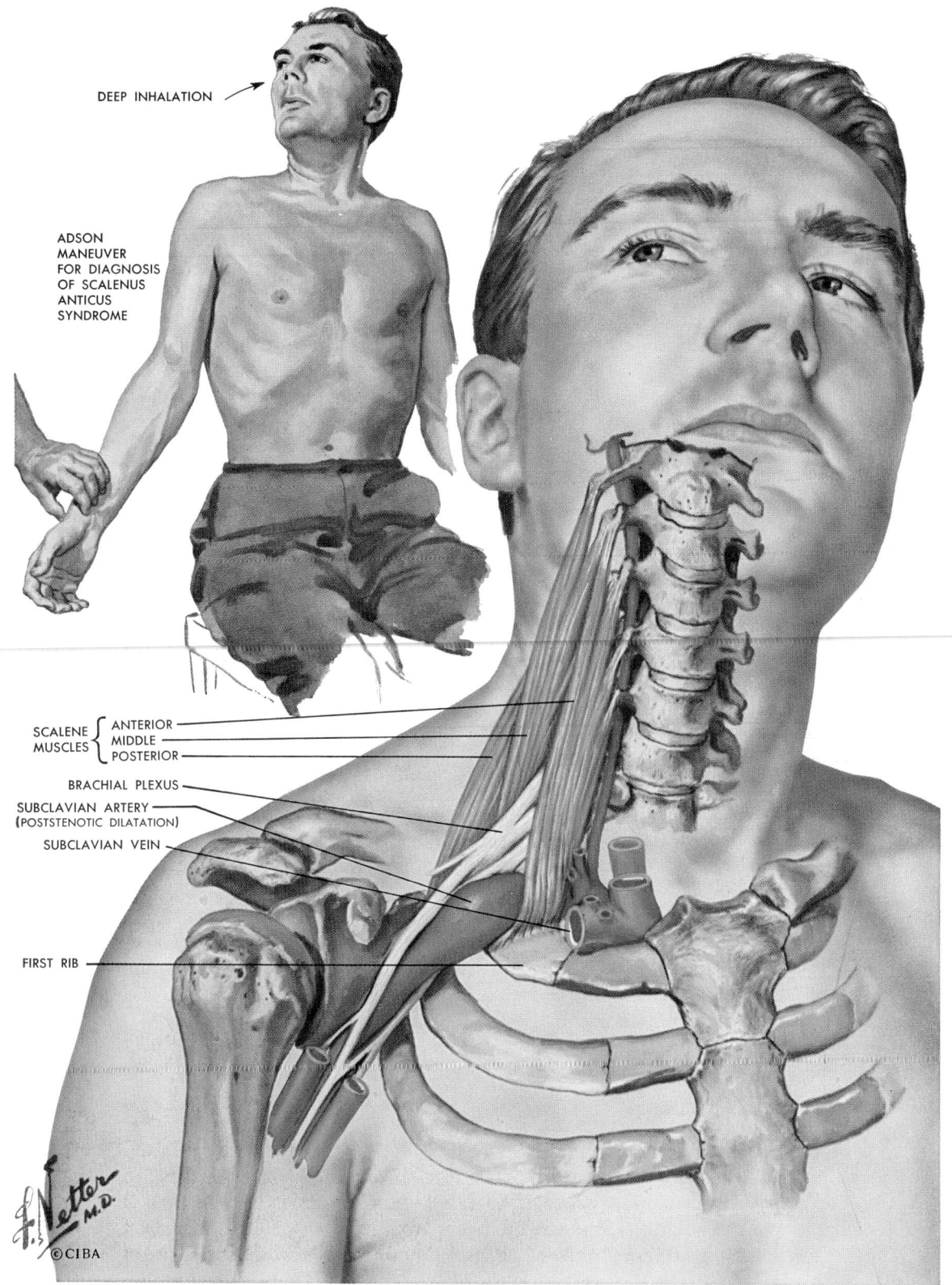

DEEP INHALATION

ADSON
MANEUVER
FOR DIAGNOSIS
OF SCALENUS
ANTICUS
SYNDROME

SCALENE { ANTERIOR
MUSCLES { MIDDLE
POSTERIOR

BRACHIAL PLEXUS

SUBCLAVIAN ARTERY
(POSTSTENOTIC DILATATION)

SUBCLAVIAN VEIN

FIRST RIB

PLATE II   ADSON MANEUVER, RELATION OF SCALENE MUSCLES WITH VESSELS AND NERVES

the brachial plexus and subclavian vessels.

3. Asymmetrical variations of the thoracic outlet can result in further pressure on the neurovascular structures.

4. Sagging and drooping of the shoulders due to postural defects can also exert tension on the nerves and blood vessels.

The relative position of the shoulder to the thorax is high in children, but at puberty, it gradually descends to the adult position. This is more pronounced in females, in whom there is greater movement in the upper part of the chest than in males.

5. Constant respiratory movements, ordinary movements of neck and upper limbs, and cervicobrachial "dragdown" when carrying weights, all put these structures under traction.

Function of the Scalene Muscles

1. Acting from above, they raise the first rib and are therefore muscles of inspiration.

2. Acting unilaterally from below, the cervical vertebral column is flexed toward the contracting side, and the chin is turned to the opposite side.

3. Acting together, they tend to flex the cervical vertebrae.

The Adson[10] or Scalene Maneuver

This maneuver, shown in Plate II, employs all of these actions in order to tense the anterior and middle scalene muscles, thus decreasing the interscalene space and increasing any existing compression of the subclavian artery and lower components (C_8 and T_1) of the brachial plexus against the first rib.

The patient is instructed to:

(1) Take and hold a deep breath.

(2) Extend his neck fully.

(3) Turn his chin toward the side being examined. (In some subjects, a greater effect upon arterial pulsation is exerted by turning the head to the opposite side. Therefore, both positions should be tried.)

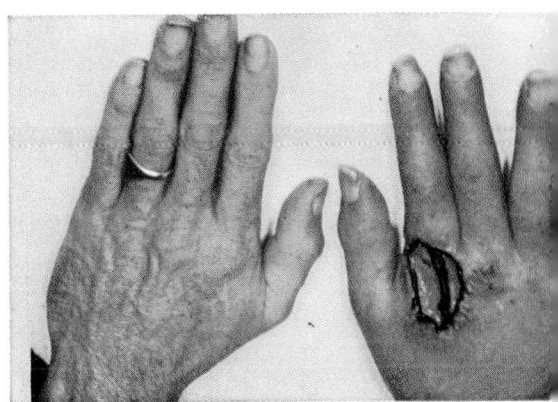

FIGURE 1-A. Scalenus-Anticus Syndrome (Case 1, a 43-year-old male). Six months before admission the patient sustained trauma to the back of the right hand. An ulcer developed, which became progressively worse.

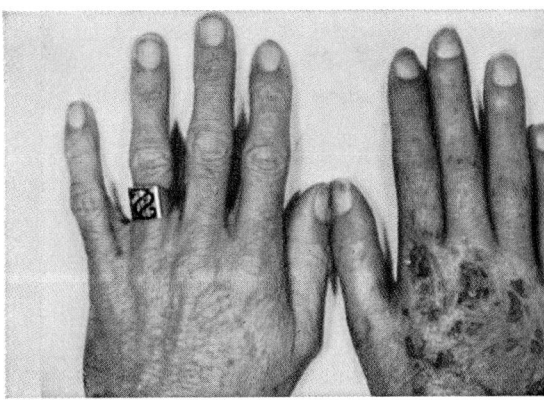

FIGURE 1-B. The same patient six weeks later, after section of the scalenus anticus muscle and an upper thoracic sympathectomy. The ulcer is almost healed; the hand is warm and free from pain and edema. (Kodachromes through courtesy of Clay-Adams, Inc.)

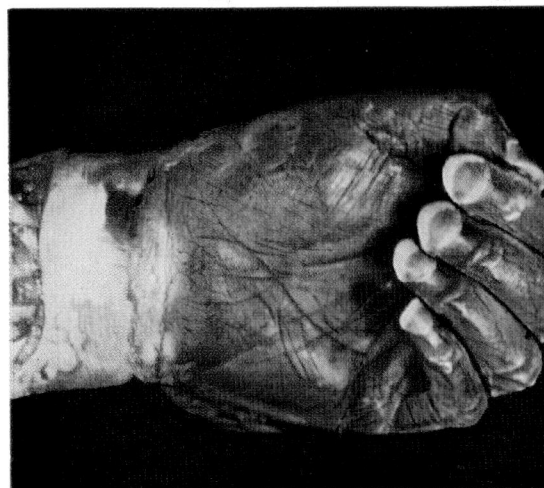

FIGURE 2. Gangrenous hand from reflex arteriospasm following an upper thoracic sympathectomy, carried out by the supraclavicular approach. This approach should not be used in a patient with vascular impairment.

The observer notes any change in the radial pulse that may be produced by this maneuver (Plate II, top). Any resulting decrease in the volume of the pulse suggests that the upper extremity symptoms previously described are caused by abnormal pressure at the interscalene triangle. However, this maneuver does *not* rule out other sources of pressure. Many cases of surgical failure may be attributed to removal of only one of several impediments to blood flow in a given patient. *As will be brought out later, it is necessary to explore thoroughly all possible areas of pressure at the time of operation, regardless of the results of the various tests.*

In Case 1, a 43-year-old Venezuelan truck driver had noted weakness and fatigue of the right arm for three years, which was aggravated by hyperabduction of the arm. One year before hospital admission, he awoke and found his right hand was cold and numb. Six months later trauma of the dorsum of the right hand led to an ulcer, which had progressively enlarged and was continually painful. He had been advised to submit to a forearm amputation.

Physical examination revealed a thin, chronically ill man who would not permit anyone to touch his right hand. There was no brachial, radial, or ulnar pulse on the right, nor could a pulsation be felt supraclavicularly. All pulses were normal in the left upper extremity. On the back of the right hand there was a large ulcer (5 cm in diameter), exposing the second metacarpophalangeal joint. The entire hand was edematous and cool, with a good deal of muscular atrophy (Figure 1-A). The oscillometric index was 0.1 at the right forearm, in contrast to a swing of 2.25 on the left.

Treatment included total abstinence from tobacco and operative exploration of the right supraclavicular fossa. Following section of the scalenus anticus muscle and fascia, the subclavian artery was found to pulsate vigorously to the lateral border of the sectioned muscle and then at that point to be thrombosed. There was no narrowing of the costoclavicular space. An upper thoracic sympathectomy was carried out through the Palumbo[12] approach (anterior transthoracic, transpleural), which affords excellent exposure of the upper thoracic ganglia.

The postoperative course was gratifying, the hand became warm, free from pain and edema, and the ulcer diminished rapidly in size so that at the time of his return to Venezuela six weeks later, it measured only 1 cm in diameter in the region of the joint (Figure 1-B).

We firmly believe that when dealing with functional or organic vascular disease of the upper extremity, under *no* circumstances should an upper thoracic sympathectomy be carried out by the supraclavicular (Telford[13]) approach. In the Telford procedure, the subclavian artery must be pulled forward and downward, and occasionally one of its branches must be divided. Even in the skilled hands of experienced neurosurgeons, serious complications, including thromboses, hemorrhage requiring ligation, and excessive reflex arteriospasm resulting in gangrene of a hand, have occurred. Figure 2 is an example of a hand which developed gangrene following the reflex spasm induced by this procedure. These complications are totally unnecessary and easily obviated when an upper thoracic sympathectomy is carried out through the anterior transthoracic approach as described by Palumbo. Another safe and excellent approach is the transaxillary one for upper thoracic sympathectomy as described by Goetz and Marr.[14]

Case 2 illustrates the fact that it is essential not only to sever the anterior scalene, but also to explore the triangle thoroughly for fibrous bands, muscle slips, or other structures which may be compressing the neurovascular bundle.

A 38-year-old white woman was admitted with the complaint of pains in the left hand, chiefly in the palm and first finger, made worse by 90-degree abduction. Her difficulty was noted for the first time seven years prior to admission. For four years there had been, in addition, pain in the left shoulder and axilla, aggravated by lifting objects from the floor and relieved by lying on her left side or by hyperabduction of the arm to 135 degrees.

An examination by an experienced neurologist ruled out disease of the spinal cord and nerve roots but suggested that pressure on the brachial plexus by a prominent firm protuberance in the left supraclavicular area might be responsible for the patient's signs and symptoms.

Examination revealed a lean, well-developed woman with unusually straight clavicles (confirmed by x-ray examination). There was a hard protuberance in the left supraclavicular area, approximately two inches lateral to the base of the neck. The left radial pulse was abolished by 135 degrees of abduction, markedly dampened by the costoclavicular maneuver, and unaltered by the scalenus-anticus maneuver.

In July, 1955, an exploration revealed a thin, poorly developed scalenus anticus muscle and a thick, broad fascial band extending from the scalenus medius, inserting into the first rib considerably more anteriorly than usual. This hard band explained the hard prominence noted preoperatively. This unusual anatomic arrangement resulted in considerable pinching of the subclavian artery and the brachial plexus (Plate VI, upper left).

The scalenus anticus was sectioned, eliminating the anterior pressure. Also the entire fascial band and scalenus medius were sectioned, thus relieving posterior and inferior pressure. This allowed adequate room for the artery and the plexus.

Immediately on awakening, the patient noted that the arm and hand were free from pain. During the 15 years which have elapsed since operation, the patient has been free from symptoms in the left arm and hand. There is no dampening of the radial pulse by any of the three maneuvers.

In this case one may speculate that the negative Adson maneuver was due to the fact that the poorly developed anterior scalene muscle failed to exert additional pressure on contraction. During the costoclavicular maneuver (which will be discussed later) the clavicle probably exerted pressure against the abnormally placed scalene muscles rather than against the first rib.

COSTOCLAVICULAR SYNDROME

Falconer and Weddell[15] defined clearly the evidence for costoclavicular compression and delineated it sharply from the scalenus anticus syndrome. In the latter, the radial pulse is dampened by the measures we have previously described. However, in the costoclavicular syndrome, pressure is exerted on the subclavian artery and vein by a backward and downward thrust of the shoulders, which narrows the space between the clavicle and first rib. This was first noticed in soldiers whose shoulders were kept in this position for long periods of time by carrying a heavy pack.

The costoclavicular area will be extensively reviewed; because in our experience, it is a major source of difficulty. Even when diagnostic studies seem to indicate otherwise, the area should be explored thoroughly.

Costoclavicular Space

This space, sometimes called the cervico-axillary canal (shown in Plate III), is a triangle bounded by:

1. Anteriorly, the inner one third of the clavicle, the underlying subclavius

muscle arising from the outer one third of the clavicle and inserting into the cartilage of the first rib and the costocoracoid ligament (Plate III top, and Plate I bottom).

2. Posteromedially, the anterior one third of the first rib and insertions of the anterior and middle scalene muscles.

3. Posterolaterally, the superior border of the scapula.

The subclavian vein lies in the inner medial angle of this interval, between the insertion of the anterior scalene muscle posteriorly and the inner end of the clavicle, with its underlying tendon of insertion of the subclavius muscle and the costocoracoid ligament inserting into the first rib anteriorly (Plate III).

The coracoclavicular fascia is a strong, thickened layer situated under the clavicular portion of the pectoralis major. It occupies the interval between the pectoralis minor and the subclavius muscles, protecting the axillary vessels and nerves. Above, it splits to enclose the subclavius muscle and clavicle, its two layers attaching to the clavicle anterior and posterior to the muscle, extending from the first rib to the coracoid process.

Predisposing Factors

Acute trauma to the subclavian artery, the subclavian vein, and the brachial plexus may result from direct fracture of the clavicle. However, there are additional mechanisms by which this bone may injure these structures. These include mal- and nonunited fractures, as well as congenital anomalies of the clavicle. Finally, there is a group of structural changes in which the retroclavicular neurovascular structures are intermittently compressed by the clavicle upon the assumption of certain postural positions. These include cervicodorsal scoliosis,[13] failure of the anterior curvature of the clavicle to develop normally, abnormalities of the first rib, hypertrophied subcla-

vius muscle, and abnormalities of the costocoracoid ligament.[16]

Functions of the Clavicle

1. Through the sternoclavicular joint, it furnishes the only direct bony connection between the upper extremity and the trunk.

2. It furnishes a bony framework for muscle origins and insertions (trapezius, deltoid, sternocleidomastoid, pectoralis major, and subclavius).

3. Since the support of the shoulder is provided mainly by muscles, particularly the trapezius, which have their origins and insertions on the clavicle, it provides the means for transmitting these muscular forces to the scapula.

4. It provides bony protection for the subclavian and axillary vessels and brachial plexus. The normal anterior curvature in its medial two-thirds provides an arch, whereby the neurovascular bundle can pass behind and beneath it to enter the axilla. In some individuals this curvature is minimal, thus narrowing the costoclavicular space.

During elevation of the arm, the clavicle rotates *backward*. In addition, when the shoulders are retracted *backward* and *downward*, the clavicle moves in this same direction. Thus both of these motions tend to narrow the costoclavicular space. The space is also narrowed by deep inspiration which raises the first rib.

The Costoclavicular Maneuver

The exaggerated military position, with the shoulders drawn downward and backward, is used to detect compression in the costoclavicular interval (Plate III).

This maneuver narrows the costoclavicular space by approximating the clavicle to the first rib, thus tending to compress the neurovascular structures that lie between. Modification or obliteration of the radial pulse, with reproduction of symptoms by this maneuver, indicates

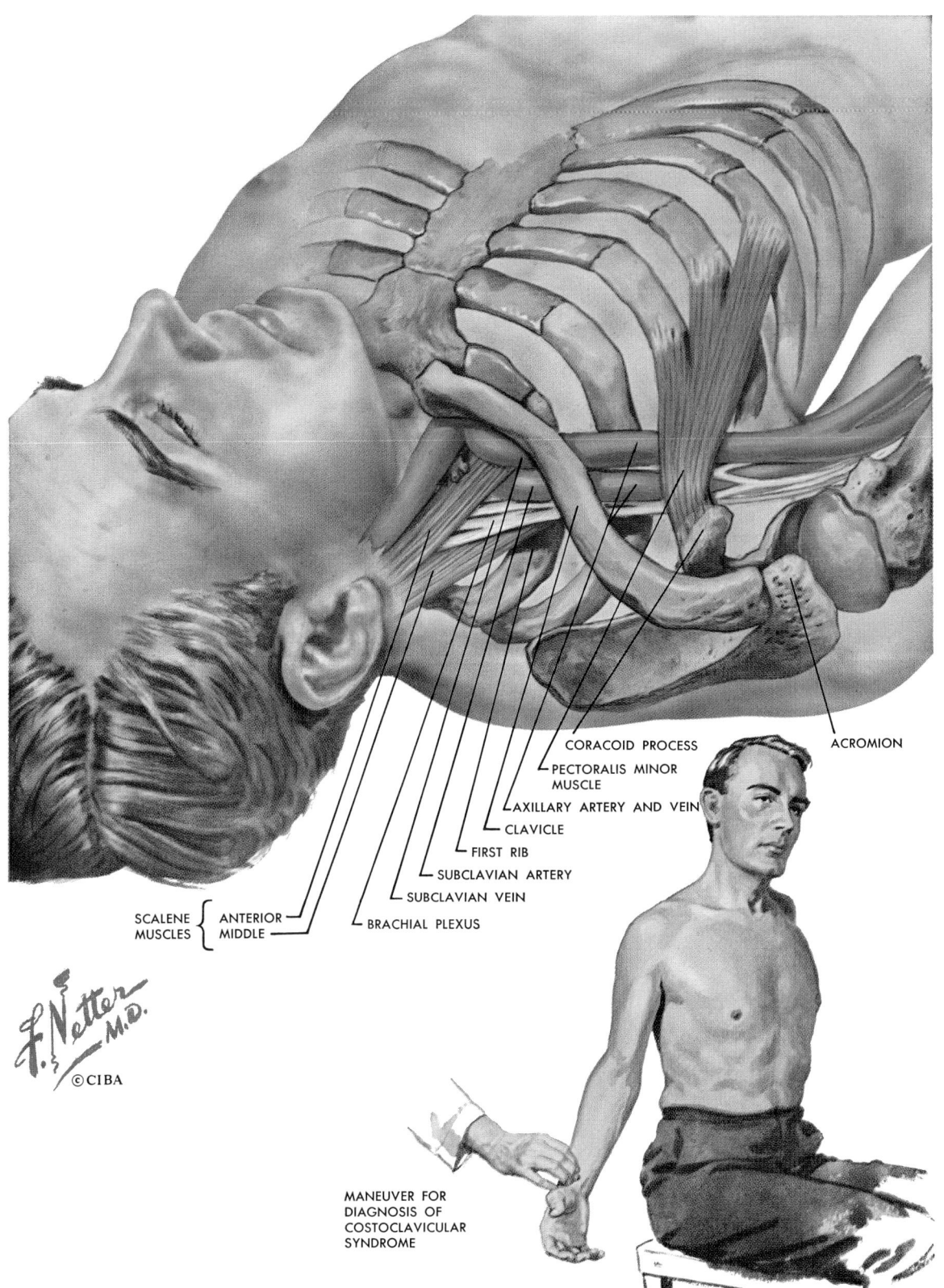

CORACOID PROCESS

ACROMION

PECTORALIS MINOR MUSCLE

AXILLARY ARTERY AND VEIN

CLAVICLE

FIRST RIB

SUBCLAVIAN ARTERY

SUBCLAVIAN VEIN

BRACHIAL PLEXUS

SCALENE MUSCLES { ANTERIOR / MIDDLE

MANEUVER FOR DIAGNOSIS OF COSTOCLAVICULAR SYNDROME

PLATE III

COSTOCLAVICULAR SPACE AND DIAGNOSTIC MANEUVER

compression in this area. It should be noted that this maneuver will cause a dampening of the pulse in many perfectly normal people. Such people do not have symptoms, because in their normal posture no pressure is present.

Special Cases

Case 3 was a 42-year-old white woman who gave a history of having sustained bilateral fractures of the clavicle and multiple fractures of the jaw 17 years prior to admission. Six weeks following the clavicular fractures, overriding was noted, and bilateral open reduction with fixation of the fragments by kangaroo tendon was performed. A satisfactory functional result was obtained on the right, but on the left side the patient noted intermittent discomfort in the region of the clavicle and shoulder.

Four months prior to admission, the patient noted that her left arm was larger than the right and that this arm fatigued more readily than the right. There was no swelling of the forearm or hand, and no paresthesias were noted. The swelling and weakness gradually increased until four days prior to admission, when, following a swim, the whole of the left arm became markedly swollen. There was extreme weakness of the extremity and a subjective sensation of coolness.

Examination revealed a malunited fracture of the left clavicle (Plate VI, right). Dilated superficial veins extended from the left arm and shoulder to the pectoral region. The entire left upper extremity was moderately swollen. Skin temperature of the arms was equal on gross testing. When lying in bed with the left arm at the side, the radial pulse was strong. However, upon sitting, which produced a modified costoclavicular maneuver, the radial pulse was obliterated by deep inspiration. Turning of the head to either side, or abduction of the left arm to 45 degrees, also obliterated the pulse. X-ray of the clavicle revealed a malunited fracture on the left, with significant overriding of the medial fragment (Figure 3-A).

At operation the patient was found to have a large number of venous collateral channels in the retroclavicular space. The subclavian vein was found to be thrombosed. The inner tip of the lateral clavicular fragment was pressing upon the subclavian artery and was apparently responsible for the intermittent compression of this vessel on deep inspiration or hyperabduction. The clavicular fragments, including periosteum, were resected (see Figure 3-B). Immediately after operation, it was possible to hyperabduct the left arm to 180 degrees without obliterating the radial pulse.

The postoperative course was uncomplicated. The arm was maintained in a position of elevation, and anticoagulant therapy was instituted and maintained for approximately one month. At the time of discharge, seven days following surgery, the left upper arm was two inches larger in circumference than the right. There was no difference in size between the left and right forearms and hands. The patient was fitted with an elastic sleeve.

During the nine-year follow-up, she had no pain in the clavicular or shoulder regions and has noted no fatigue or paresthesias in the left upper extremity. It is her impression that the collateral veins over the left shoulder have become slightly more prominent. There has been no evidence of clavicular regeneration.

The left arm remains slightly larger than the right. Turning the head, depressing the shoulders, deep inspiration, and hyperabduction do not dampen the left radial pulse. Figure 3-C shows the patient four years postoperatively.

Case 4 was a 47-year-old white woman who had first noted pain, numbness, tingling, and weakness in the left hand and arm five years prior to admission. At that time she had been studied at another hos-

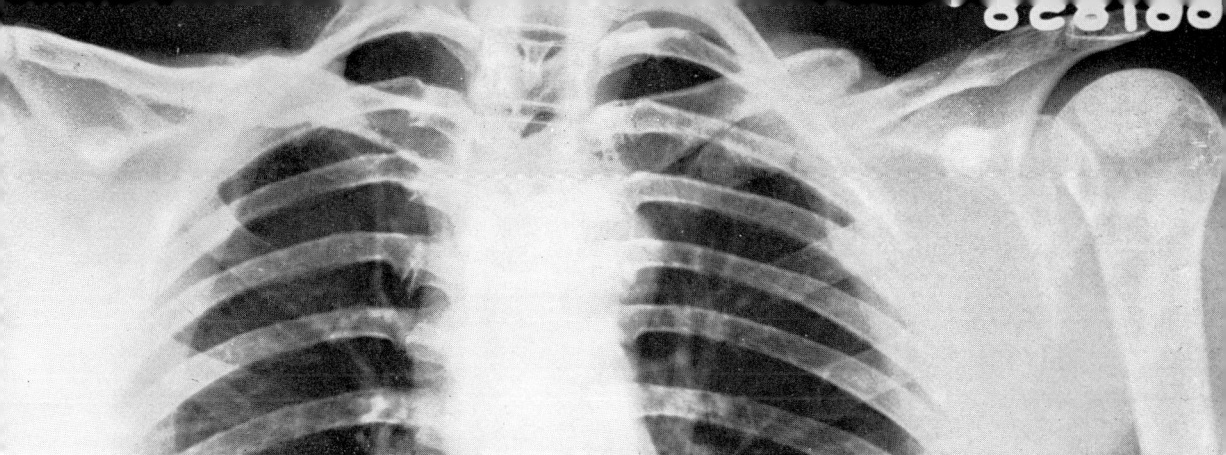

FIGURE 3-A. A bilateral clavicular fracture was sustained 17 years previously by a 42-year-old woman (Case 3). Four months before admission the left arm became swollen and tired easily. On sitting up, turning the head to either side, or abducting the arm, the pulse became obliterated. X-ray showed a malunited fracture on the left.

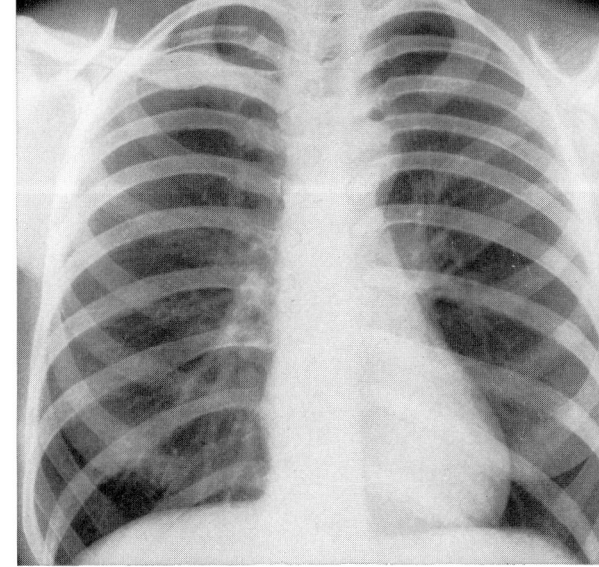

FIGURE 3-B. At surgery the subclavian vein was found to be thrombosed. The inner tip of the lateral clavicular fragment was pressing on the artery, apparently causing intermittent compression. The clavicular fragments, including periosteum, were resected.

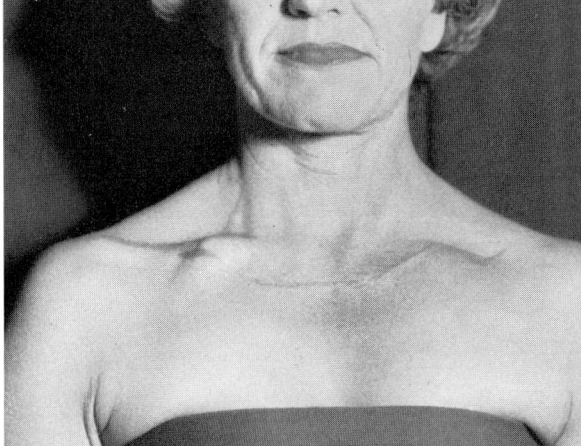

FIGURE 3-C. The same patient shown four years postoperatively. The left arm is still slightly larger, but turning of the head, depressing the shoulders, and hyperabduction do not dampen the left radial pulse.

pital, and conservative therapy was recommended. The symptoms had improved during the following seven months. Five months prior to admission, similar symptoms occurred for the first time in the right arm.

Examination revealed an absence of all major arterial pulsations in both arms. The hands were not cold, and there was no pallor. Oscillometric studies showed no pulsations in either arm or forearm. There was a palpable defect in the middle third of both clavicles. X-rays of the clavicles revealed a congenital absence of the middle third of the bone bilaterally.

Subtotal resections of the medial and lateral fragments of both clavicles, including the periosteum, were performed. Anterior scalenotomy with mobilization of the subclavian artery was also carried out on both sides. The subclavian arteries were found to be thrombosed. On both sides, the medial tip of the lateral segment of the clavicle pressed on the artery.

Following removal of the clavicular fragments on the right (Figure 4), the symptoms on that side cleared within one week. At one time, feeble radial pulsations were felt by a number of observers.

At the time of discharge, following removal of the left clavicle, the patient was asymptomatic. She was followed by her family physician in Venezuela for 18 months and remained in good health, with normal use of the upper extremities.

The two preceding cases illustrate the difference between arterial and venous thromboses. It is our impression that unless operated *very* promptly, a venous thrombosis seldom canalizes. While circulatory improvement from collaterals may sustain function and relieve symptoms, the arm rarely, if ever, returns completely to normal. On the other hand, in a few cases arterial thromboses do become canalized. Of 15 such cases of arterial thrombosis, we feel confident that four have recanalized, six have developed excellent collateral circulation with a weak pulse, and in five the pulse is still absent, suggesting only slight to moderate development of collateral vessels.

FIGURE 4. Patient's (Case 4) symptoms were produced by bilateral thrombosis of subclavian arteries, secondary to congenital absence of middle third of both clavicles. X-ray appearance after removal of the right clavicular fragment.

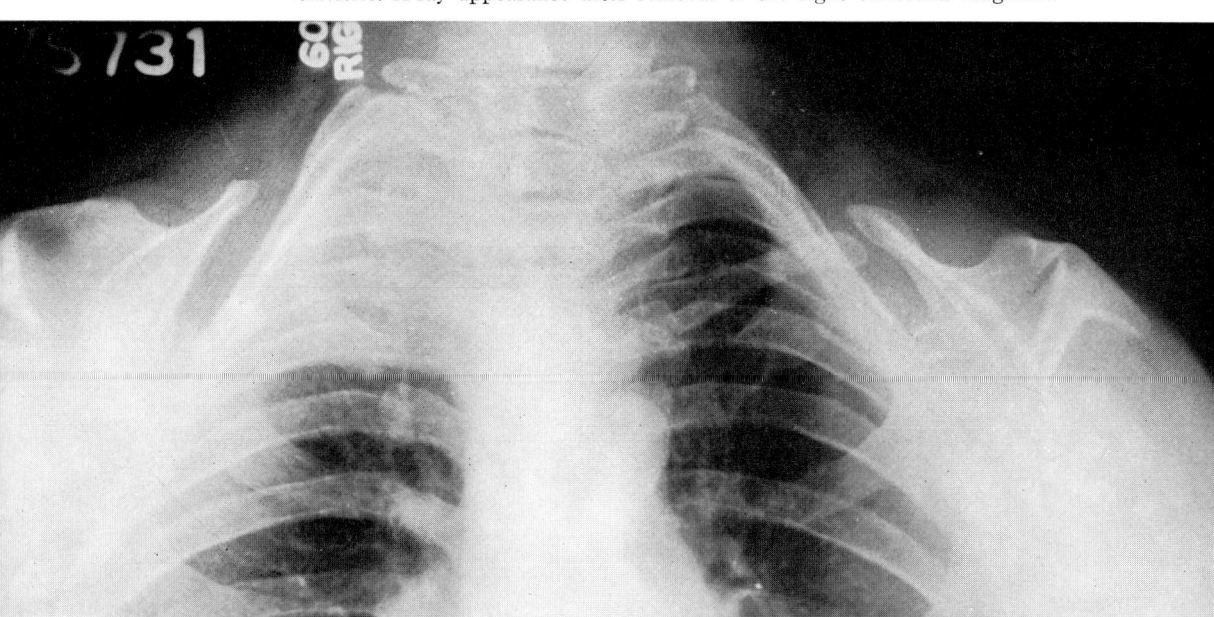

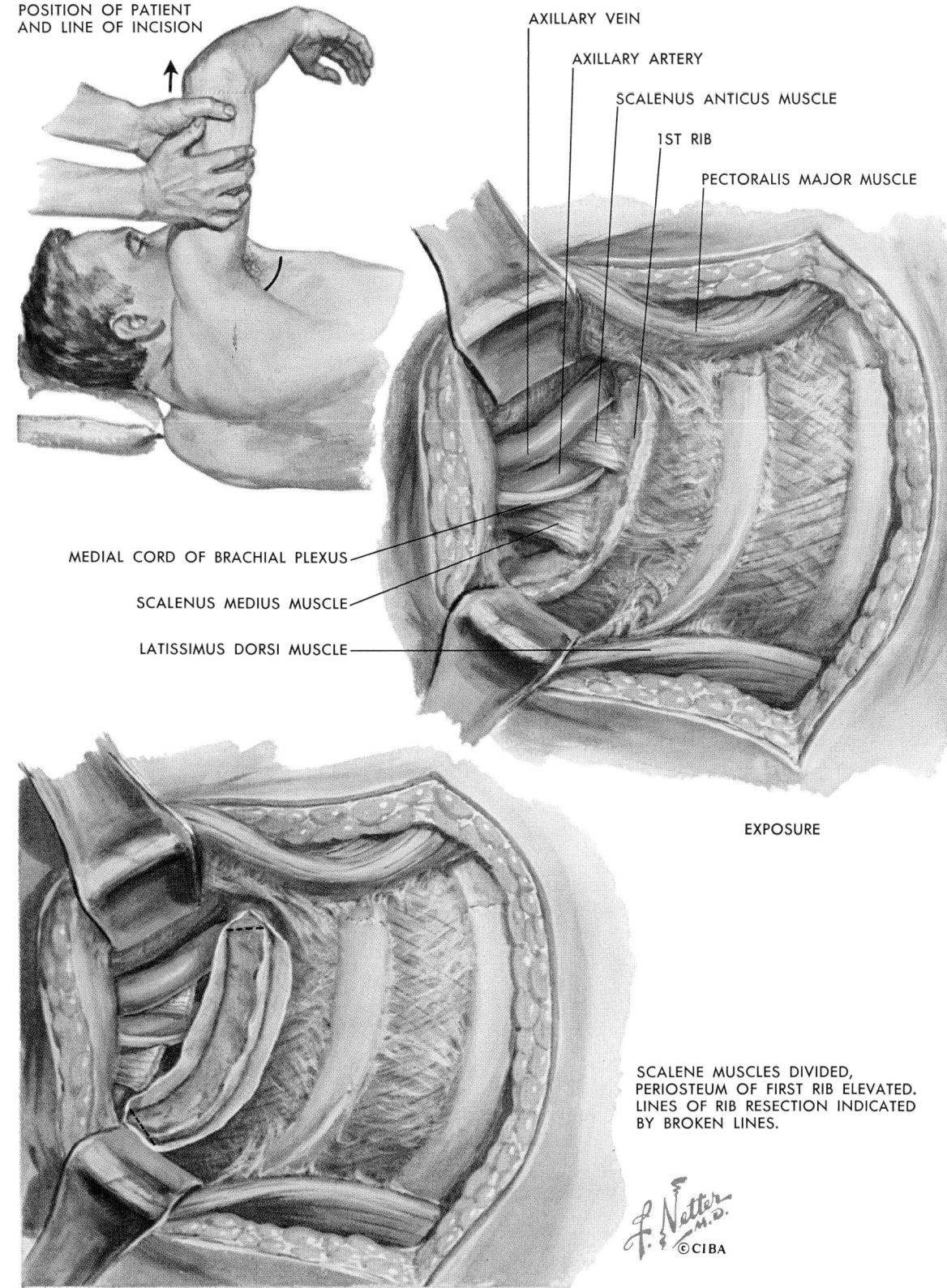

POSITION OF PATIENT
AND LINE OF INCISION

AXILLARY VEIN

AXILLARY ARTERY

SCALENUS ANTICUS MUSCLE

1ST RIB

PECTORALIS MAJOR MUSCLE

MEDIAL CORD OF BRACHIAL PLEXUS

SCALENUS MEDIUS MUSCLE

LATISSIMUS DORSI MUSCLE

EXPOSURE

SCALENE MUSCLES DIVIDED,
PERIOSTEUM OF FIRST RIB ELEVATED.
LINES OF RIB RESECTION INDICATED
BY BROKEN LINES.

PLATE IV

RESECTION OF FIRST RIB (TRANSAXILLARY APPROACH)

Presently, we believe that the best operation for the majority of patients suffering from compression of the nerves and vessels in the thoracic outlet is transaxillary resection of the first rib (Plate IV). Included in the procedure is section of the scalenus anticus and medius muscles at their insertion to the first rib. Roos and Owens[2] and Sanders[3] deserve great credit in developing this procedure. In contrast to their writings, however, we believe there are important exceptions where other procedures should be selected when specific indications exist.

1. For correction of the costoclavicular syndrome when the clavicle is abnormal due to a congenital malformation or as a result of improper healing following fracture, then total claviculectomy with complete removal of the periosteum to prevent regeneration is the operation of choice. In some instances, section of the scalenus anticus should be included. The functional result is excellent and the appearance cosmetically acceptable.

2. When the cervical-rib syndrome is paramount, then the supraclavicular approach with excision of the rib and sectioning of the scalenus anticus is highly satisfactory.

3. For intermittent or complete obstruction of the subclavian vein which requires surgical relief, we prefer the operation designed by McCleery and Kirtley[17] which includes section of the scalenus anticus and partial excision of the subclavius muscle and costocoracoid ligament. If a recent thrombosis has occurred, then transbrachial extraction of the thrombus with a Fogarty catheter with maintenance of continuity by careful suture of the aperture in the vein should be combined with the procedure outlined above to prevent reformation of a thrombus.

If signs of arterial or neurological involvement accompany the venous lesion, then transaxillary resection of the first rib with concomitant section of the scalenus anticus and medius muscles should be the operative approach. The McCleery-Kirtley procedure will therefore have only limited application.

Case 5, a powerfully built 16-year-old weight lifter, was examined for the first time three months following the development of a swollen right arm noticed upon awakening one morning. For one week there was cyanosis of the entire right upper extremity with increase in swelling and pain.

Phlebogram performed at that time showed obstruction of the entire axillary vein with a large collateral from the cephalic to the jugular vein. The measurements showed a 3.5 cm increase in arm circumference and a 2 cm increase at the forearm.

Transaxillary resection of the first rib with section of the scalenus medius and anticus muscles was carried out.

Reexamination two years later showed the arm and forearm circumferences to be only 1 cm larger on the right over the left. He had been completely asymptomatic, playing college football without limitation. Clinically, venous pressure in the two upper extremities was normal.

4. For reconstruction of the subclavian artery, we prefer wide exposure of the vessel with proximal and distal control and insertion of a vein graft. Such exposure is best obtained by removal of the clavicle and its periosteum and division of the scalenus anticus muscle. For exposure of the axillary vessels, detachment of the pectoralis major and minor tendons may be included.

OBSTRUCTION OF SUBCLAVIAN VEIN

Case 6 was a 32-year-old white woman who had noticed swelling of the left arm, aching, and heaviness without significant pain for a period of two weeks. In May,

1956, she was treated by bed rest, elevation of the left arm, moist warm packs, and anticoagulants, with pronounced improvement. She was discharged in two weeks, maintained on Dicumarol for four weeks, and did well for one more week, when she experienced a recurrence of the swelling with bluish discoloration of the arm. This episode followed the washing of her child's hair, which required 90-degree abduction of her arm.

On readmission to the hospital, examination showed the venous pressure in the left arm to be approximately 15 cm higher than in the right arm. There was tenderness along the medial aspect of the arm and in the axilla. The scalenus-anticus maneuver was positive, dampening the radial pulse; whereas the hyperabduction and costoclavicular maneuvers were without effect on the pulse. On the right side all three tests were negative.

Conservative measures were employed, and there was improvement for ten days, at which time an operative procedure was performed, consisting of resection of the subclavius muscle and the costocoracoid ligament with section of the scalenus anticus muscle. At the completion of these procedures, it was possible to pass the index finger between the clavicle and the first rib. The subclavian vein was thrombosed at this point. By the fifth postoperative day the venous pressure in the left hand was estimated to be normal, and the arm was asymptomatic. The patient was discharged on the seventh postoperative day. Anticoagulants were continued postoperatively for two months.

When last seen, 14 years postoperatively, she was asymptomatic, and the only residual abnormality was a one and one-half cm increase in circumference of the left arm compared with the right. The forearm, wrist, and hand were of equal dimension, and the venous pressure was equal bilaterally.

This last case illustrates the complicated diagnostic problems encountered in these compression syndromes and a possible reason for failure after a single corrective measure. Because of the negative hyperabduction and costoclavicular tests and the positive scalene maneuver, one might have been tempted to undertake only an anterior scalenotomy, whereas the actual obstruction was between the clavicle and first rib.

Development of an intra-arterial and an intravenous catheter by Fogarty and his associates[18] must be regarded as an outstanding advance. With minimal training in their use, vascular surgeons have utilized these catheters for the extraction of emboli and thrombi from vessels of the arterial and venous systems consistently and from regions far from the surgically exposed vessels.

Pertinent to this monograph is the extraction of thrombi from the subclavian vein via a small opening in the brachial vein. This maneuver, in conjunction with correction of the thoracic-outlet problem by transaxillary resection of the first rib or the removal of a portion of the subclavius muscle and costocoracoid ligament plus section of the scalenus anticus muscle, constitutes the ideal procedure in patients with acute thrombosis of the axillosubclavian vein.

From an analysis of several venograms of patients suffering from so-called "effort thrombosis" of the axillary vein (Figure 5), it seems evident that the point of obstruction is at the site where the vein passes between the costocoracoid ligament and subclavius muscle anteriorly and the first rib posteriorly (Plate I, bottom). This may be readily demonstrated in the cadaver, and we have also confirmed this as being the point of costoclavicular pressure in several patients. That this area is the site of intermittent obstruction may be observed in angiocardiography when the arm is abducted to 135 degrees. Figure 6 (A, B, C, and D) shows the marked

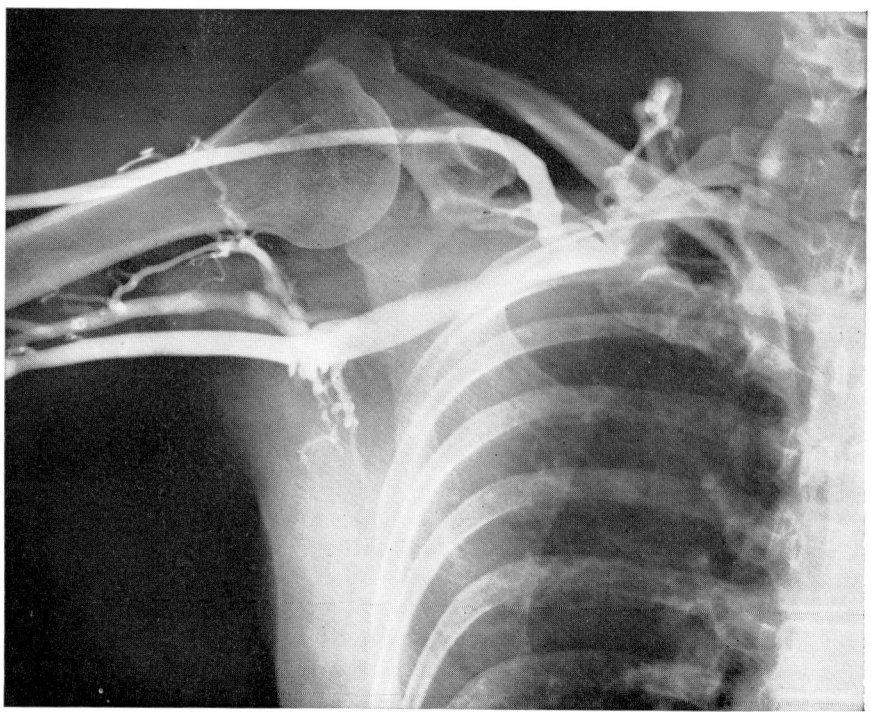

FIGURE 5. An analysis of venograms indicates the point of obstruction in the so-called "effort thrombosis" is where the vein passes between the costa-coracoid ligament and subclavius muscle anteriorly and first rib posteriorly.

delay in emptying of a normal axillary and subclavian vein in a patient who was studied for a possible cardiac lesion. This concept was first pointed out by Lowenstein[16] in 1924. His sound conclusions were based on careful dissection studies on 36 cadavers.

As pointed out by McCleery *et al*[17] in 1951, a second point of pressure may exist between the scalenus anticus muscle posteriorly and the clavicle and subclavius muscle anteriorly. In this condition, it may be necessary to remove the costocoracoid ligament and subclavius muscle and also to divide the scalenus anticus muscle.

HYPERABDUCTION SYNDROME

In 1945, Wright[18] first described a syndrome characterized by neurovascular symptoms in the upper extremities following repeated and prolonged assumption of the position of hyperabduction. The postural attitude responsible for the symptoms was one in which the arms were brought together above the head, with the elbows flexed. This position is frequently assumed in sleep and to lesser degree is practiced in certain occupations, such as grease-pit mechanics and painters. With wider recognition of the syndrome, it has been extended to include neurovascular symptoms resulting from lesser degrees of hyperabduction.

Wright described two potential sites of compression of the subclavian vessels and the brachial plexus in the hyperabduction syndrome. One site is the point at which the neurovascular structures pass beneath the tendon of the pectoralis minor muscle and under the coracoid process. The second site of compression is the retroclavicular space between the clavicle and first rib, which is diminished

20

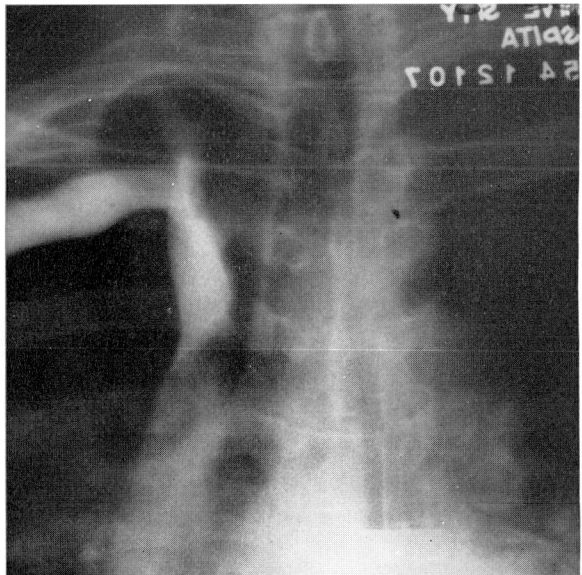
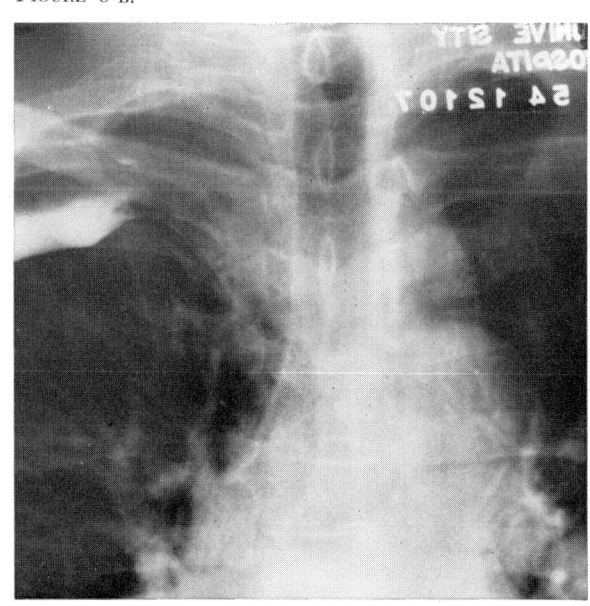

FIGURES 6-A, 6-B, 6-C, AND 6-D. Pictures taken at 1, 10, 20, and 28 seconds after the intravenous injection of a radiopaque dye in a patient being studied for a cardiac lesion. These serial angiograms show the delay in emptying of a normal axillary and subclavian vein, when the arm is abducted 135 degrees.

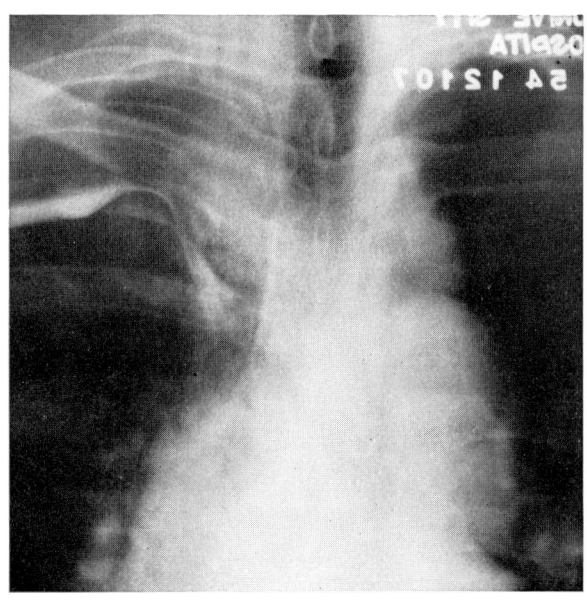
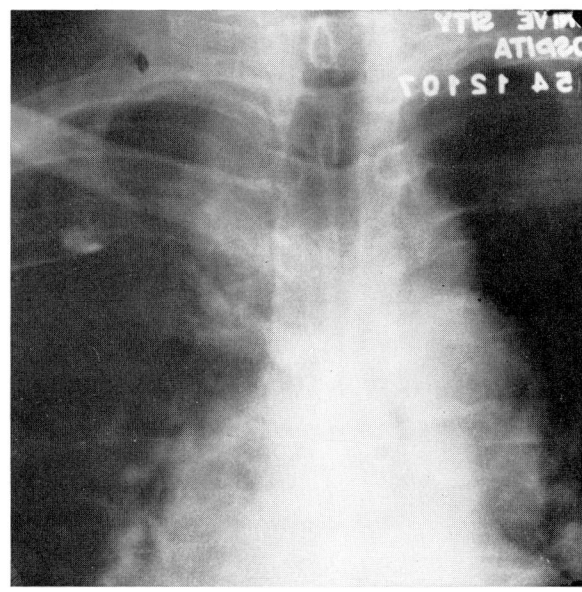

FIGURE 6-C.

FIGURE 6-D.

to a variable degree by hyperabduction.

We have been particularly impressed with the importance of the pectoralis minor tendon as a cause of symptoms and the value of its division in alleviating the vascular compression that occurs during hyperabduction.

During the dissection of cadavers for illustration of this article, we found that when the arm is hyperabducted and the artery, vein, and nerve somewhat fixed by the pectoralis minor tendon, the humeral head may also exert pressure against them.

Anatomy of Hyperabduction

The term hyperabduction describes the full range of normal scapulohumeral motion, enabling the hand to move from a position at the side of the body through an arc of 180 degrees (Plate V).*

When the arm is undergoing abduction to 180 degrees, five anatomic features are involved in relation to the problem of cervicobrachial-compression syndromes.

1. The neurovascular components are pulled around the pectoralis minor tendon, the coracoid process, and the head of the humerus as though across a pulley.

2. As abduction proceeds, the coracoid process moves *downward,* thus exaggerating the pulley effect on vessels and nerves.

3. The clavicle moves upward 30 degrees and *backward* 35 degrees at the sternoclavicular joint. In some cases this also narrows the costoclavicular space.

4. The subclavius and the pectoralis minor muscles and the costocoracoid ligament become increasingly taut.

5. When the arm is fully abducted to 180 degrees, the components of the brachial plexus and axillary vessels are bent

to form a 90-degree angle, subjecting the axillary artery and vein to maximum compression against the axillary "pulley" previously described.

The radial pulse may be dampened by this maneuver in many perfectly normal people in whom absence of symptoms may be explained by the fact that they rarely assume this abnormal position. However, when this maneuver produces typical symptoms, it suggests the desirability of operative intervention, and corrective measures should be considered.

Case 7, a 39-year-old white female, had noted redness and swelling of the right arm and a sensation of tightness in the muscles of the arm aggravated by exercise for three months. She consulted a surgeon who reported the presence of erythema of the right arm and a one-inch increase in its circumference on comparison with the left arm. The veins of the right arm were more prominent than those of the left. The blood pressure was essentially the same in both upper extremities. X-ray films of the cervical spine did not reveal a cervical rib. A diagnosis of scalenus anticus syndrome had been made, and a right anterior scalenotomy was performed without relief of symptoms.

When seen a month later, the patient gave the additional history that when she combed her hair or abducted the right arm to 90 degrees or more in the performance of household duties, the arm became heavy and tired quickly.

Abduction of the right arm to 90 degrees resulted in complete obliteration of the radial pulse. The scalenus anticus and costoclavicular maneuvers did not dampen the radial pulse. It was felt that the patient had a thrombosis of the subclavian vein and the hyperabduction syndrome. The right pectoralis minor tendon was divided. Immediately postoperatively the right arm could be abducted to 180 degrees without dampening of the radial pulse.

Examination one month following

---

*As has been pointed out by Beyer and Wright,° "while hyperabduction is accepted in anatomic terminology, it is neither ideal nor entirely logical, but it is still considered to be better than any other available term."

operation revealed that she had regained full use of the right arm. The heavy sensation and tired feeling had completely cleared. The right arm remained approximately one inch greater in diameter than the left, a residual of thrombosis of the subclavian vein. Thus the relief of compression beneath the pectoralis minor tendon resulted in excellent function, in spite of the unchanged venous thrombosis. A follow-up letter nineteen months later stated that she had no further trouble with the right arm.

Case 8, a 43-year-old white electrical worker, was admitted in January, 1957. He had been in excellent health until six months prior to admission, when he developed brown spots on the tip of the right index finger, which subsequently ulcerated, and the finger became swollen. A diagnosis of Raynaud's disease was made, and within two months the process progressed to involve the third finger. On exposure to cold, the fingers of the right hand blanched and became painful. One week before admission, he was exposed to severe cold, and marked pain developed in the fingers of his right hand. His heavy smoking was stopped only at the time of admission to the hospital.

Physical examination showed a firm nodule located in the right supraclavicular area near the clavicle. On this side a strong brachial pulse and moderate radial pulse were present. The day after admission, the radial pulse disappeared. Hyperabduction and costoclavicular maneuvers markedly weakened the brachial pulse. The index and middle fingers of the right hand showed gangrene of their tips and small areas of superficial necrosis of the tips of the fourth and fifth fingers (see Figure 7). X-ray of the chest and clavicular area showed an abnormal bony enlargement of the first rib on the right, both medially and laterally, in the region of the clavicle (Plate VI, lower right).

At operation, after the scalenus anticus muscle had been divided, it was obvious there was marked narrowing of the space between the clavicle and first rib due to the bony prominence on the first rib. In order to make room for the subclavian artery, the clavicle was completely removed along with its periosteum. Postoperatively the patient made a rapid recovery. By the fourth postoperative day an ulnar pulse could be felt, becoming strong by the tenth postoperative day. The radial artery remained a thrombosed cord. The result has been excellent during the 13-year follow-up.

CARPAL-TUNNEL SYNDROME

Over the past 20 years the carpal-tunnel syndrome[20] has been increasingly recognized as a cause of pain and paresthesia involving the flexor aspect of the wrist and those fingers supplied by the median nerve. The term now encompasses all conditions producing irritation or, particularly, compression of the median nerve within the carpal tunnel (Figure 8).

Diagnosis of the syndrome is almost always established by noting the presence of one or more of the three major clinical signs: (1) hypesthesia restricted to median-nerve distribution in the hand; (2) Tinel's sign, a tingling sensation radiating into the hand on percussing the median nerve at the wrist; or (3) Phelan's sign, reproduction or exaggeration of symptoms after holding the wrist in complete flexion for 30 to 60 seconds. Atrophy of the thenar muscles is often seen, but this usually does not appear early.

Electrodiagnostic studies to evaluate motor and sensory conduction of the median and ulnar nerves are mandatory for identification of the site of compression when symptoms suggest a neurological basis. On several occasions the carpal-tunnel syndrome has been the offending mechanism accounting for discomfort in the arm and shoulder areas secondary to

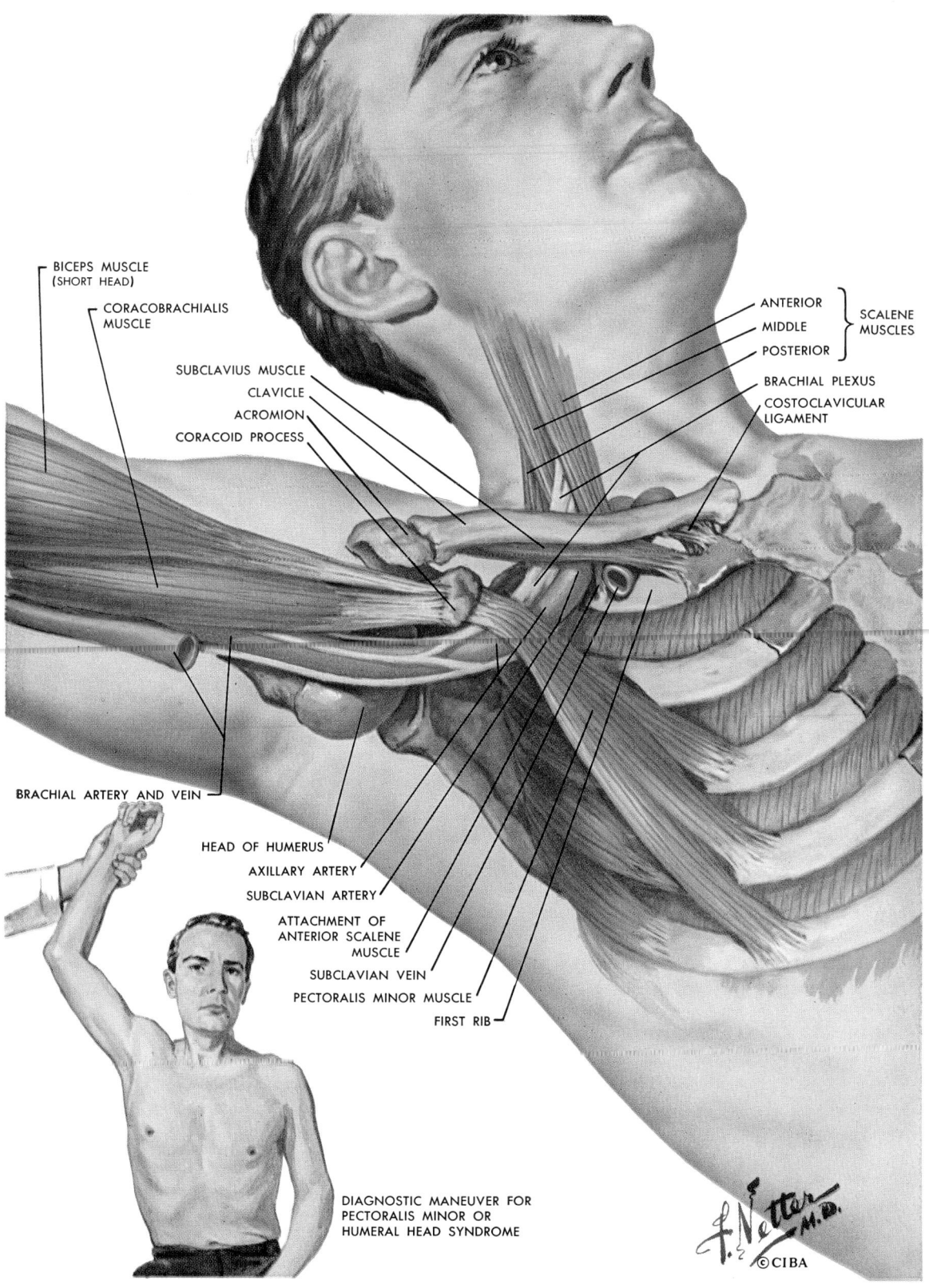

BICEPS MUSCLE
(SHORT HEAD)

CORACOBRACHIALIS
MUSCLE

SUBCLAVIUS MUSCLE

CLAVICLE

ACROMION

CORACOID PROCESS

ANTERIOR

MIDDLE — SCALENE MUSCLES

POSTERIOR

BRACHIAL PLEXUS

COSTOCLAVICULAR
LIGAMENT

BRACHIAL ARTERY AND VEIN

HEAD OF HUMERUS

AXILLARY ARTERY

SUBCLAVIAN ARTERY

ATTACHMENT OF
ANTERIOR SCALENE
MUSCLE

SUBCLAVIAN VEIN

PECTORALIS MINOR MUSCLE

FIRST RIB

DIAGNOSTIC MANEUVER FOR
PECTORALIS MINOR OR
HUMERAL HEAD SYNDROME

f. Netter M.D.
©CIBA

PLATE V PRESSURE EXERTED BY PECTORALIS MINOR IN HYPERABDUCTION SYNDROME

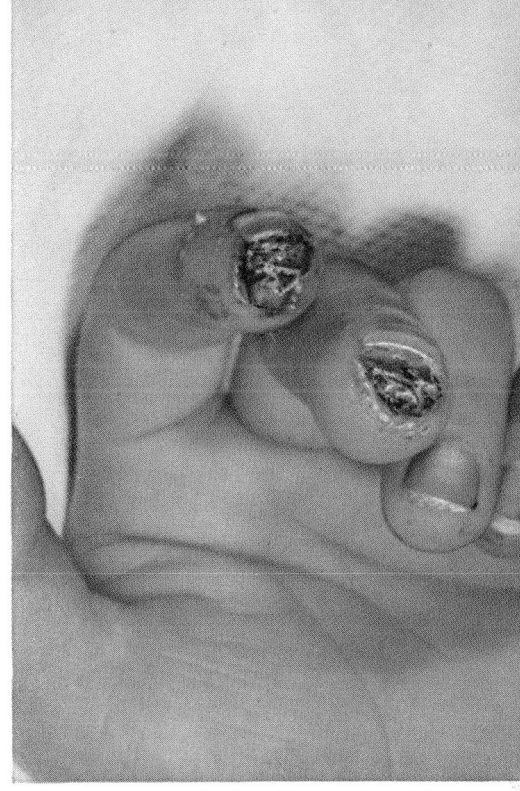

Figure 7. Ulcerated second and third finger tips due to pressure caused by the bony enlargement of the first rib (Case 8). (Kodachrome courtesy of Clay-Adams, Inc.)

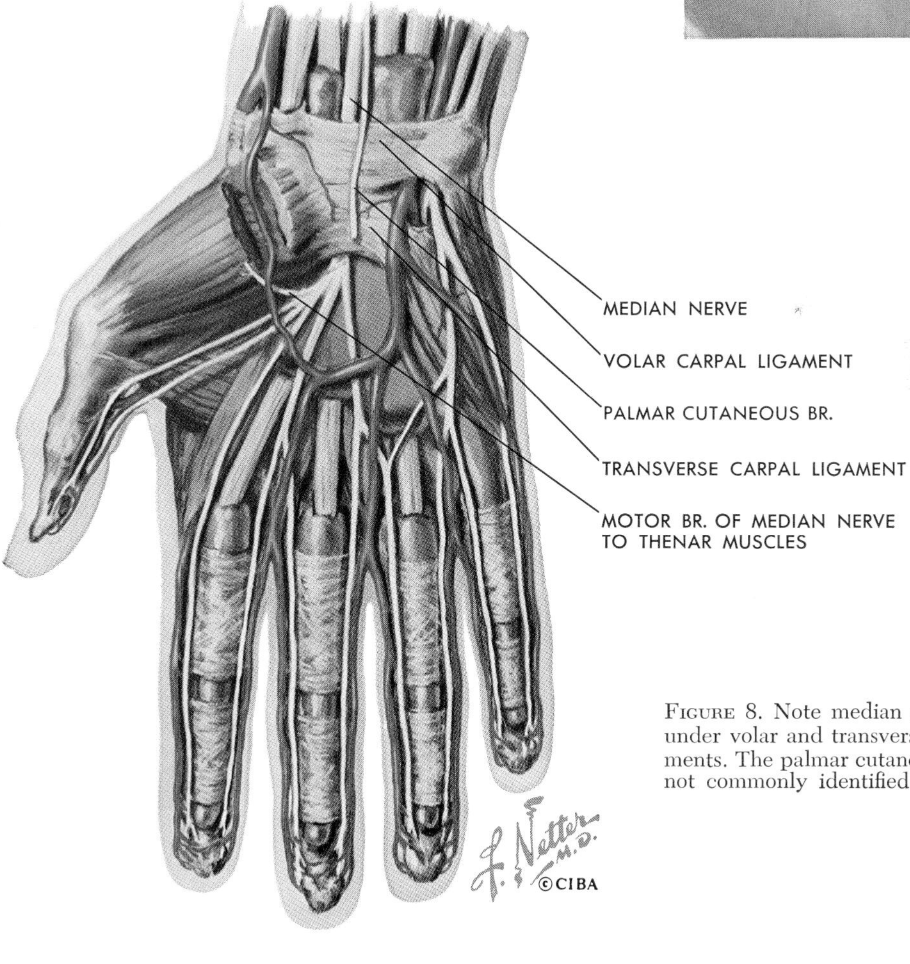

MEDIAN NERVE

VOLAR CARPAL LIGAMENT

PALMAR CUTANEOUS BR.

TRANSVERSE CARPAL LIGAMENT

MOTOR BR. OF MEDIAN NERVE TO THENAR MUSCLES

Figure 8. Note median nerve passing under volar and transverse carpal ligaments. The palmar cutaneous branch is not commonly identified at operation.

25

those experienced in the hand. Of 118 patients with 140 upper extremities operated upon, there have been 17 patients with 22 carpal-tunnel compressions requiring section of the transverse carpal ligament and neurolysis of the median nerve. As evidence of the accuracy of the electrodiagnostic studies performed by Dr. Joseph Goodgold of the Institute of Rehabilitation, New York University, each and every patient has obtained an excellent result. Conversely, where suspicion of the carpal-tunnel involvement has not been confirmed by such studies, other sites of compression have been sought and symptoms relieved by a conservative and/or operative management.

Case 9, a 50-year-old housewife, was first examined by us on January 5, 1968 with a history of paresthesias of both hands and swelling and pounding of the left forearm and hand. A neurologist, one month earlier, had diagnosed a thoracic-outlet syndrome and recommended a conservative therapeutic trial. We concurred in this program. However, four months later the patient returned and complained of discomfort in the right middle and fourth fingers.

Examination revealed significant atrophy of the right thenar eminence and a cooler right hand than left. For the first time, a carpal-tunnel syndrome was considered, and electrodiagnostic studies showed profound interference with the motor and sensory functions of the median nerve distal to the wrist. Less significant changes were noted on the left side.

Following section of the right transverse carpal ligament with unroofment of the median nerve, she became asymptomatic. Two years later the thenar musculature had returned to normal with excellent conduction of the median nerve. Because of symptomatic and electrodiagnostic progression of compression of the left median nerve, we sectioned the left transverse carpal ligament in September, 1970, thus

achieving an equally good result.

This patient is of considerable interest, because several physicians, including us, were in error regarding the correct diagnosis for too many months. She, as well as a few other patients, points up the need for accurate electrodiagnostic tests to rule in or out the carpal-tunnel syndrome.

Phlebography in conjunction with pressure measurement has been helpful in identifying those patients with intermittent compression of the subclavian vein. The catheter is passed to the right auricle and gradually withdrawn to the axillary region recording the pressure and the "A" wave. If there is substantial narrowing in the interval between the costocoracoid ligament and the first rib, then there will be a pressure gradient noted and disappearance of the "A" wave. With the catheter in the distal axillary vein, a phlebogram is made. When thrombosis of the subclavian vein has occurred, then only a phlebogram will be made.

Case 10, a 33-year-old carpenter, was first examined on February 11, 1964 complaining of aching discomfort of the right arm and dorsum of hand following an active day's work. Involvement was worse at night with tingling of all five fingers. Some relief was noted by lying in the prone position with the arm hanging towards the floor.

Past history was significant only in that the patient was left handed and had had a lumbar laminectomy four years earlier with relief of low-back syndrome.

Examination revealed a heavily muscled man with negative positional signs on the right side. Venous pressure was questionably elevated. Studies by venous catheterization showed a pressure of 150 mm saline distal to the costocoracoid ligament and 100 mm proximally. Figure 9 shows flattening of the "A" wave in the axillary vein. Phlebography (Figure 10-A) demonstrated profound stenosis of the subclavian vein by the costocoracoid ligament superiorly and by the first rib inferiorly.

At operation a markedly thickened costocoracoid ligament was excised along with a portion of the subclavius muscle and section of the scalenus anticus muscle performed. Postoperative studies revealed abolition of the gradient across the first rib and phlebography showed a full subclavian venous channel (Figure 10-B).

For 12 months he was completely relieved of all symptoms in the right arm, but following an operation on his knee, he again experienced aching in his arm and some swelling of the hand and forearm.

He was restudied and found to have a normal phlebogram and venous pressure. On this occasion electrodiagnostic examination revealed marked conduction delay of the median nerve by the transverse carpal ligament on the right and minor changes on the left. Cortisone injection relieved the discomfort temporarily. In view of progression of discomfort, section of the transverse carpal ligament with unroofing of the median nerve was performed on March 3, 1966, with an excellent result for the past four years.

This patient is one of five individuals who have had combined thoracic-outlet and carpal-tunnel syndromes. In all but one patient, there was an interval of one or more years between the two difficulties. Whether this is coincidental or related in some unclear fashion, we are not certain.

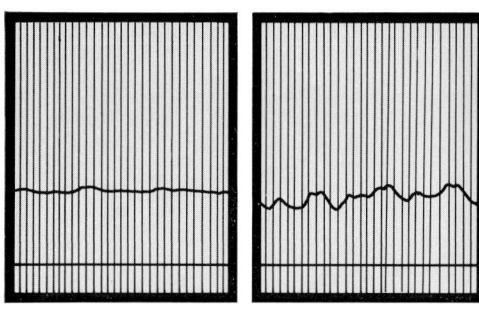

PREOPERATIVE   POSTOPERATIVE

FIGURE 9. Note preoperative flattening of A wave with return to normal after operation.

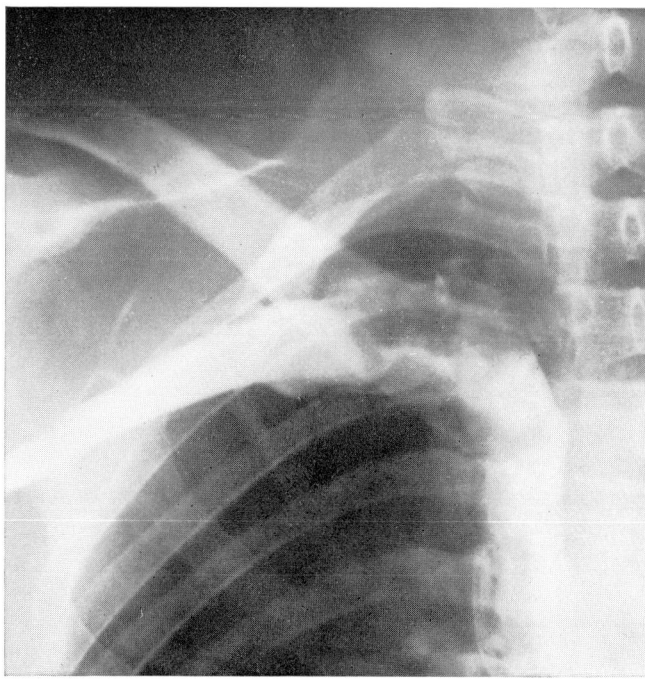

FIGURE 10-A. Profound stenosis of subclavian vein caused by costocoracoid ligament and first rib.

FIGURE 10-B. Phlebogram shows full subclavian venous channel postoperatively (Case 9).

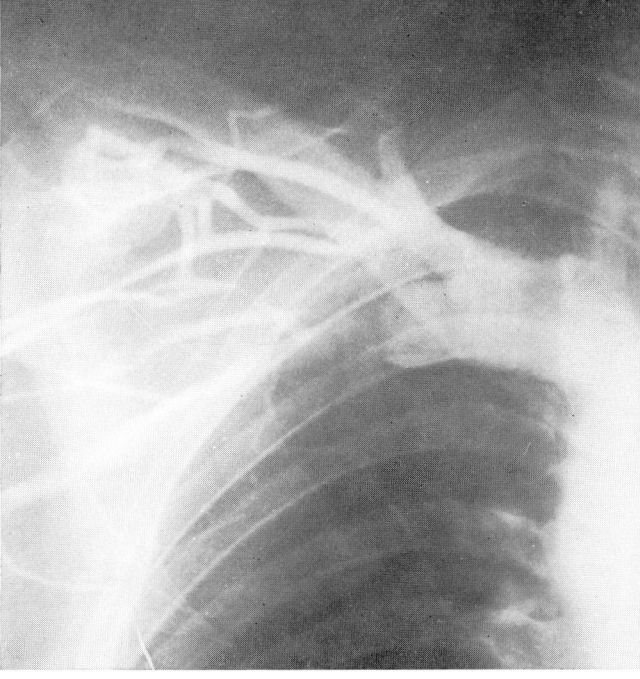

27

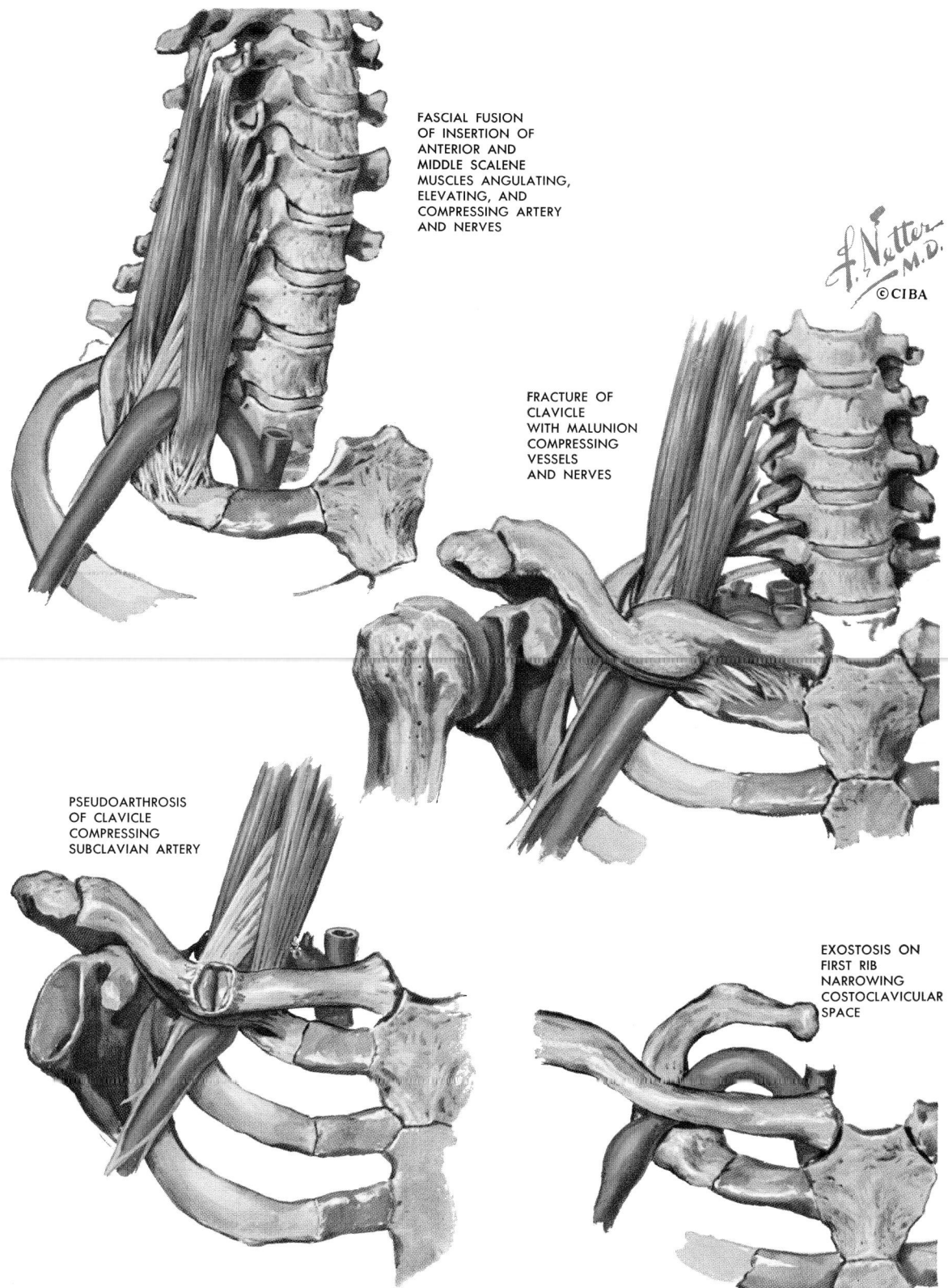

FASCIAL FUSION OF INSERTION OF ANTERIOR AND MIDDLE SCALENE MUSCLES ANGULATING, ELEVATING, AND COMPRESSING ARTERY AND NERVES

FRACTURE OF CLAVICLE WITH MALUNION COMPRESSING VESSELS AND NERVES

PSEUDOARTHROSIS OF CLAVICLE COMPRESSING SUBCLAVIAN ARTERY

EXOSTOSIS ON FIRST RIB NARROWING COSTOCLAVICULAR SPACE

©CIBA

PLATE VI

STRUCTURAL ABNORMALITIES CAUSING COMPRESSION

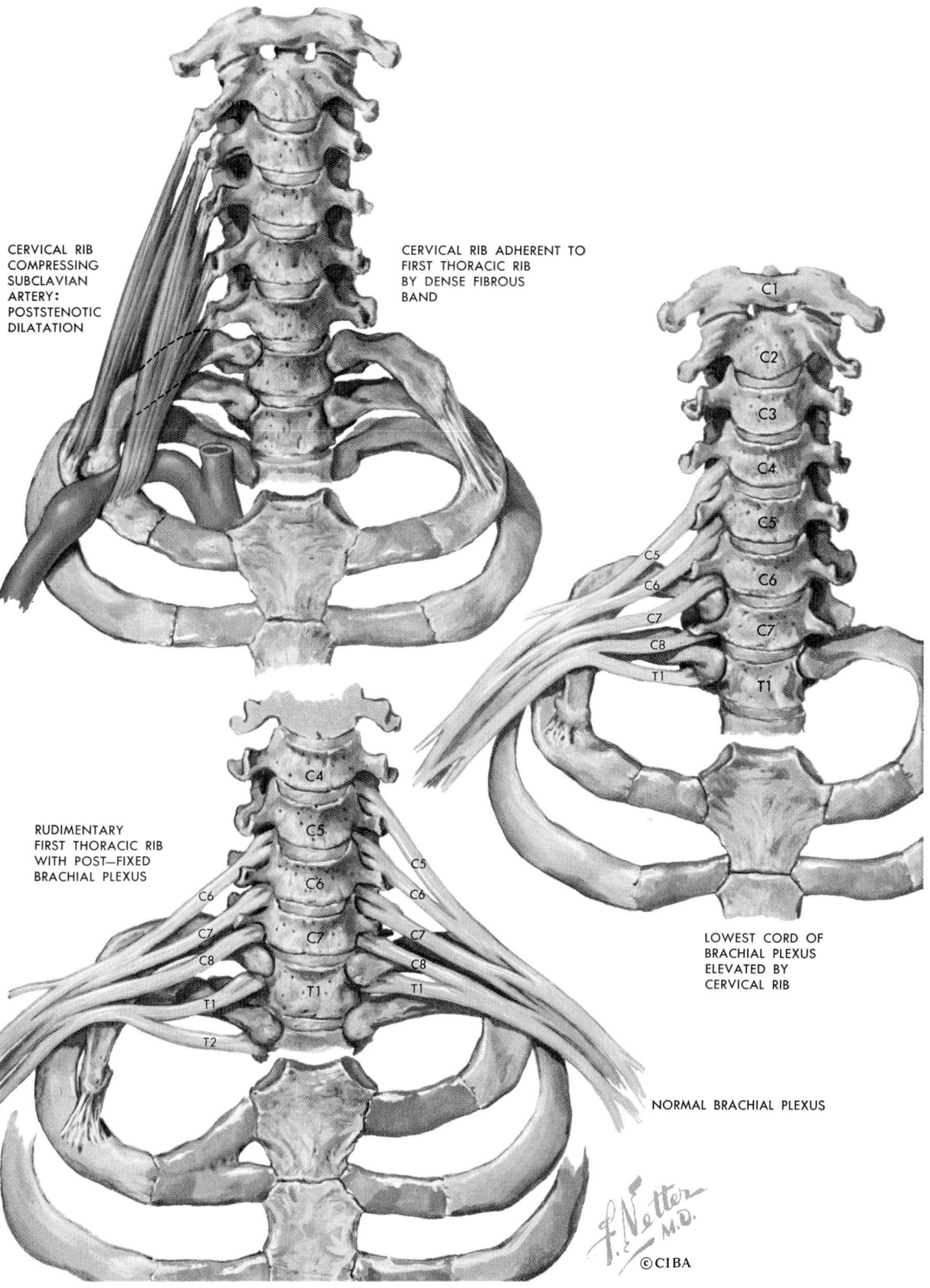

CERVICAL RIB
COMPRESSING
SUBCLAVIAN
ARTERY:
POSTSTENOTIC
DILATATION

CERVICAL RIB ADHERENT TO
FIRST THORACIC RIB
BY DENSE FIBROUS
BAND

RUDIMENTARY
FIRST THORACIC RIB
WITH POST—FIXED
BRACHIAL PLEXUS

LOWEST CORD OF
BRACHIAL PLEXUS
ELEVATED BY
CERVICAL RIB

NORMAL BRACHIAL PLEXUS

PLATE VII COMPRESSION CAUSED BY CONGENITAL RIB ABNORMALITIES

In the differential diagnosis of the compression syndromes, it is not only important to decide which mechanical factor is at fault; it is also necessary to differentiate certain other lesions which cause pain and paresthesias in the shoulder, arm, and hand, and hence suggest one of the syndromes we have discussed. One must therefore rule out *protruded cervical disc, cervical arthritis, cord tumors, and exostoses of the laminae* which may cause pressure on various roots of the cervicobrachial plexus and lead to symptoms which, on superficial consideration, may suggest one of the syndromes previously described. In this connection it is well to remember that the neurologic manifestations of the compression syndromes are usually confined to involvement of the eighth cervical and first thoracic roots and not to any of the others. A protruded cervical disc, on the other hand, usually involves C_5 or C_6. Involvement due to cervical arthritis tends to be more diffuse.

In addition, in the various shoulder-girdle-compression syndromes, the subclavian-axillary artery and/or vein is usually involved intermittently by pressure or persistently by thrombosis. Studies to determine the integrity of their vascular function, such as venous pressure and oscillometry, are most helpful in arriving at a correct differential diagnosis.

The *shoulder-hand syndrome*, described so clearly by Steinbrocker,[21] must be understood and distinguished from the shoulder-girdle syndromes. This syndrome is characterized by the presence of a primary lesion which causes pain, such as a subdeltoid bursitis or a coronary occlusion. Because of the pain, the shoulder and arm are immobilized spontaneously by the patient. This leads to atrophy and later to overactivity of the sympathetic nervous system. This excessive sympathetic flow results in a cold, sweaty, painful hand, which in turn may become stiff and atrophic with fibrosis of the joints.

It is obvious that the mechanism of production of this syndrome is entirely different, and therapy is completely dissimilar to that in conditions we have described. In common, however, they both have pain in the shoulder, arm, and hand.

Other conditions which should be investigated include: sclerodactylia associated with myocardial ischemia, scleroderma, thromboangiitis obliterans, pernio, migratory thrombophlebitis, diffuse vasculitis, sympathetic dystrophy, posttraumatic osteoporosis, herpes zoster (postherpetic), posthemiplegia dystrophies, Dupuytren's contracture, causalgia, peripheral neuritis, syringomyelia, crutch palsy, dermatomyositis, and nodular panniculitis.

TREATMENT

From the therapeutic viewpoint, it should be emphasized that conservative measures should be employed in most patients and surgical intervention reserved for those who fail to respond satisfactorily or who demonstrate a critical arterial or venous impairment when first seen.

In many cases improved posture and avoidance of positions which increase the pressure are worthy of trial. During this period attention should be given to treatment of residual neuritis, myositis, or trophic changes by appropriate medical and physical therapy.

Those with the hyperabduction syndrome who habitually sleep with arms upraised may be able to adopt another sleeping posture if gauze is tied about the wrists and attached to the foot of the bed, allowing only enough slack to permit bringing the arms as high as the chest.

In the selection of patients for a surgical procedure, it is of the greatest importance to assess the patient's mental and emotional patterns and to be certain that there is clear-cut physical evidence of objective interference with the function of elements of the neurovascular bundle. Otherwise, failure may follow any surgical procedure. Pains in the shoulders and arms have many causes, and emotional tension is one of them. One must be particularly cautious where Workmen's Compensation factors are involved, as well as when dealing with neurotics, particularly where the history suggests hysteria or hypochondriasis.

In patients in whom the maneuvers that we have described produce a definite diminution or obliteration of the pulse or in those with gross evidence of venous obstruction, such as a larger circumference of the affected arm, one is tempted to advise surgery at once. As several of these cases illustrate, where abnormal compression occurs, even though transient and occasional, there is always the risk of complete vascular occlusion by a thrombus. This possibility is certainly decreased by removal of the compression.

After complete arterial occlusion has occurred, one may be faced with emergency surgery. Furthermore, only in an occasional case will the pulse wave ever be completely restored simply by removing the source of compression. In most such cases complete restoration of blood flow can be achieved only by a reconstructive procedure.

Arteriographic studies are useful in identifying the site of stenosis or occlusion in the subclavian and axillary arteries. The catheter is passed by the Seldinger technique from a femoral artery to the origin of the subclavian artery on the appropriate side and identification of the inflow and outflow tracts ascertained. These data are vital in planning a suitable procedure for arterial reconstruction.

Case 11, a 78-year-old widow, experienced progressively severe pain in the left shoulder and hand for two months. The hand was also noted to be cold and pal-

lid. A stellate-ganglion block produced no benefit. Past history was unremarkable regarding heart disease and diabetes. Examination revealed a cold, pallid left hand and no radial, brachial, or axillary pulse. Two ulcerations 15 by 10 mm were noted in the left axilla.

A left subclavian angiogram with the catheter passing through the left femoral artery was positive for occlusion of the left subclavian artery 3 cm beyond its origin (Figure 11). The block extended for 2 cm, then an isolated segment of axillary artery was patent for 6 cm. The angiogram showed small collateral vessels for the remainder of the arm above the elbow. No dye was demonstrable in the forearm and hand.

A saphenous vein bypass graft was inserted into the patent subclavian near the vertebral artery to the proximal axillary artery. Resection of the clavicle provided excellent exposure.

During the follow-up of one year, there has been a feeble left radial pulse, the graft pulsates strongly, and the hand is warm and of good color with a good grip.

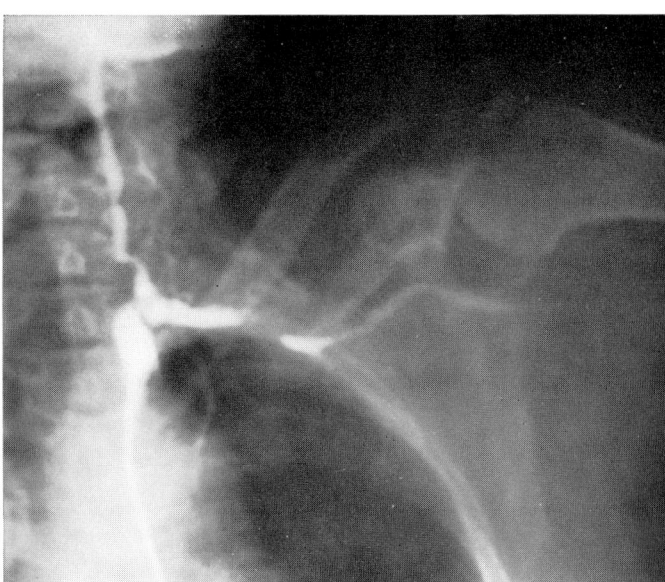

Figure 11. Angiogram showing occlusion of left subclavian artery in Case 11.

SUMMARY

Knowledge of the surgical anatomy of the thoracic outlet is basic to an understanding of the several bony, fascial, and muscular structures capable of interfering with the functions of the neurovascular bundle. That these factors are also dynamic must be considered.

Whereas clinical examination was formerly the chief basis for selecting patients for appropriate surgical intervention, we currently have several excellent diagnostic procedures, such as phlebography, arteriography, and electrodiagnostic tests, to improve the selection of patients in whom an appropriate surgical procedure will lead to a successful outcome. Favorable operative results will be observed in a large majority of those patients culled from a much vaster group whose therapeutic regimen is conservative. Except for emergencies, we believe that careful selection of patients for operative intervention is the cornerstone for a high degree of surgical success in patients with the thoracic-outlet syndrome.

BIBLIOGRAPHY

1. Rob CG, Standeven A: Arterial occlusion complicating thoracic outlet compression syndrome. Brit Med J 2:709, 1958
2. Roos DB, Owens JC: Thoracic outlet syndrome. Arch Surg 93:71, 1966
3. Sanders RJ, Monsour JW, and Baer SB: Transaxillary first rib resection for the thoracic outlet syndrome. Arch Surg 97:1014, 1968
4. Willshire WH: Supernumerary first rib, clinical records. Lancet 2:633, 1860
5. Gruber W: Uber die Halsrippen des Menschen mit vergleichend anatomischen Bemerkungen. Mem Acad imp d sc St. Petersburg Vol 12, 1869
6. Murphy JB: Case of cervical rib with symptoms resembling subclavian aneurysm. Ann Surg 41:399, 1905
7. Naffziger HC, Grant WT: Neuritis of the brachial plexus mechanical in origin: The scalenus syndrome. Surg, Gynec & Obst 67:722, 1938
8. Ochsner A, Gage M, and DeBakey M: Scalenus anticus (Naffziger) syndrome. Am J Surg 28:669, 1935
9. Beyer JA, Wright IS: Hyperabduction syndrome with special reference to its relationship to Raynaud's syndrome. Circulation 4:161, 1951
10. Adson AW: Cervical ribs: Symptoms, differential diagnosis for section of the insertion of the scalenus anticus muscle. J Internat Coll Surgeons 16:546, 1951
11. Raaf J: Surgery for cervical rib and scalenus anticus syndrome. JAMA 157:219, 1955
12. Palumbo LT: Anterior transthoracic approach for upper thoracic sympathectomy. AMA Arch of Surg 72:659, 1956
13. Telford ED, Mottershead S: Pressure at the cervicobrachial junction. J Bone and Joint Surg 30B:249, 1948
14. Goetz RH, Marr JAS: Importance of second thoracic ganglion for sympathetic supply of upper extremities, with description of 2 new approaches for its removal in cases of vascular disease; preliminary report. Clin Proc 3:102, 1944
15. Falconer MA, Weddell G: Costoclavicular compression of the subclavian artery and vein: Relation to the scalenus anticus syndrome. Lancet 2:539, 1943
16. Lowenstein PS: Thrombosis of the axillary vein: An anatomic study. JAMA 82:854, 1924
17. McCleery RS, Kesterson JE, Kirtley JA, et al: Subclavius and anterior scalene muscle compression as a cause of intermittent obstruction of the subclavian vein. Ann Surg 133:588, 1951
18. Fogarty TJ, Cranley JJ, Krause RJ, et al: A method for extraction of arterial emboli and thrombi. Surg, Gynec & Obst 116:241, 1963
19. Wright IS: The neurovascular syndrome produced by hyperabduction of the arms. Am Heart J 29:1, 1945
20. Phelan GS: Reflections on 21 years' experience with the carpal-tunnel syndrome. JAMA 212:1365, 1970
21. Steinbrocker O, Spitzer N, and Freidman HH: The shoulder-hand syndrome in reflex dystrophy of the upper extremity. Ann Int Med 29:22, 1948

The first issue of CLINICAL SYMPOSIA appeared in the spring of 1948 and has been followed by over 100 issues in the succeeding 22 years. The Editor and guiding light over this entire span was J. HAROLD WALTON, M.D., who with the last issue has officially — albeit reluctantly — retired to rest on his well-deserved laurels.

My association with Dr. Walton and CLINICAL SYMPOSIA began with Volume 3 in 1951 and continued for 3 years, when other responsibilities within CIBA intervened until last year. So it is with humility and enthusiasm that I take over the helm for a voyage I hope will be as successful as his.

RICHARD H. ROBERTS, M.D.

SECTION D

CIBA

SYPHILIS

SYPHILIS

Prepared in cooperation with the U.S. Public Health Service with its publication, *Syphilis, A Synopsis* (PHS No. 1660) as principal resource.

RICHARD H. ROBERTS, M.D., *Editor*

J. HAROLD WALTON, M.D., *Editor Emeritus*

LARAINE GRAY, *Editorial Assistant*

CIBA PHARMACEUTICAL COMPANY

DIVISION OF CIBA-GEIGY CORPORATION

SUMMIT, NEW JERSEY 07901

THE CIBA COLLECTION OF MEDICAL ILLUSTRATIONS
Frank H. Netter, M.D.

Beginning with its first volume eighteen years ago, the CIBA Collection of Medical Illustrations continues to enjoy an almost "unheard-of" reception from members of the medical community. The remarkable illustrations by Dr. Frank Netter and text discussions by select specialists make these books unprecedented in their educational, clinical, and scientific value.

Volume 1   NERVOUS SYSTEM
"... a beautiful bargain ... and handsome reference work."
Psychological Record

Volume 2   REPRODUCTIVE SYSTEM
"... a desirable addition to any nursing or medical library."
American Journal of Nursing

Volume 3/I   DIGESTIVE SYSTEM (Upper Digestive Tract)
"... a fine example of the high quality of this series."
Pediatrics

Volume 3/II   DIGESTIVE SYSTEM (Lower Digestive Tract)
"... a unique and beautiful work, worth much more than its cost." *Journal of the South Carolina Medical Association*

Volume 3/III   DIGESTIVE SYSTEM (Liver, Biliary Tract and Pancreas)
"... a versatile, multipurpose aid to clinicians, teachers, researchers, and students ..." *Florida Medical Journal*

Volume 4   ENDOCRINE SYSTEM and Selected Metabolic Diseases
"... another in the series of superb contributions made by CIBA ..." *International Journal of Fertility*

Volume 5   HEART
"The excellence of the volume ... is clearly deserving of highest praise." *Circulation*

In the United States, copies of all CIBA Collection books may be purchased from the Publications Section, CIBA Pharmaceutical Company, Division of CIBA-GEIGY Corporation, Summit, New Jersey 07901. In other countries, please direct inquiries to the nearest CIBA-GEIGY office.

SYPHILIS

Prepared in cooperation with the U.S. Public Health Service with its publication, *Syphilis, A Synopsis* (PHS No. 1660) as principal resource.

Control of syphilis requires a combination of factors, including a high index of suspicion, clinical acumen, laboratory tests, diagnosis, treatment, case reporting, and epidemiology. In addition to interviewing patients for sexual contacts and follow-up by trained health department personnel, the epidemiologic (preventive) treatment of sexual contacts exposed to infectious syphilis, even though negative on initial examination, is essential to successful control.

Compared with many other maladies of man, syphilis should not be a difficult disease to eradicate. Its causative organism, *Treponema pallidum,* is not borne by food, air, water, or insect, nor is there any extrahuman reservoir of infection. In fact, about the only way for a person to contract it is through the closest and most intimate relationship with someone who has it. Moreover, that "someone" must not only have syphilis, but have it in an infectious stage, a period comprising only a relatively short segment of the entire span of the infection.

When infectious, syphilis is relatively easy to detect, diagnose, treat, and cure. With teamwork between private physician and health officers, a lasting victory over the treponeme of syphilis is inevitable.

TREPONEMA PALLIDUM

Belonging to the order *Spirochaetales* and the family *Treponemataceae, T. pallidum* is the organism responsible for human syphilis. Other treponemes pathogenic to man are *T. pertenue* (yaws) and *T. carateum* (pinta). *T. pallidum* is a thin, delicate organism with tapering ends. It varies from about 5 to 15 microns in length and is of a uniform cylindrical thickness of approximately 0.25 micron. The organisms usually exhibit 6 to 14 spirals (Figure 1). They are actively motile, motion being produced by corkscrew rotation rather than by flagella. The usual method of division is thought to be binary transverse fission, although some authorities claim that longitudinal division may occur (Figure 2).

NATURAL COURSE OF SYPHILIS

The disease is transmitted through direct contact with an infectious lesion. Spirochetes pass through intact mucous membranes and abraded skin, following which they are carried by the bloodstream to every organ of the body. The infection is systemic a few hours after exposure, although clinical and serologic evidence of the disease is lacking for a time.

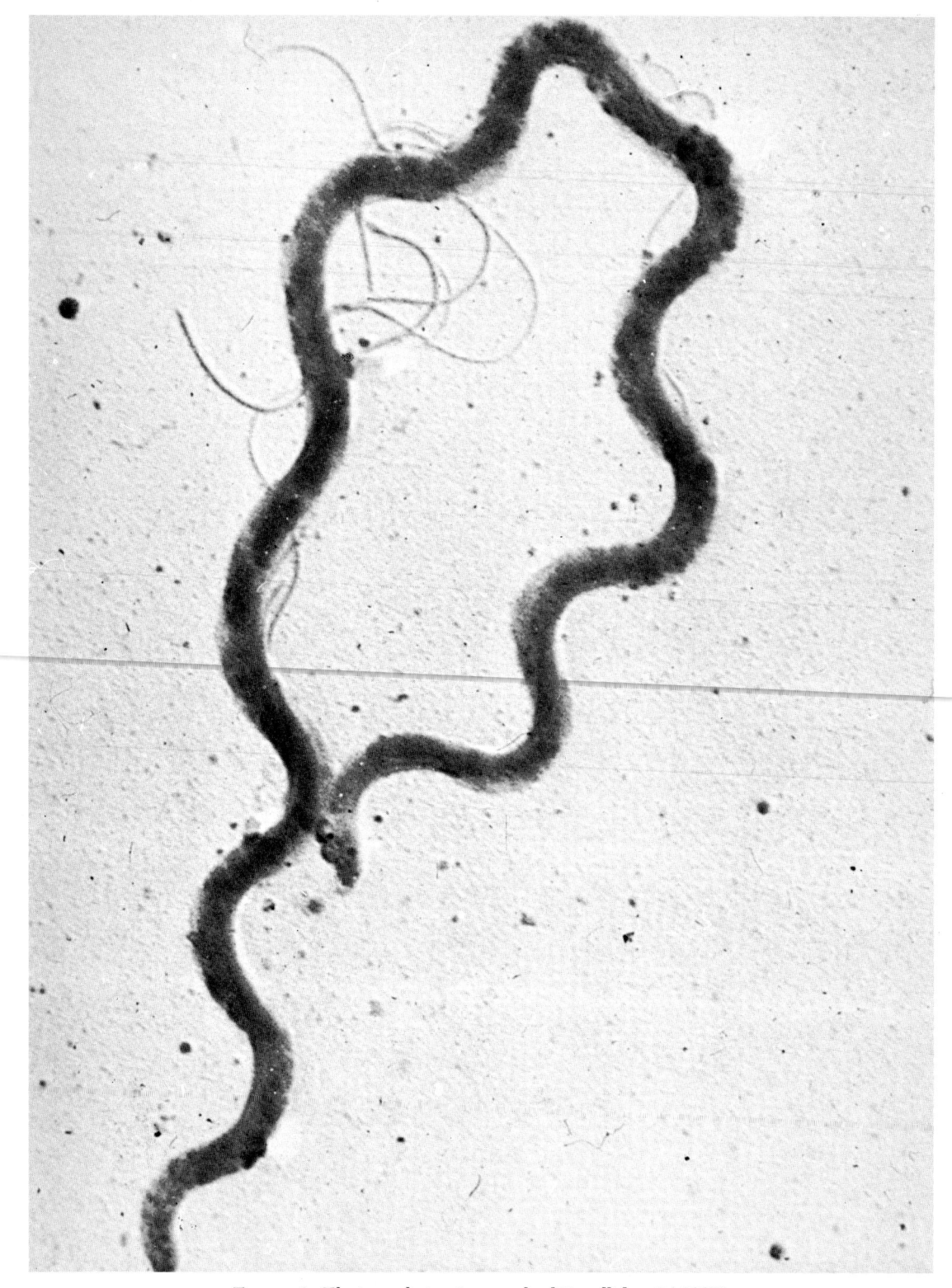

FIGURE 1. Electron photomicrograph of *T. pallidum* 34,000X.

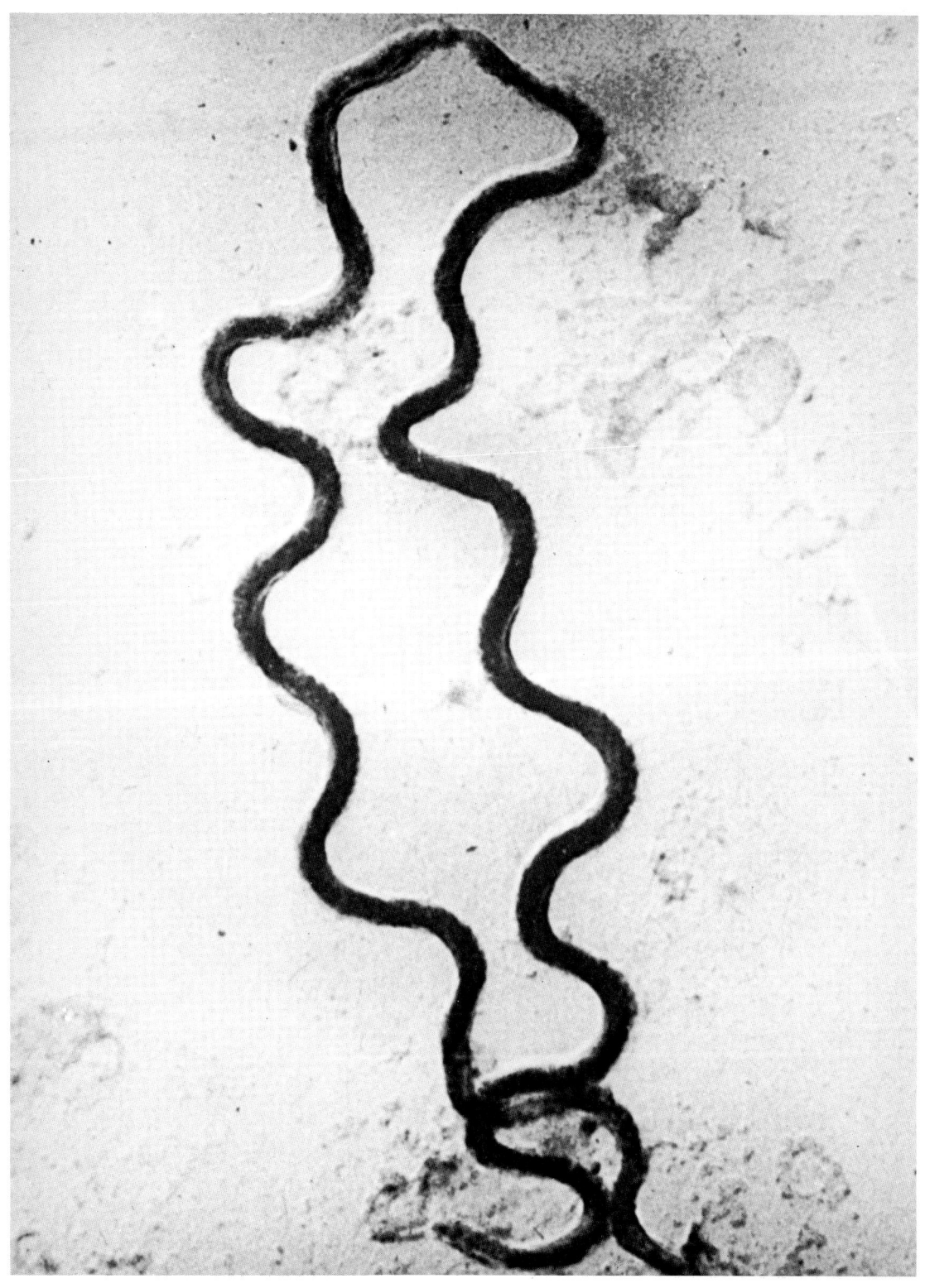

FIGURE 2. Electron photomicrograph of *T. pallidum* suggesting binary transverse fission 36,000X.

From 10 to 90 days (usually 3 to 4 weeks) after exposure, a primary lesion, the chancre, develops at the portal of entry. This persists 1 to 5 weeks and then heals spontaneously. Serologic tests for syphilis (STS) are usually nonreactive when the chancre first appears, becoming reactive during the next 1 to 4 weeks.

About 6 weeks later (2 weeks to 6 months), a localized or generalized cutaneous eruption may appear. Sometimes this secondary stage may precede the healing of the chancre. In other cases, it may be so minimal or transient that it is never clinically apparent. As with primary syphilis, healing occurs spontaneously in 2 to 6 weeks. Then a quiescent or latent stage ensues during which no clinical signs or symptoms are present. Approximately one quarter of cases will experience at least one cutaneous relapse after the secondary eruption has healed. Serologic tests during this stage are invariably reactive. Hence, the stages of secondary syphilis and early latency fluctuate until certain immunologic changes take place, usually after one year of infection. During these stages, STS are invariably reactive, and these tests are the only means of recognizing an infected individual during the latent stage.

As defined by the World Health Organization, latent syphilis is divided into two periods:

Early latent (duration under 4 years).

Late latent (duration 4 years and more). However, from an *epidemiologic* point of view, only early latent syphilis of under 1 year's duration produces sufficient infectious syphilis to warrant interviewing and contact investigation.

Statistically, the WHO definition is employed. After 4 years of infection, relapsing infectious lesions similar to those of

secondary syphilis are very rare. Latency may last a lifetime or be followed in a few or many years by lesions of late syphilis.

Untreated

Of individuals with untreated syphilis, approximately one third will develop late destructive lesions (late benign, 17%; cardiovascular, 10%; CNS, 8%), and up to 23% of the entire group can be expected to die primarily as a result of the disease. Cardiovascular complications cause 80% of the deaths, with most of the remainder resulting from CNS involvement. The other two thirds go through life with minimal or no physical inconvenience, although more than half of these will remain serologically positive for life. Unfortunately, we have no means of predicting which patients will develop the lesions of late syphilis and which will not.

Treated

Treatment changes both the clinical course and serologic pattern of the disease. (1) With adequate treatment before the appearance of the chancre, it is probable that no lesion will appear, and that the STS will remain nonreactive. (2) With treatment during the seronegative primary stage, the STS usually remains nonreactive; and the chancre heals rapidly. Occasionally, the STS may become transiently reactive. (3) Treatment during the seropositive primary stage effects rapid healing of the chancre, and the STS usually becomes nonreactive within 12 months. (4) If therapy is delayed until the secondary stage, 90 to 95 percent of patients adequately treated will become serologically nonreactive within 18 months. (5) Effects of treatment after the secondary stage are variable, but as a rule, the sooner the infected person is treated, the more marked and rapid will be the serologic response. Individuals infected 2 years or more before treatment may remain seroreactive for life, despite optimal doses of penicillin and clinical cure.

Prior to the 1940's, most physicians were well trained in didactic syphilology and had the opportunity to observe many clinical cases. Since the advent of penicillin, most physicians have graduated with an inadequate knowledge of the many faces of syphilis. Without a high index of suspicion on the part of the physician, this "great imitator" will go undiagnosed and continue its path of destruction. Remember too that there is no isolated case of infectious syphilis. Every case of primary and secondary syphilis is directly related to at least one additional case and therefore requires urgent epidemiologic investigation.

History and Physical Examination

An accurate history is important and often essential to the diagnosis and treatment of syphilis. One should speak in the language of the layman, for all venereal diseases have their own, often colorful, names in lay terms. The routine medical history should cover chief complaint, present illness, past and social history, and system review. Such a history should include:

Previous infection (bad blood, lues, haircut, or other venereal disease).

Remembered signs and symptoms (prior lesions of skin and genitalia, eye complaints, hair loss, etc).

Parental or family infection (blood tests, stillbirths, etc).

Previous STS (premarital, employment, hospitalization) and lumbar puncture.

Treatment which might be antiluetic ("hip and arm" shots).

Recent antibiotics (drug reactions).

The necessity of a careful and complete physical examination, including neurological evaluation and a routine STS, cannot be overstressed. The patient should be completely unclothed, and all cutaneous surfaces, including the mucous membranes and anogenital region, inspected in a good light, preferably daylight.

Darkfield Examination

Because *T. pallidum* is not stained readily by ordinary laboratory methods and is so similar to other spirochetes which inhabit the mouth and genitalia of nonsyphilitic persons, it is essential to examine the organism in the living state. *T. pallidum* is so narrow that the ordinary light microscope does not permit sufficient resolution to visualize the organism. However, this can be accomplished by use of darkfield microscopy. The technic is not difficult, but differentiation of *T. pallidum* from other spiral organisms requires careful study and considerable experience.

The darkfield microscope differs from other microscopes chiefly in use of a darkfield condenser, which blocks out the central rays of light and directs the peripheral rays from the side upon the object under study. Thus, light does not enter the objective directly, but only those rays directed upward by the object pass into the eyepiece. The organism appears bright against a black background, just as dust particles become visible when a ray of sunshine enters a darkened room.

In collecting specimens for examination, plastic or rubber gloves should be worn to protect the examiner from accidental infection. The surface of the suspected lesion should be cleansed carefully

7

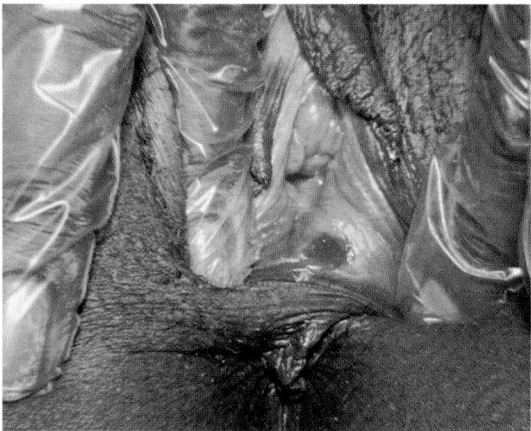

FIGURE 3. Primary syphilis: Chancre of fourchette.

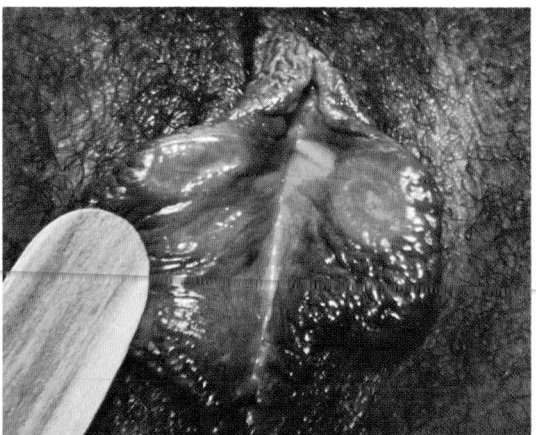

FIGURE 4. Primary syphilis: Multiple primary chancres of labia minora.

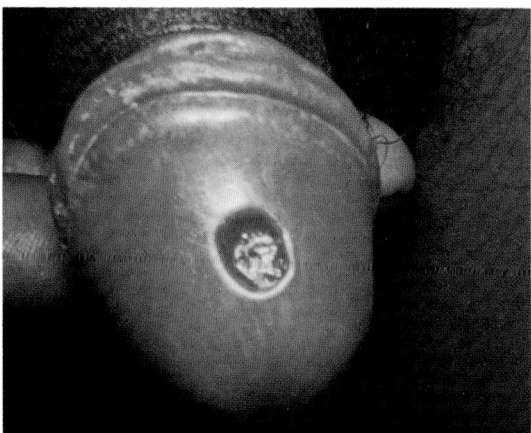

FIGURE 5. Primary syphilis: Chancre of the glans.

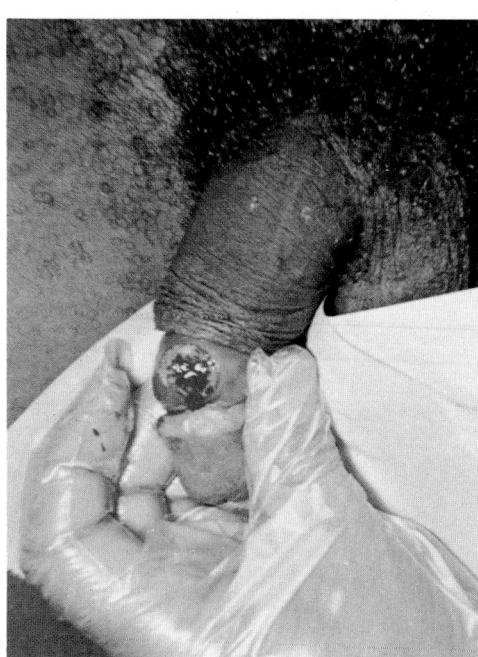

FIGURE 6. Primary syphilis: Typical chancre located at coronal sulcus.

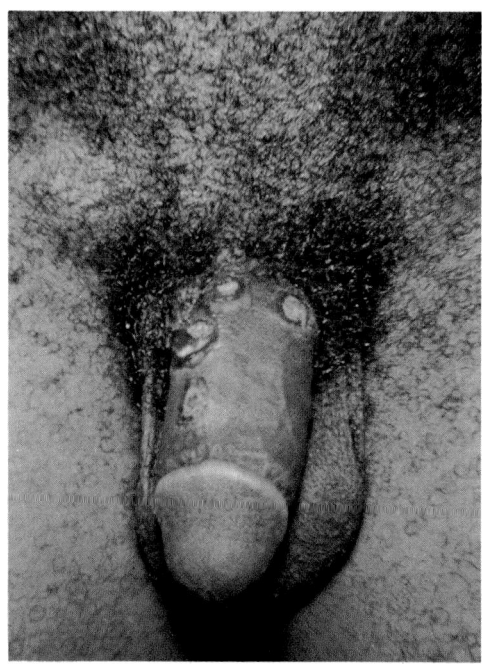

FIGURE 7. Primary syphilis: Multiple primary chancres of penile shaft.

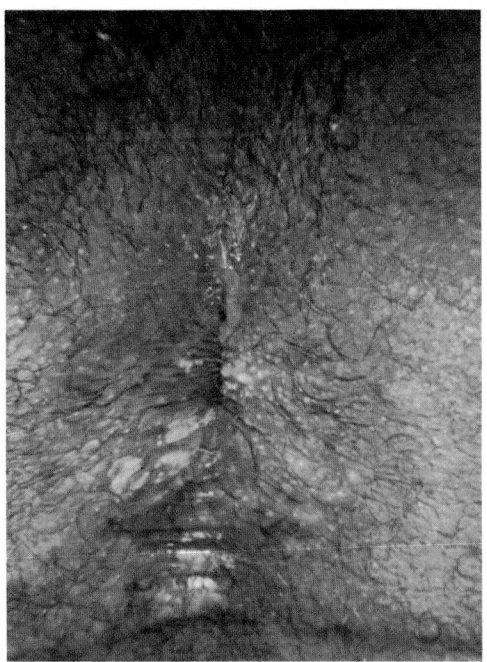

FIGURE 8. Primary syphilis: Anal chancre in a homosexual male.

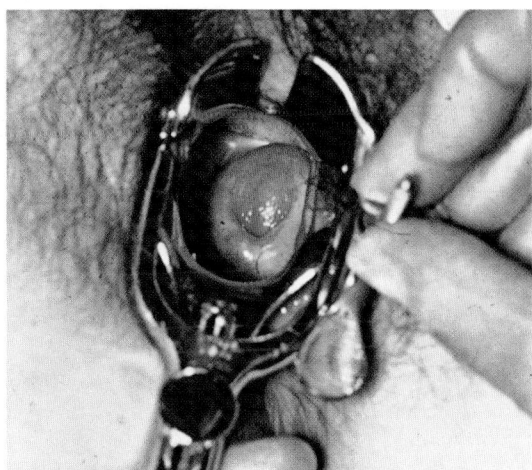

FIGURE 10. Primary syphilis: Primary lesion of cervical os.

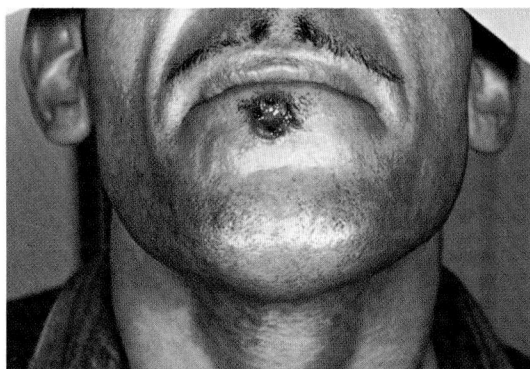

FIGURE 11. Primary syphilis: Typical Hunterian chancre on lower lip.

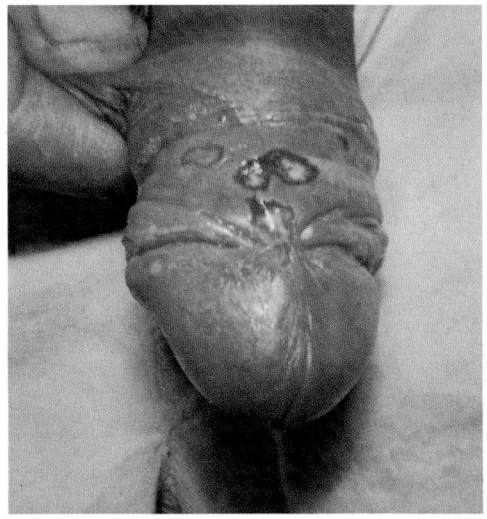

FIGURE 9. Differential diagnosis: Chancroidal ulcers.

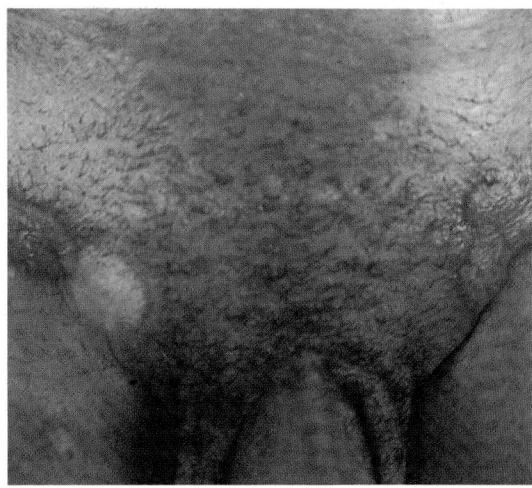

FIGURE 12. Differential diagnosis: Granuloma inguinale with both active and healed areas.

9

with saline, dried, then gently abraded to the point of bleeding. When clear serum exudes, a drop is picked up directly on the surface of a glass slide and a cover slip placed over it. Should there be any appreciable delay before examination, cover the edges of the cover slip with petroleum jelly.

T. pallidum can be identified by its morphologic characteristics and its motions. The latter consist of a slow forward and backward movement, rotation about the long axis like a corkscrew, and a slight bending, twisting, or undulation from side to side. Exercise care in identifying organisms from the mouth or moist areas of the genitalia, since saprophytic spirochetes from these areas may be morphologically identical to *T. pallidum.*

Spinal-Fluid Examination

The only means of diagnosing neurosyphilis accurately and evaluating its treatment is by spinal-fluid examination. Not infrequently, neurosyphilis can be demonstrated months or even years before development of subjective or objective neurologic evidence of the disease. In early forms of syphilis, spinal-fluid examination is most meaningful 6 months to 1 year after treatment; in latent and late forms, examination should precede treatment. A diagnosis of latent syphilis cannot be made unless asymptomatic neurosyphilis is excluded by a negative cerebrospinal-fluid examination.

Clinical Signs

From 10 to 90 days (average 21 days) following infection, a sore or chancre develops at the site where treponemal invasion occurred. Chancres are usually single lesions, but multiple lesions are not rare (Figures 3 through 7). The lesion is usually an eroded papule that is decidedly firm and indurated, the surface being crusted or ulcerated. The size varies from a few millimeters in diameter to 1 or 2 cm. The border surrounding the lesion is frequently raised and firm. When free of other infectious agents, the chancre is typically painless, although extragenital chancres may be painful. Lymphatic glands draining the involved area are frequently enlarged, hard, and painless (satellite bubo). Darkfield examination of fluid obtained by needle aspiration of a bubo can be diagnostic in cases where sufficient fluid cannot be obtained from the chancre itself, where the patient has applied topical medications to his lesion, or where the chancre is hidden. In women, examination by speculum is required to detect chancres in the vagina or on the cervix, where they may vary in appearance from an erosion to a deep ulceration resembling carcinoma (Figure 10).

Primary lesions are by no means confined to the genitalia. Extragenital chancres may be seen on the lips, tongue, tonsil, nipple, fingers, and anus (Figures 8 and 11). In recent years, the last-named site has become increasingly recognized as a result of homosexual transmission. Even without treatment, the chancre will heal completely within 4 to 6 weeks. If the lesion has been present for 4 weeks, nearly all reagin tests will be reactive.

Differential Diagnosis

Any genital lesion should be considered suspect until ruled out clinically and by specific procedures.

Chancroid — These lesions are usually multiple, soft, tender erosions or ulcerations with a grayish base (Figure 9). Both the lesions and associated adenopathy, often more pronounced on one side, are quite painful. While darkfield examination is negative, *H. ducreyi* may be demonstrated from the lesion by direct stained smear or by culture. Occasionally, false-positive, low-titered STS may be noted.

Granuloma Inguinale — This disease is characterized by a soft, painless, raised, raw beef-colored, smooth, granulating lesion (Figure 12). Darkfield and STS are negative, and no significant adenopathy occurs. The pathognomonic Donovan bodies (*Calymmatobacterium granulomatis*, formerly *Donovania granulomatis*) are best demonstrated by direct tissue-spread smears stained with such dyes as Wright's stain. Biopsy may demonstrate the causative organisms and rule out carcinoma.

Lymphogranuloma Venereum — The initial lesion is a small, transient, rarely seen vesiculo-ulcer. The patient usually shows unilateral, painful, inguinal adenopathy. *T. pallidum, C. granulomatis,* and *H. ducreyi* should be excluded by specific studies. A rising titer detected by complement-fixation tests against the causative psittacosis-like virus organism, *Chlamydial* (formerly *Bedsonia*) *lymphogranulomatis,* is diagnostic.

Herpes Progenitalis — This viral process is usually manifested by grouped, painful, vesicular lesions. History usually reveals recurrent lesions at the same site. A smear will demonstrate typical "balloon" cells. This virus is easily isolated directly from lesions where this laboratory service is available.

Carcinoma — Usually the lesion has been present for a considerable period. Diagnosis is established by biopsy.

Scabies — Pruritic vesicles with burrow formation are highly suggestive, and find-ing the mite in the burrow diagnostic. The burrow may provide a break in the skin for inoculation of *T. pallidum.*

Lichen Planus — Genital lesions are usually annular or the typical polygonal, flat-topped, violaceous papules. They may be pruritic and may be single or multiple. STS are nonreactive.

Psoriasis — This disease often presents an erythematous or erythematosquamous plaque on the glans. Removal of the scale produces pinpoint bleeding. STS are nonreactive.

Drug Eruptions — The genital region is a frequent site of "fixed" dermatitis medicamentosa. Antipyrine, phenolphthalein, phenacetin, barbiturates, salicylates, sulfonamides, and antibiotics are among the most common offenders. STS are usually nonreactive.

Aphthosis — Along with oral and ocular lesions, aphthosis appears as round to polycyclic, painful, mucous-membrane erosions on the genitalia.

Deep Mycotic Infections — Deep fungi may produce chancriform genital lesions. Diagnosis is based on potassium hydroxide preparations, culture, and biopsy. STS are nonreactive.

Reiter's Syndrome — This syndrome consists of nonspecific urethritis, mucopurulent conjunctivitis, and polyarticular arthritis. However, superficial lesions of the glans may occur.

In differential diagnosis, syphilis can be ruled out by:

(1) Darkfield examination studies, combined with:

(2) Serologic reagin tests, both qualitative and quantitative, and

(3) Specific treponemal tests, particularly the FTA-ABS (see Serologic Interpretation) if the above are equivocal. But remember that:

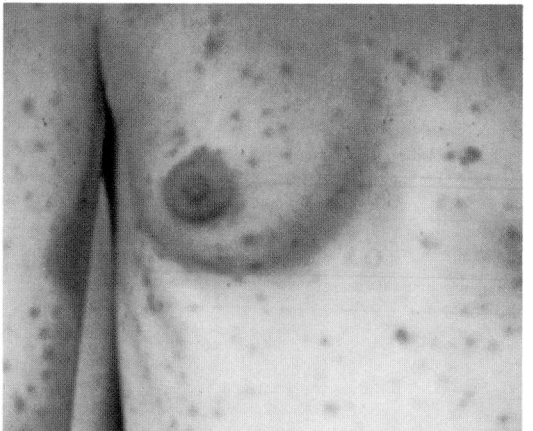

Figure 13. Secondary syphilis: Extensive papulosquamous rash on body.

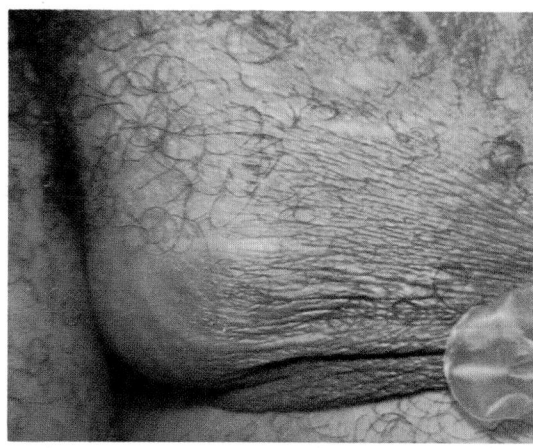

Figure 16. Secondary syphilis: Annular squamous lesions of scrotum.

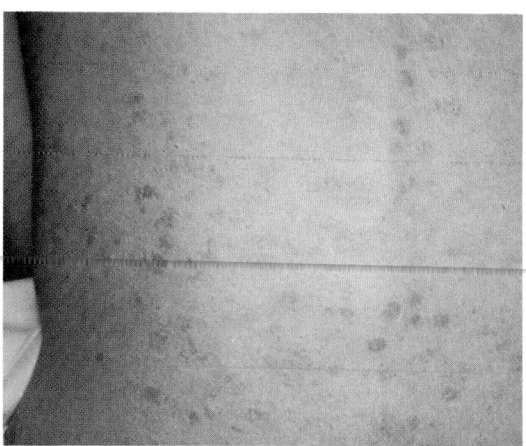

Figure 14. Secondary syphilis: Secondary lesions resembling pityriasis rosea.

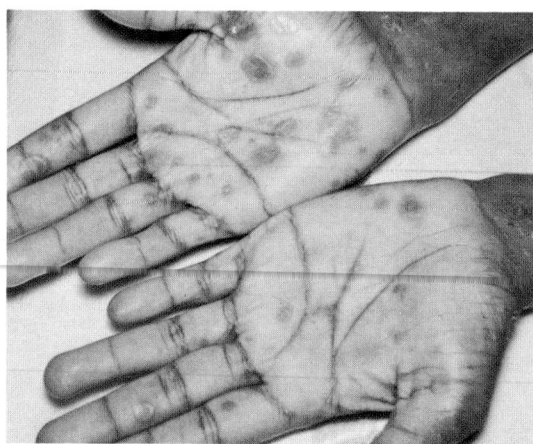

Figure 17. Secondary syphilis: Papulosquamous syphilids of wrists and palms.

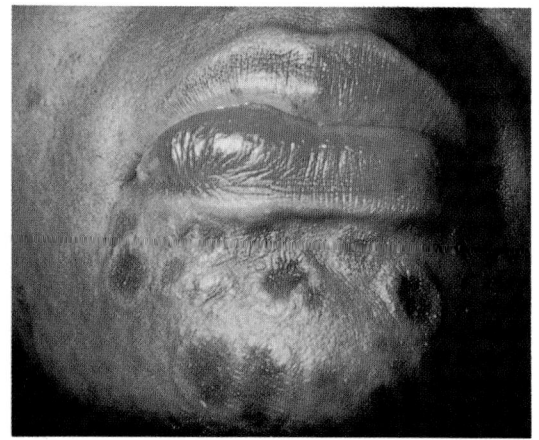

Figure 15. Secondary syphilis: Typical "nickel and dime" lesions.

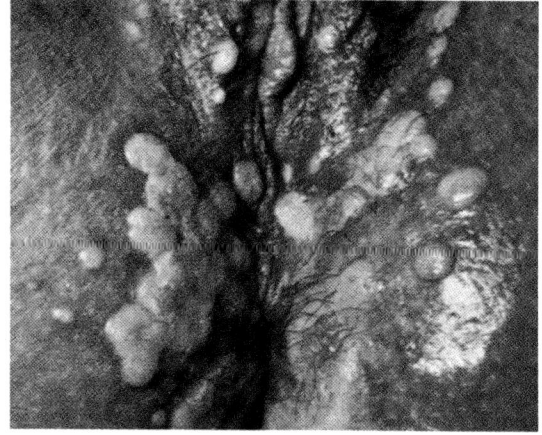

Figure 18. Secondary syphilis: Condylomata lata involving vulva and anal region.

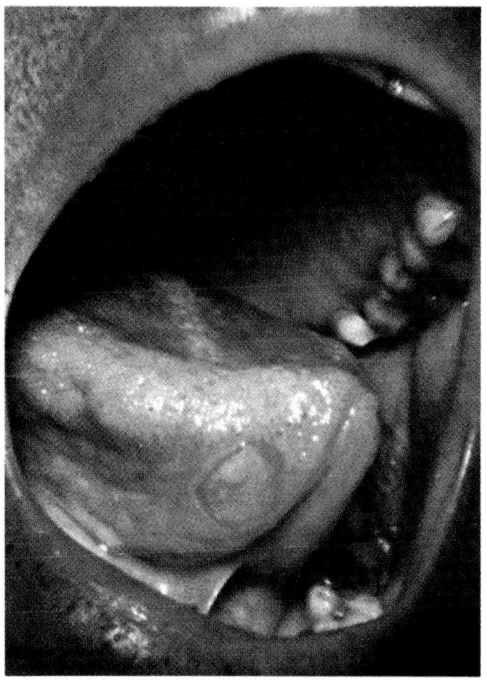

FIGURE 19. Secondary syphilis: Mucous patch of tongue.

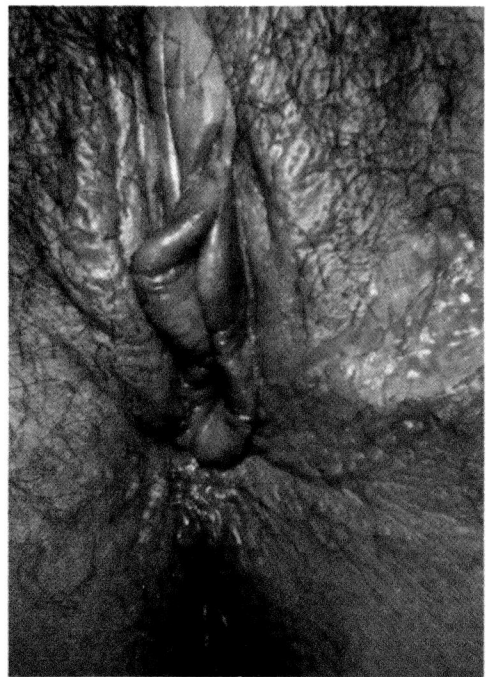

FIGURE 20. Secondary syphilis: Coexistent chancre and secondary vulvar mucosal lesions.

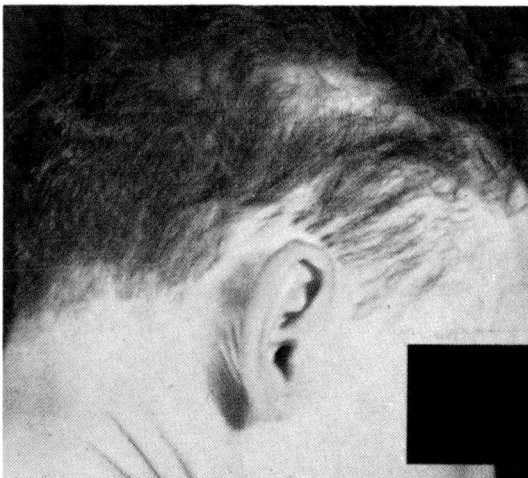

FIGURE 21. Secondary syphilis: Alopecia of scalp.

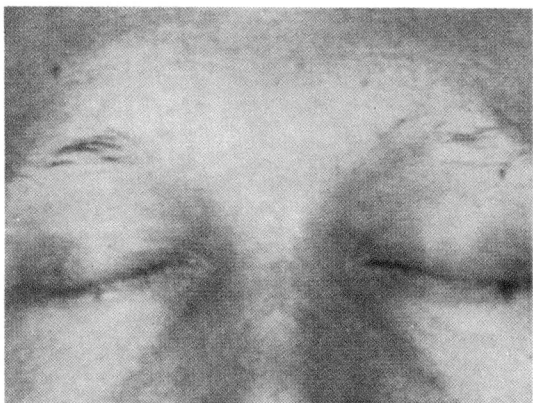

FIGURE 22. Secondary syphilis: Eyebrow alopecia.

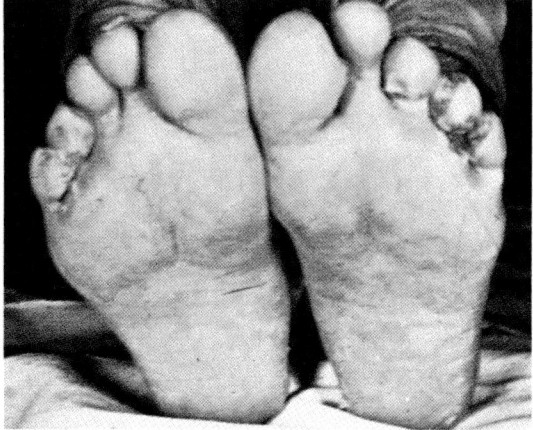

FIGURE 23. Secondary syphilis: Moist papules developing in intertriginous areas of toes.

13

(4) Many nonvenereal genital diseases mimic primary syphilis.

(5) Extragenital chancres are not uncommon.

(6) Other venereal and nonvenereal disease may coexist with primary syphilis.

SECONDARY SYPHILIS

Clinical Signs

Secondary syphilis is quite varied in its clinical manifestations and may involve any cutaneous or mucosal surface of the body, as well as any organ. Although iritis and constitutional symptoms may be present, diagnosis of secondary syphilis is suspected primarily on the basis of the skin and mucous-membrane lesions. The skin lesions are bilaterally symmetrical and may be macular, papular, follicular, papulosquamous, or pustular (Figures 13 through 18). They are seldom pruritic and usually dry. Vesiculobullous lesions do not occur in adults, but may be seen in neonatal congenital syphilis.

In secondary relapsing syphilis, lesions tend to be arciform and may be asymmetrical. "Moth-eaten" scalp alopecia beginning in the occipital hair is characteristic, and loss of eyelashes and the lateral third of the eyebrows may occur (Figures 21 and 22). Moist papules occur most frequently in the anogenital region, mouth, and intertriginous surfaces (Figure 23). Lesions of the mouth (Figure 19), throat, and cervix (mucous patches) frequently occur in secondary syphilis. Occasionally, secondary lesions appear while the chancre is still present (Figure 20). An extremely important concomitant finding is generalized lymphadenopathy. Splenomegaly is occasionally present.

Whenever feasible, it is preferable to diagnose secondary syphilis on the basis of a positive darkfield and a reactive STS. As a rule, *T. pallidum* may be obtained from any mucous or cutaneous secondary lesion, but most easily from a moist one. Failure to demonstrate the organism does not, however, rule out the diagnosis. Drying of the lesions, improper darkfield microscopy, use of topical medications, antiseptics, or soaps, and systemic antibiotics may result in failure to find the organisms. In practice, the diagnosis may be established without a positive darkfield if characteristic lesions are present and the STS reactive in high titer. A history of a recent primary lesion is helpful.

The nontreponemal serologic tests are uniformly reactive during this stage, and most of the treponemal serologic tests are also reactive.

Differential Diagnosis

Pityriasis Rosea—Erythematous, maculopapulosquamous lesions occur along the lines of skin cleavage, usually sparing the distal parts of the extremities, head and neck, and mucous membranes. The body eruption is often preceded for one or more weeks by a single lesion, the herald patch. Darkfield negative, STS nonreactive.

Psoriasis—Erythematous, maculopapulosquamous lesions commonly appear on the scalp, elbows, knees, chest, back, and buttocks. The nails and intertriginous areas may be involved. Pinpoint bleeding results from manual removal of scales. A history of chronicity is usually obtained. Darkfield negative, STS nonreactive.

Lichen Planus—Violaceous, papular, pruritic lesions occur most commonly on wrists, ankles, and sacral areas. Genital and oral lesions may occur. Darkfield negative, STS nonreactive.

Tinea Versicolor — Brown, superficial,

scaly lesions, which may be erythematous, are typical. Scrapings for spores and hyphae are positive.

Drug Eruptions—Skin lesions may be of any type. History of drug use is of utmost importance.

"Id" Eruptions — Lesions are diversified, but may be papulosquamous, macular, or vesicular. Dermatophyte infection, bacterial infection, and/or eczematous processes can usually be found in other parts of the body. Darkfield negative, STS nonreactive.

Perlèche — The fissured split papules occurring at the angles of the mouth in secondary syphilis mimic the fissuring occasionally associated with cheilitis, hypovitaminosis, and oral moniliasis. STS negative.

Parasites — Scabies and pediculosis infestations are suggested by excoriated papules and pustules often found in intertriginous areas. Pruritus is severe. Demonstration of the parasite is diagnostic. Darkfield negative, STS nonreactive.

Iritis and Neuroretinitis — When these conditions are part of the secondary syphilis syndrome, they are accompanied by other recognizable lesions. The STS will be reactive.

Condylomata Acuminata—These verrucous acuminate lesions, which are of viral origin, are most frequently seen around the glans, vulva, and rectal regions. Darkfield examination may reveal large numbers of saprophytic treponemes, but no *T. pallidum*. STS are nonreactive.

Acute Exanthemata—Epidemic, generalized, morbilliform, occasionally petechial eruptions associated with fever and other constitutional symptoms are the usual manifestations. Darkfield negative, STS usually nonreactive.

Infectious Mononucleosis — The generalized eruption (present in about 10 percent of cases), lymphadenopathy, and inflamed throat closely resemble secondary syphilis. Very rarely some of the STS are reactive, and the spleen may be markedly enlarged. Careful darkfield examination of lesions may be necessary to exclude syphilis. Atypical lymphocytes in the blood smear and a positive heterophile agglutination test establish the diagnosis.

Alopecia — The nonscarring temporary hair loss of secondary syphilis (described above) is usually associated with other characteristic cutaneous lesions. STS are uniformly reactive and darkfield examination of moist lesions occurring elsewhere will be positive for *T. pallidum*. Toxic and traumatic alopecia, as well as alopecia areata, may be ruled out by history, examination of the hair, negative darkfield, and nonreactive STS.

Any of the above conditions can occur concurrently with syphilis.

EPIDEMIOLOGY

Every case of infectious syphilis must be considered the source of a potential epidemic. Since no case exists in isolation, the disease occurs because a personal interchange of the infecting organism took place through some form of intimate physical contact with another person. Control procedures, therefore, must take into account medical as well as social considerations, and both normal and deviate behavior.

Syphilis epidemiology is simple in theory, but complex in application. The busy physician will find it difficult, if not impossible, to involve himself deeply in this demanding and time-consuming process. All state health departments, and many local units, have personnel specially

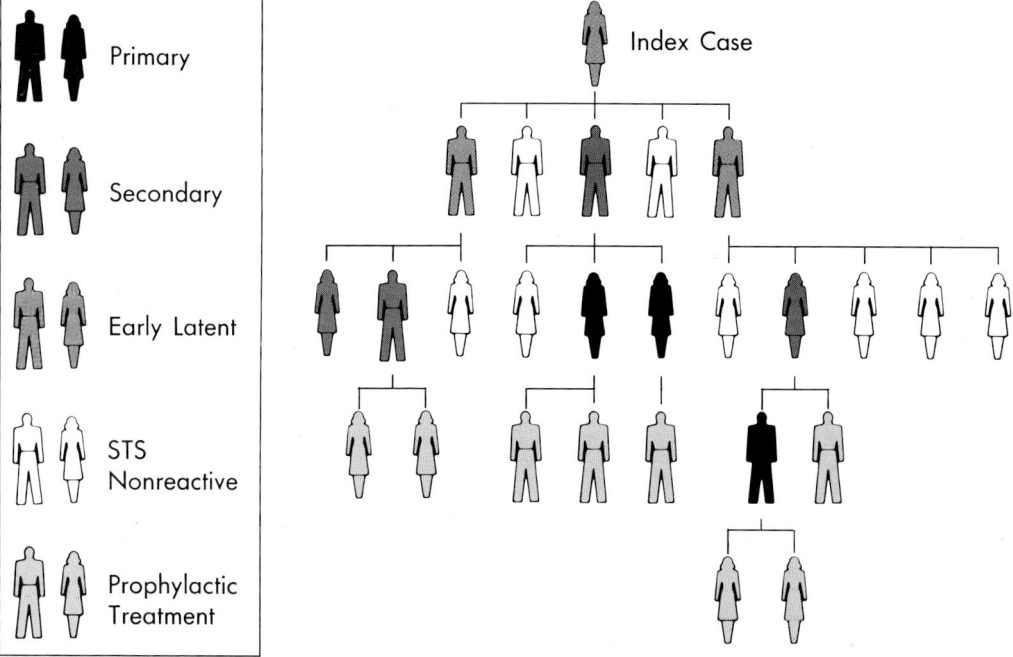

The index case was brought to medical attention through a routine reactive serologic test. Prophylactic treatment was administered to all named sexual contacts who were clinically negative and serologically non-reactive on initial examination, but who were within the critical 90-day incubation period following exposure.

FIGURE 24. The arrest of a syphilis outbreak through prophylactic treatment.

trained to handle the great variety of personal and social problems related to sexual behavior and venereal disease. They are schooled in interviewing and investigation technics, thus ensuring confidentiality and bringing to treatment the maximum number of infected contacts.

Patient Interview

Promptly upon diagnosis, the patient should be interviewed to elicit not only sexual contacts, but also a select group of persons known by the patient to be syphilis suspects or associates. The interview must also serve as an information-giving process to inform the patient about his disease.

As a rule of thumb, patients with primary syphilis should be interviewed to determine sexual contacts during the three months prior to onset of symptoms; those with secondary syphilis, 6 months; and those with early latent syphilis, 12 months. The exact interview period will be determined by examining the available medical and epidemiologic information. If all named contacts are examined and found not to be infected, the interview is incomplete.

Contact Tracing

The average patient may be expected to name three or four contacts, and more is not unusual. Any one of these contacts not found and examined may develop the disease, pass it on to other persons, and later become afflicted with the damaging late manifestations.

The mobility of today's population demands rapid exchange of information between geographic areas to ensure prompt examination and treatment of

TABLE 1

CHARACTERISTIC	EARLY SYPHILIS	LATE SYPHILIS
Infectivity	Yes	No, except in pregnant female.
Darkfield	Positive	Negative
Reinfection	Can occur after adequate treatment.	Rare even after adequate treatment.
Destructive lesions	No	Yes
Serologic tests	Reactive, often with high titer, reverting to negative, or with marked fall to low titer, after treatment.	Usually reactive, often with low titer, with little or no change after treatment. High titers are frequently associated with gummas and paresis.

infected contacts. Furthermore, those contacts located, but found to be not infected at the time of first examination, should be given prophylactic (epidemiologic, preventive) treatment (Figure 24).

If the patient is known to have been exposed to "lesion" syphilis, it is foolish to wait for the disease to develop to the clinical or reactive serologic stage, meanwhile allowing reinfection of treated patients and infection of additional persons.

LATENT AND LATE SYPHILIS

Latent Syphilis

By definition, latent syphilis is that stage of the disease where there are no clinical signs or symptoms of syphilis; the spinal fluid is negative; and STS are reactive. All syphilis is latent at some time during its course, and some cases may be virtually latent for the duration of the disease or the life of the patient. A clinical diagnosis of latency does not preclude the possibility of infectiousness, or of developing gummatous lesions, cardiovascular abnormalities, or of neurosyphilis. Should one of these become apparent, the diagnosis is no longer latent syphilis.

The diagnosis is made on the basis of repeated reactive STS in the absence of concurrent disease which may produce a false positive. A treponemal test is often indicated to establish the syphilitic nature of the serologic-test reactivity. A history of exposure, of early lesions, of previous reactive serologic tests, or of antecedent treatment is helpful, if elicited, and may help in classification as early or late.

After an infection has persisted for more than 4 years, it is rarely communicable, except in the case of the pregnant woman. In addition, if after 4 years the spinal fluid is normal, it will probably remain so.

Late Syphilis

From beginning to end, syphilis is essentially a vascular disease, with the exception of the gumma, which is probably a hypersensitivity phenomenon. Aside from gummas, the lesions of late syphilis are produced by obliterative endarteritis of terminal arterioles and small arteries, and by the resulting inflammatory and necrotic changes.

Practical differentiations may be made between lesions of early and late syphilis (see Table 1).

Untreated late syphilis may present a

TABLE 2

TYPE OF LATE SYPHILIS	FREQUENCY (PERCENT)
Latent	60-70
Neurosyphilis (Symptomatic) . . .	8
Late Benign Syphilis	17
Cardiovascular Syphilis	10

broad range of signs and symptoms, varying from none apparent to those indicating severe damage to one or more body systems. The most usual types and their incidence may be found in Table 2.

These divisions, however, are not mutually exclusive. Examples:

(1) Of patients with late benign syphilis, about 13 percent have cardiovascular involvement, and another 10 percent neurosyphilis.

(2) Of patients with cardiovascular syphilis, about 12 percent have associated neurosyphilis.

(3) Of patients with neurosyphilis, about 15 percent have associated cardiovascular syphilis.

Neurosyphilis

All neurosyphilis is asymptomatic at some time during its course, and it is rare for it to occur in "pure" forms. In all types, the essential changes are the same: obliterative endarteritis, usually of terminal vessels, with associated parenchymatous degeneration, which may or may not be sufficient at the time of examination to produce symptoms.

Neurosyphilis may be arbitrarily divided into the following groups, depending on the type and degree of CNS pathology: Asymptomatic; meningovascular; and parenchymatous, consisting of paresis and tabes dorsalis.

Asymptomatic Neurosyphilis — The patient is usually seen because of a reactive STS with no signs or symptoms of CNS involvement. However, examination of the cerebrospinal fluid is abnormal, with an increase in cells, total protein, and a reactive VDRL or Kolmer complement-fixation test.

Meningovascular Neurosyphilis — Present are definite signs and symptoms of CNS damage resulting from cerebrovascular occlusion, infarction, and encephalomalacia with focal neurologic signs varying with the size and location of the lesion. The spinal fluid is always abnormal, with an increase in cells, in protein, and a reactive VDRL or complement-fixation reaction.

Parenchymatous Neurosyphilis — This form of neurosyphilis presents as paresis or tabes dorsalis.

PARESIS: While the signs and symptoms of paresis may be myriad, they are always indicative of widespread parenchymatous damage. Personality changes range from minor to frankly psychotic. Focal neurologic signs are frequent. The CSF is invariably abnormal, with cells and protein increased, and the VDRL or complement-fixation test reactive.

TABES DORSALIS: The typical signs and symptoms of tabes dorsalis are those of posterior column degeneration, with ataxia, areflexia, paresthesias, bladder disturbances, impotency, and lancinating pain. Spinal-fluid findings are abnormal in 90 percent of cases and blood serology reactive in 75 percent. Gastric or abdominal "crises" frequently begin with vomiting, which may lead to serious electrolyte disturbances and abdominal pain. Trophic joint changes (Charcot's joints) result from loss or impairment of the sensation of pain. The knee joint is most commonly affected, and severe degeneration is common (Figure 25). Loss of deep pain sensation may be associated with perforating ulcers on the soles or toes (mal perforans) as shown in Figure 26.

Optic atrophy is a serious complication of neurosyphilis and should be looked for in every patient; examination of the peripheral fields is imperative in every suspected neurosyphilitic. Pupillary changes may be seen in both forms of late neurosyphilis, the classic being the Argyll-Robertson pupil, which is small, irregular, and fails to react to light, but responds normally to convergence.

The signs and symptoms of paresis and tabes dorsalis frequently coexist (taboparesis) in the same patient.

Examination of the Spinal Fluid—Three tests of the spinal fluid are essential for the diagnosis of neurosyphilis and its intelligent follow-up:

(1) Cell count: More than 4 lymphocytes is abnormal.

(2) Total protein: Protein is always elevated in active neurosyphilis. Since "normal" values vary from laboratory to laboratory, know your laboratory's normal. Individuals, too, may vary considerably, but a total protein of more than 40 mg% is usually abnormal.

(3) Kolmer or VDRL spinal-fluid tests: A reactive spinal fluid Kolmer or VDRL is virtually always an indication of CNS syphilis, but not necessarily of its activity. False-positive reactions in the spinal fluid are exceedingly rare.

The presence of reagin in the spinal fluid is the only pathognomonic finding, since any meningeal irritation may result in increased cells and protein. Only in late tabes dorsalis would one consider the diagnosis of neurosyphilis in the face of negative reagin findings. Conversely, even in the absence of clinical signs and symptoms, a positive reagin test indicates asymptomatic neurosyphilis. Following

adequate treatment, years may elapse before the test becomes nonreactive. As a rule, the cell count returns to normal first, followed by the protein.

The degree of activity is indicated by the increased numbers of lymphocytes and increased protein. When investigating the spinal fluid, beware of the bloody tap! Small quantities of reactive blood serum in spinal fluid can produce a positive Kolmer or VDRL reaction, and red cells may be mistaken for white cells.

As an historical note, colloidal tests of spinal fluid (colloidal gold), once widely employed, are of no diagnostic significance and unreliable as a guide to activity. They are without value in the management of neurosyphilis.

Cardiovascular Syphilis

The lesions are usually caused by medial necrosis of the aorta, with aortic dilatation often extending into the valve commissures. The essential signs are those of aortic insufficiency or saccular aneurysm of the thoracic aorta. Careful clinical evaluation of hypertension, arteriosclerosis, and previous rheumatic heart disease is essential.

Saccular aneurysm of the thoracic aorta is pathognomonic of cardiovascular syphilis. Aortic insufficiency with no other valvular lesions in a middle-aged person with reactive STS should be considered cardiovascular syphilis until proved otherwise. In cardiovascular syphilis, STS are usually reactive.

Late Benign Syphilis

The term "benign" is used because the lesions (gumma) of late benign syphilis seldom result in total physical incapacity or death. When such gummas occur in the brain or other vital organs, the word

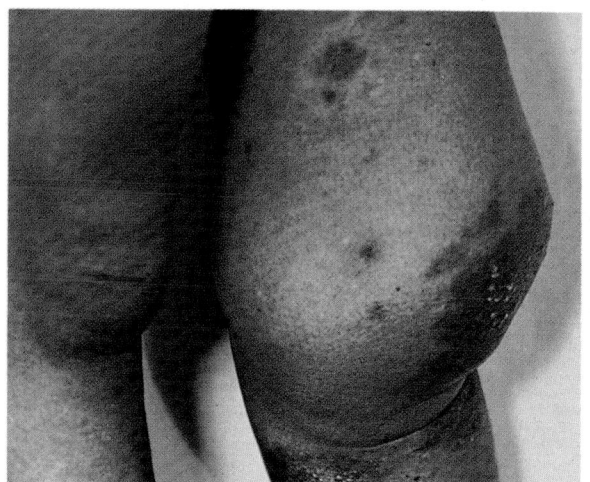
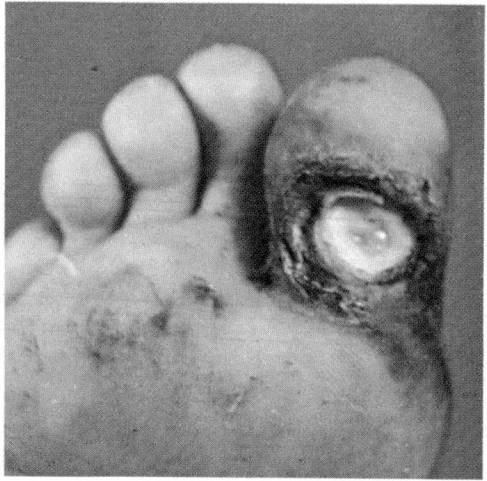

FIGURE 25. Late syphilis: Charcot knee in tabes dorsalis of longstanding.

FIGURE 26. Late syphilis: Perforating ulcer of great toe (mal perforans) in tabes dorsalis.

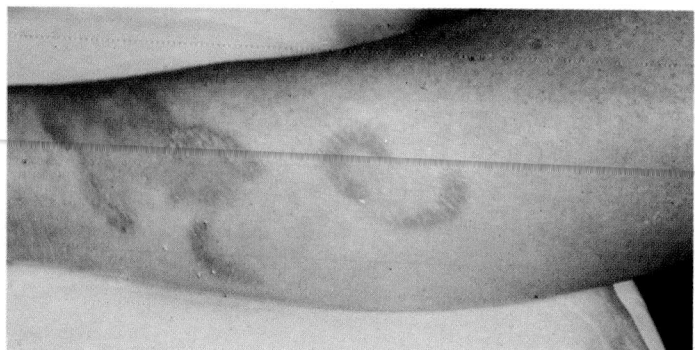

FIGURE 27. Late syphilis: Gummas of the arm.

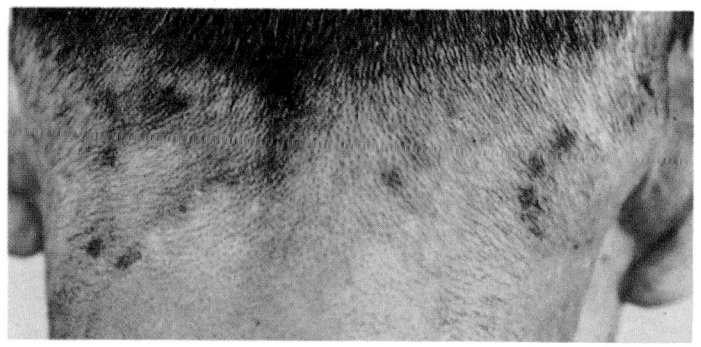

FIGURE 28. Late syphilis: Gummas of the scalp.

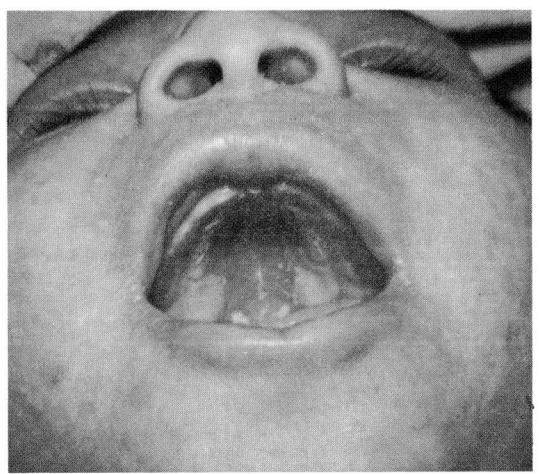

FIGURE 29. Congenital syphilis: Infant demonstrating mucous patches and skin lesions.

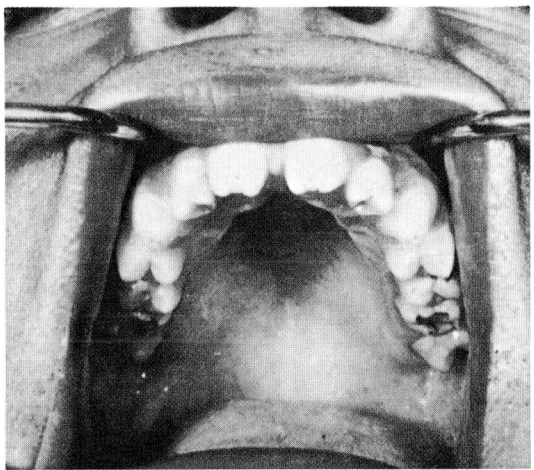

FIGURE 31. Congenital syphilis: Hutchinson's teeth. Note notched edges and "screwdriver" shape of central incisors.

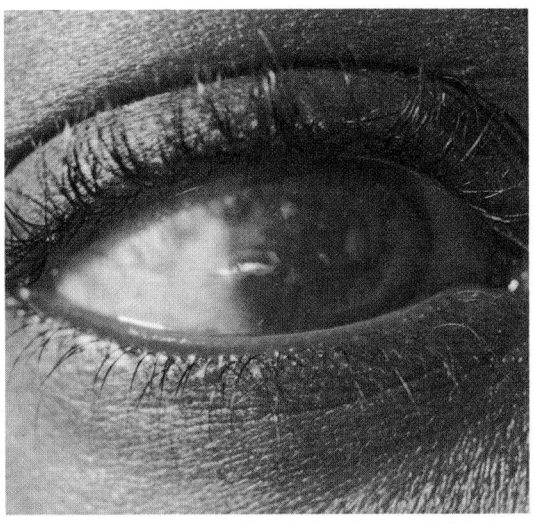

FIGURE 30. Congenital syphilis: Interstitial keratitis causing blindness.

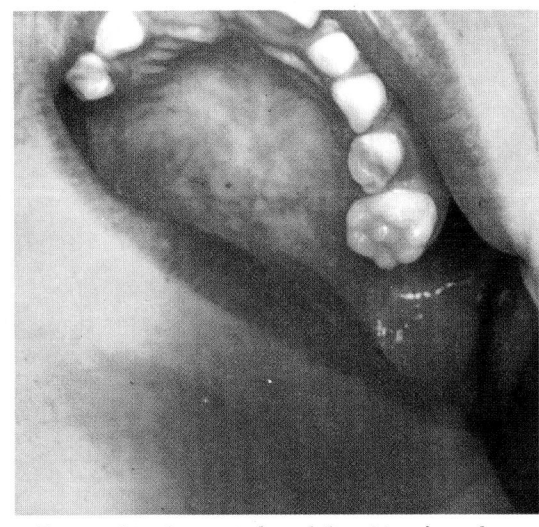

FIGURE 32. Congenital syphilis: Moon's molar.

"benign" is misleading and inaccurate.

As mentioned before, gummas are probably the result of hypersensitivity reactions to treponemal infection. The most common sites are skin, bone, and liver, but many other organs can be involved. Skin lesions may be solitary or multiple, tend to form circles or segments of circles, are destructive and chronic, and tend to heal centrally while extending peripherally (Figures 27 and 28).

Bone lesions are usually marked by periostitis with associated new bone formation, or by gummatous osteitis, with bone destruction. The cardinal signs are pain, swelling, and bony tumor, usually

21

affecting the skull, tibia, and clavicle.

In late benign syphilis, STS are almost always reactive and usually of high titer.

Syphilis in Pregnancy

After the 18th week of gestation, when Langhans' cell layer of the early placenta has atrophied, the treponeme may cross the placenta to infect the fetus. Pregnancy while the mother is in the primary or secondary stage of syphilis frequently terminates in a stillbirth, whereas pregnancy occurring during the later stages of syphilis may result in a clinical spectrum from a fulminating fatal congenital syphilis to an uninfected child.

Adequate treatment of the mother before the 18th week of pregnancy prevents infection of the fetus. Because penicillin crosses the placental barrier, treatment of the mother after the 18th week will also cure the fetus. A woman adequately treated and followed with quantitative STS, and with no evidence of reinfection, does not need to be retreated with each subsequent pregnancy. However, when any doubt exists about the adequacy of previous treatment or the presence of active infection, a course of treatment should be given to prevent congenital syphilis.

Congenital Syphilis

Congenital syphilis is divided into stages similar to those of acquired syphilis. Since *T. pallidum* is introduced directly into the fetal circulation, there is no primary stage.

The *early stage of congenital syphilis* is characterized by the appearance of signs and symptoms before the age of two years. The earlier the onset, the poorer the prognosis. Among the more important signs:

(1) Cutaneous lesions: Shortly after birth, the skin lesions are frequently vesicular or bullous, progressing to superficial crusted erosions. When developing later, the lesions are often papulosquamous with a generalized symmetrical distribution like that of acquired syphilis and may form typical condylomata lata.

(2) Mucous-membrane lesions: The nose and pharynx are often involved to produce heavy mucoid discharge referred to as the "snuffles." Hemorrhagic nasal discharge in the newborn is characteristic of syphilis. Both skin and mucous-membrane lesions (Figure 29) teem with spirochetes, rendering these lesions and secretions extremely infectious. A positive diagnosis can be made by darkfield examination.

(3) Bone: Although only 15 percent of infants show clinical signs, almost 100 percent will show radiologic evidence of osteochondritis of the long bones after the first month of life. Dactylitis results from involvement of the phalanges.

(4) Anemia: A self-limited, hemolytic anemia is common.

(5) Hepatosplenomegaly: Two thirds will show this sign, which may be associated with a low-grade icterus.

(6) Central nervous system: Up to one half of infants may have abnormal spinal fluid, although the incidence of clinical manifestations is much lower.

The late stage of congenital syphilis is defined as that persisting beyond two years of age. In about 60 percent, the disease is latent with no manifestations other than reactive STS. The signs may be produced by continued activity or may be the so-called "stigmata" resulting from previous infection.

(1) Interstitial keratitis: Near puberty, the cornea develops a ground-glass appearance with vascularization of the adjacent sclera (Figure 30). The condition becomes bilateral and leads to blindness.

(2) Hutchinson's teeth: Because of poor development of the middle denticle, the permanent upper central incisors develop a barrel-shaped, notched appearance and are smaller than normal. X-ray study permits diagnosis, even while unaffected deciduous teeth are in place (Figure 31).

(3) Mulberry or Moon's molars: The first molars may show maldevelopment of the cusps (Figure 32).

(4) Eighth-nerve deafness: This sign is not common, but may be seen at puberty or even into middle age.

(5) Neurosyphilis: The congenital syphilitic may show the same manifestations as those seen in acquired syphilis. Tabes dorsalis is uncommon, paresis being more frequent than in the adult.

(6) Bone: Involvement may be sclerotic to produce sabre shin (Figure 34) and frontal bossing, or it may be lytic (gummatous) and produce destruction (saddle nose). Perforation of the hard palate (Figure 33) is highly suggestive of congenital syphilis. Any part of the skeletal system may be involved.

(7) Cutaneous lesions: Rhagades (Figure 35) may result from infantile syphilitic rhinitis, but are rarely seen. Gummas may involve skin or other organs, as in acquired syphilis.

(8) Cardiovascular lesions: Rare, but reported.

(9) Clutton's joints: Painless hydrarthrosis, usually of the knees (Figure 36), rarely involves the elbows or other large joints.

Interstitial keratitis, eighth-nerve deafness, and Clutton's joints are often associated with each other near puberty. This triad does not respond well to penicillin and is thought to be a hypersensitivity phenomenon rather than a purely spirochetal involvement of the structures.

Serology in Pregnancy and the Newborn

Both reagin and treponemal antibodies, as well as those antibodies responsible for a false-positive reaction, will cross the placenta. If the mother has a reactive STS, so will the newborn. The higher the titer of the mother's blood, the greater the chance of reactivity in the newborn. If the mother has a high titer, the infant will probably have a high titer. In the case of passive transfer of antibody, the child's titer should not exceed the mother's, and the child's reactive STS should revert to negative by 3 to 4 months of age. If it does not become nonreactive, active infection is strongly suggested. A rising titer is diagnostic.

If the mother is infected late in pregnancy, both mother and child may be nonreactive at delivery. In that case, clinical signs and a rising titer in the ensuing weeks will confirm the diagnosis.

A new test has been described for the detection of congenital syphilis. This test, the FTA-ABS-IgM, is based on the knowledge that IgM antibodies are too large to cross the placental barrier and are normally absent in the newborn. The presence of IgM antibody against the *T. pallidum* in the neonatal period establishes the diagnosis of active infection in the infant.

Pregnancy, in itself, is a rare cause of false-positive reactions. However, a false positive, as occurring in the general population, may also be seen in pregnancy.

SEROLOGIC INTERPRETATION

Human infection with *T. pallidum* stim-

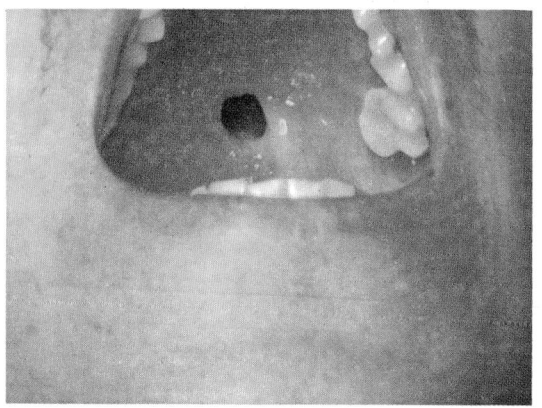

FIGURE 33. Congenital syphilis: Perforation of hard palate resulting from gummatous destruction.

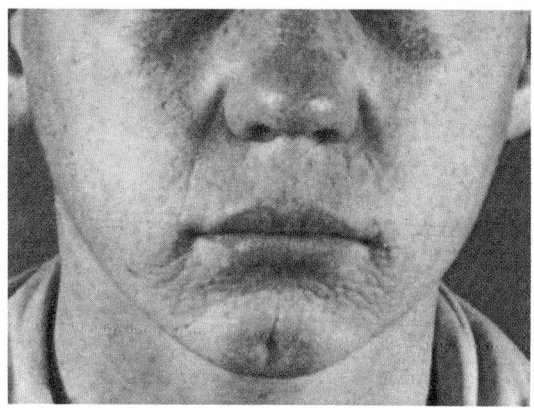

FIGURE 35. Congenital syphilis: "Rhagades" facial disfigurement resulting from persistent syphilitic rhinitis of infancy.

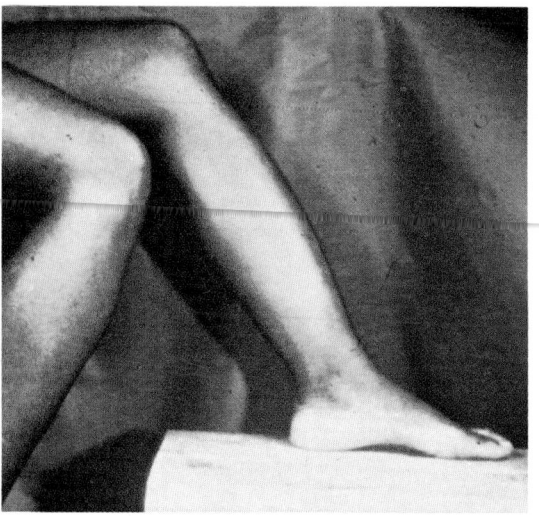

FIGURE 34. Congenital syphilis: Osteoperiostitis of the tibia resulting in "sabre shins."

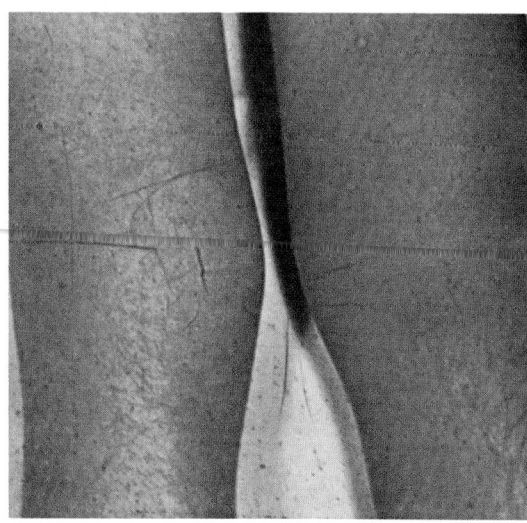

FIGURE 36. Congenital syphilis: Clutton's joints.

ulates the host's defense mechanisms and provokes a complex antibody response. The detection of one or more of these antibodies is the basis for serologic testing. The ideal single test should be (1) easily and quickly performed, (2) highly sensitive and specific, and (3) readily reproducible in different laboratories. Although more than 200 tests have been described, no ideal test is currently available. The physician should select two or three tests, familiarize himself with them, and thus be able to diagnose syphilis in nearly any stage.

The *sensitivity* of a test refers to its ability to be reactive in the presence of syphilis, while the *specificity* of a test refers to its ability to be nonreactive in the absence of the disease. Some highly sensitive tests are particularly suited for screening purposes; other tests are highly specific and assist in making problem diagnoses.

Classification

All STS depend on the reaction of antibody with antigen. The tests may be classified by the type of antigen used. Nontreponemal or reagin tests are performed with extracts of normal tissue or other sources. Treponemal tests employ treponemes or treponemal extracts to detect antibody.

TABLE 3

Partial Classification of Tests for Syphilis

I. NONTREPONEMAL ANTIGEN TESTS

    Flocculation
        Venereal Disease Research Laboratory
        (VDRL) Slide
        Kahn Standard
        Kline
        Mazzini

    Complement Fixation
        Kolmer

    Agglutination
        Rapid Plasma Reagin

II. TREPONEMAL ANTIGEN TESTS

    Complement Fixation
        Reiter Protein Complement Fixation
        Kolmer with Reiter Protein Antigen
        Treponema pallidum Complement
        Fixation
        Treponema pallidum Cryolysis Protein

    Agglutination
        Treponema pallidum Agglutination

    Immobilization
        Treponema pallidum Immobilization
        (TPI)

    Immunofluorescence
        Fluorescent Treponemal Antibody
        (FTA-200)
        Fluorescent Treponemal Antibody
        Absorption (FTA-ABS)

The indicator system employed allows a further classification of the treponemal and nontreponemal tests (Table 3). For example, the antibody (reagin) that reacts with purified beef heart extract (cardiolipin-lecithin) binds complement and prevents hemolysis of sensitized erythrocytes (the indicator system). The test is nontreponemal; the reaction is demonstrated by complement fixation. An example of a nontreponemal complement-fixation test is the Kolmer.

When antibody reacts with treponemes dried and fixed on a microscopic slide, the reaction may be demonstrated by the reaction of antisera to human immune globulin conjugated with a fluorescent dye. The Fluorescent Treponemal Antibody Absorption (FTA-ABS) test is a treponemal immunofluorescent test.

Nontreponemal Antigen Tests

Unless specifically noted to the contrary, use of the terms "serology," "serologic test," "STS," or "serologic reaction" in this article refers to nontreponemal antigen tests. While these tests are not absolutely specific or sensitive for syphilis, their performance is quite practical, they are widely available, and their findings are undoubtedly indicative of possible infection.

The original Wassermann test was a complement fixation using an extract of the liver of a syphilitic stillborn as the antigen. However, normal liver extract served equally well, and the test that eventually developed was a nontreponemal STS. Although some still use the term "Wassermann" for any nontreponemal STS, the test is no longer performed, and the term should be dropped.

Reactive nontreponemal tests confirm the diagnosis in the presence of early- or late-lesion syphilis; offer a diagnostic

TABLE 4

Comparative Sensitivity of Nontreponemal and Treponemal Tests in Untreated Syphilis

| STAGE | APPROXIMATE PERCENT OF SERUMS EXPECTED TO GIVE REACTIVE TEST RESULTS | | | | |
| | NONTREPONEMAL TESTS | | TREPONEMAL TESTS | | |
	VDRL SLIDE	KOLMER	FTA-200	TPI	FTA-ABS
Primary	76	65	40	53	86
Secondary	100	100	95	98	100
Early Latent	95	95	90	94	99
Late Latent	72	65	68	89	96
Late (Tertiary)	70	60	77	93	97

clue in latent, subclinical syphilis; are an effective tool for detecting cases in epidemiologic investigations; and are superior to the treponemal tests for following response to therapy. The likelihood of obtaining a reactive VDRL or Kolmer test is shown in Table 4. Reagin is first detected in the serum at approximately 4 to 6 weeks after infection or 1 to 3 weeks after the chancre appears.

Serial quantitative STS may reveal a dynamic process. A rising titer may indicate a recent infection, reinfection in an adequately treated patient, relapse of an inadequately treated patient, or an acute false-positive reaction. Adequate treatment of early syphilis is shown by a decline in titer (Table 5).

Titers should become nonreactive in 6 to 12 months following treatment for primary syphilis and in 12 to 18 months after therapy for secondary syphilis. Treatment of a late or latent infection usually has little or no effect on the titer and should not be used to gauge adequacy of therapy. The posttreatment titer in early latent syphilis may follow the course of either secondary or late latent syphilis. If the titer rises persistently (by at least 2 tube dilutions), it must be concluded that the disease remains active, and retreatment must be initiated. (One-tube variation is within the limits of laboratory error.)

Careful attention must be paid to every reactive or weakly reactive STS. Many cases of untreated late latent or late syphilis will produce only weakly reactive results with undiluted serum. On the other hand, the titer is usually high (16 dils or greater) in secondary syphilis. A high titer does not necessarily mean early syphilis (or even syphilis, for that matter), but it is strong evidence. Some of the highest titers recorded have been in late visceral or cutaneous syphilis or in nonsyphilitic diseases; eg, hemolytic anemia or systemic lupus erythematosus.

Certain special tests have been developed for rapid screening of sera. One of these is the Rapid Plasma Reagin (RPR) test. A modified VDRL antigen is used, and the test is made sensitive by the addition of choline chloride. Blood is collected in anticoagulant tubes, centrifuged,

TABLE 5

Typical Serologic Response to Therapy in Syphilis

| STAGE | DAYS AFTER THERAPY | QUALITATIVE METHODS | | QUANTITATIVE METHOD |
		VDRL SLIDE	KOLMER[1]	VDRL SLIDE
I. PRIMARY	0	R	R 4+	R 2 dils
SYPHILIS.	32	R	4+	2 dils
	62	R	4+	2 dils
	96	WR	R 2+	WR 0 dils
	118	N	N	N
	165	N	N	N
	239	N	N	N
II. SECONDARY	0	R	R 4+	64 dils
SYPHILIS.	34	R	4+	32 dils
	65	R	4+	16 dils
	91	R	4+	4 dils
	118	R	R 3+	4 dils
	180	WR	R 1+	WR 0 dils
	245	N	N	N
	299	N	N	N
	348	N	N	N
III. EARLY LATENT	0	R	R 4+	32 dils
SYPHILIS.	2	R	4+	16 dils
	36	R	4+	16 dils
	66	R	4+	8 dils
	100	R	4+	4 dils
	147	R	4+	8 dils
	203	R	R 3+	2 dils
	266	WR	3+	WR 0 dils
	349	N	R 1+	N
	428	N	N	N
	510	N	N	N
IV. LATE LATENT	0	R	R 4+	8 dils
SYPHILIS.	9	R	4+	8 dils
	94	R	4+	4 dils
	178	R	4+	4 dils
	255	R	4+	8 dils
	360	R	4+	4 dils
	537	R	4+	2 dils
	709	R	4+	4 dils
	888	R	R 3+	2 dils
	1,061	WR	3+	WR 0 dils
	1,366	WR	3+	WR 0 dils
	1,651	WR	3+	WR 0 dils

SYMBOLS: N = nonreactive; WR = weakly reactive; R = reactive; dils = abbr. for dilutions – the reciprocal of the highest titer giving a fully reactive test.

[1] In qualitative tests, numbers refer to the intensity (1-4) of the reaction in undiluted serum.

EXAMPLE	0	2	4	8	16	32	64	128	256
(a)	4+	4+	4+	4+	4+	4+	2+	0	0
(b)	R	R	R	R	R	R	WR	N	N
(c)	R	R	R	WR	N	N			
(d)	WR	N	N						
(e)	N	WR	R	R	R	R	R	R	N

and tested immediately without heating the plasma.

The "RPR" antigen has been adapted to perform a similar test on the plasma portion of a microhematocrit determination (Plasmacrit or PCT test). After reading the packed-cell volume, the capillary tube is divided, and the plasma expressed for testing. The PCT test has been especially useful in blood-bank operation to exclude donors before collection, in screening hospital admissions, and since capillary specimens are used, in testing infants. The Unheated Serum Reagin (USR) test is a further modification of the RPR test.

Reporting of Nontreponemal Antigen Tests

The results of qualitative tests for syphilis are customarily reported as *reactive* (positive, 4+), *weakly reactive* (weakly positive, 3+, 2+, or 1+), or *nonreactive* (negative). Quantitative results may be obtained by diluting the serum in geometrical progression to an end-point. The titer is usually expressed as the highest dilution in which the test is fully reactive. In examples (a) and (b) above, the specimen was fully reactive at a dilution of 1 to 32 (1:32), which may also be expressed as "32 dils." Example (c) would be reported as reactive at 4 dils; example (d) weakly reactive, 0 dils.

Excessive production of antibody (particularly in the secondary stage of syphilis) occasionally results in the prozone phenomenon. This occurs with complement-fixation or flocculation tests. Undiluted specimens will give a nonreactive or weakly reactive result. Testing at higher dilutions, however, gives reactive test results. In example (e), a prozonal reaction, the result would be reported as R 128 dils.

A few laboratories still report Kahn or Kolmer tests by multiplying the last reactive dilution by 4 and calling the product "Kahn units" or "Kolmer units," or simply "KU."

Treponemal Antigen Tests

Treponemal tests are primarily employed as confirmatory tests in diagnostic problem cases, patients in whom the clinical, historical, or epidemiologic evidence of syphilis is equivocal.

The *Treponema pallidum* Immobilization (TPI) test, while time consuming, technically difficult, and very expensive to perform, has been the standard by which all treponemal tests are judged.

The Fluorescent Treponemal Antibody (FTA) tests are the most recent and most promising tests to date. The best of these tests is the Fluorescent Treponemal Antibody Absorption (FTA-ABS) test, which is now widely available and, because of its increased sensitivity and specificity, is the confirmatory test of choice. It becomes reactive earlier than the TPI in early syphilis and is about 5 percent more sensitive in late latent or late syphilis. The patient's serum is diluted with an extract of non-pathogenic treponemes (Reiter), which absorb "group" treponemal antibodies, but leave "specific" antibodies in the syphilitic serum. The antigen employed is dead *T. pallidum* (Nichols strain). If the serum contains antibodies, they will adhere to and cover the organism. This is then treated with fluorescein-tagged antibody to human globulin. If the globulin (syphilitic antibody) coats the treponeme, the tagged material will react with it, and the treponeme will fluoresce when viewed under ultra-violet light.

Recently the FTA-ABS test has been automated, greatly increasing the number of tests that can be performed.

False-Positive Reactors

All normal sera may contain minute amounts of reagin and thus may produce false-positive STS. The sensitivity of non-treponemal tests is altered by varying the proportion of the reagents, temperature, mixing time, and other physiochemical variables. For these reasons, about one quarter of all false-positive reactions are technical in origin, the titers rarely exceeding weakly reactive or reactive at 1 dil. Repeating the STS will often produce negative reactions.

Repeatedly reactive STS accompanied by nonreactive treponemal tests (eg, FTA-ABS) characterize the false-positive reactor. The duration of reagin activity arbitrarily determines whether the false-positive reaction is acute (less than 6 months) or chronic (6 months or longer).

Acute false-positive reactions are found in persons suffering from many viral or bacterial infections or who have had certain vaccinations and immunizations. Titers are generally less than 8 dils, the reaction persisting for a few weeks to a few months.

Chronic false-positive reactions are less frequent than technical or acute false positives. They may be associated with collagen or autoimmune diseases, malaria, leprosy, or heroin addiction.

TREATMENT

Even after 25 years, the causal treponeme has not developed any measurable resistance to penicillin, and it continues as the best and most effective treatment of syphilis. Any of the following preparations may be employed satisfactorily in the treatment of any stage of syphilis:

(1) Benzathine penicillin G.

(2) Procaine penicillin G with 2 percent aluminum monostearate (PAM).

(3) Aqueous procaine penicillin G.

For instance, in primary and secondary syphilis:

Rx: Benzathine penicillin G: 2.4 million units total (1.2 million units in each buttock) intramuscularly at one clinic session.

or: PAM: 4.8 million units total usually given 2.4 million units at first session, as above, and 1.2 million units in each of 2 subsequent injections 3 days apart.

or: Aqueous procaine penicillin G: 4.8 million units as total given 600,000 units daily for 8 days.

These preparations must be administered intramuscularly. Oral penicillin is *not* recommended. See Table 6 for dosage schedules and follow-up.

When patient sensitivity to penicillin precludes the use of this drug, then erythromycin, tetracycline, chlortetracycline, oxytetracycline, and demethylchlortetracycline are the best alternate choices. In

TABLE 6

Summary of the Management of Syphilis

STAGE	TREATMENT	FOLLOW-UP POSTTREATMENT	
		SEROLOGY	DISCHARGE[1]
Primary and Secondary..	2.4 million units benzathine penicillin G, half in each buttock, single session.	1st, 3rd, 6th, 12th months.	End of 1 year.
Latent, both Early and Late	If no spinal fluid examination: Total: 6.0 million units benzathine penicillin G. Initial: 3.0 million units, then 1.5 million units at 7-day intervals x 2. If spinal fluid examination is non-reactive: Total: 2.4 million units in single dose.	As above, then every 6 months for 2nd year.	End of 2 years.
Syphilis in Pregnancy[2]....	As above depending on stage.	Monthly until delivery, then as for appropriate stage.	End of 1-2 years, depending on stage.
Subsequent pregnancies. No change in titer[2]......	No treatment indicated.	Initial visit and monthly until delivery.	
Early Congenital (under 2 years)[3]......................	50,000 units benzathine penicillin G/Kg body weight in a single dose.[4]	Same as primary or secondary.	End of 1 year.
Late Congenital (over 2 years)[3]: Under 12 years: weight 70 lb. or less[3]	Same as early congenital.	Plus every 6 months for 2 years.	End of 2 years.
12 yr. or older but weight more than 70 lb.	Same as comparable adult stage.	Same	End of 2 years.
Neurosyphilis ....⎫ Cardiovascular Syphilis .. ⎬ Late Benign Syphilis ......⎭	Total: 6.0-9.0 million units benzathine penicillin G. Initial: 3.0 million units, then 3.0 million units every 7 days x 1 or 2.	Every 3 months for 1st year. Every 6 months for 2nd year.	End of 2 years.

[1] A spinal fluid examination is suggested at the time of discharge for all patients with other than primary or secondary syphilis as discharge patients should have either negative serologic tests for syphilis or fixed low titers. Neurosyphilis patients should have a spinal fluid examination at each follow-up visit.
[2] Retreatment is indicated if there is any doubt concerning adequacy of previous treatment.
[3] An appropriate medical specialist should be consulted regarding treatment of the complications of congenital syphilis.
[4] Aqueous procaine penicillin G is probably the preferred form of penicillin in the treatment of very small infants because of the local irritant effect occasionally observed with benzathine penicillin G.

NOTE: When penicillin is contraindicated, use: Tetracycline or Erythromycin: 750 mg every 6 hours for 10-15 days. In pregnancy, erythromycin for a full 15 days is preferred. The infant should be followed clinically and serologically for 3-4 months following birth. Tetracycline has been reported to cause dental staining and deformity when used in pregnancy and young children.

early syphilis, the recommended total dosage for demethylchlortetracycline is 20-30 grams; if another tetracycline or erythromycin is given, the dosage should be 30-40 grams. Treatment should be given 4 times daily in equally divided oral doses and extended over a period of 10-15 days. If these alternate broad-spectrum antibiotics are employed, close follow-up of the syphilitic patient is imperative for the reasons mentioned earlier. This is especially true in pregnant females. It is also imperative that a spinal-fluid examination be done as part of follow-up after this type of therapy. In late syphilis, cardiovascular syphilis, or neurosyphilis, the total dosage should be doubled if any of these broad-spectrum antibiotics are used in treatment.

Preventive Treatment

While every effort should be made to establish a diagnosis before administering preventive treatment to someone known to have been exposed to infectious syphilis, do not wait for clinical or serologic signs to appear. Such delay permits reinfection of treated patients and infection of additional patients. Adequate preventive treatment (2.4 million units of benzathine penicillin G) will destroy all treponemes of a contact with incubating syphilis, abort the disease in its prodromal stage, and render the patient incapable of spreading it to others.

Jarisch-Herxheimer Reaction

This reaction, known in older literature as therapeutic shock, is believed to be caused by the rapid release of antigenic materials from lysed treponemes. It is noted after the first injection of any treponemicidal agent and is evidence of the efficacy of the medication rather than a manifestation of an allergic reaction. Local and general reactions may occur. The local reaction consists of an intensification of the lesions. In primary syphilis, the chancre may become edematous with increase in size of the satellite bubo. A faint secondary rash may become prominent. Systemically, the temperature may rise to 102° and rarely to 104°. These reactions usually occur within 12 hours after initiation of treatment, lasting a few hours and rarely more than 24. Herxheimer reactions are most marked in stages when treponemes are abundant. The ambulant patient should be informed that he may experience a self-limited febrile period following initial therapy. Antipyretics and analgesics are helpful in reducing discomfort.

Usually the Herxheimer reaction is benign and indicates a favorable response to treatment, although in late syphilis it may be more severe. Regardless of severity, treatment should not be discontinued. The physician must be aware of this reaction and not confuse it with an allergic reaction, thus mislabelling the patient as penicillin sensitive.

Allergic Problems

Unfortunately, skin tests for penicillin hypersensitivity leave much to be desired as predictors of reactions. At present, alternate therapy should be given to patients with a past history of penicillin sensitivity.

Allergic reactions may be immediate (humoral), delayed (cellular), or delayed-immediate (serum sickness). Clinically, the immediate reactions are characterized by urticaria, angioneurotic edema, pruritus, or deep shock. The delayed type may take the form of contact dermatitis, rashes, bullous eruptions, and exfoliative dermatitis. Serum sickness may result when the antigen is retained long enough to function both as the sensitizing and challenging antigen. Patients with serum sickness will have fever, arthralgias, urticaria, and maculopapular skin eruptions occurring some 7 to 12 days after injection.

With the exception of anaphylaxis (see below), allergic reactions are generally successfully treated by antihistaminic agents in milder cases and corticosteroids in the more severe.

Anaphylaxis is an immediate hypersensitivity where the antibody is thought to be fixed on the mast cells or basophils. On reacting with the antigen, histamine, serotonin, and other pharmacologically active substances are released from the carrier cell. They in turn react on such "end-organ" tissues as smooth muscle, connective tissue, and blood vessels.

A shock-like state may develop and be life-threatening. All patients should be closely observed for 20 minutes after penicillin injection. Adequate facilities for emergency treatment should be immediately available.

REPRINTS AVAILABLE

In the United States, reprints of CLINICAL SYMPOSIA without advertising may be purchased from the Publications Section, CIBA Pharmaceutical Company, Division of CIBA-GEIGY Corporation, Summit, New Jersey 07901. In other countries, please direct inquiries to the nearest CIBA-GEIGY office.

SECTION E

C I B A

CHEST TRAUMA

EMIL A. NACLERIO, M.D., F.A.C.S.

Attending Thoracic Surgeon, Department of Surgery, Harlem Hospital Center,
College of Physicians and Surgeons of Columbia University, and
Columbus Hospital, New York, New York

INTRODUCTION

The chest contains the most vital of life-sustaining organs, the heart and the lungs. Therefore, any trauma to the chest, that seriously compromises the function of these organs, is an immediate threat to survival. Unless these injuries are treated on-the-spot or within a short period of time, death often occurs rapidly.

Many of these injuries have a way of happening at unpredictable times and in out-of-the-way places, often hours away from a specially trained physician, or even an ambulance. To wait for expert care when seconds or minutes count is tantamount to issuing a death sentence.

In these situations, the lives of over 80 per cent of patients with critical but reversible chest problems can be saved with the mere application of a few simple measures.

Therefore, if lives are to be saved, all physicians, and their paramedical associates, must become familiar with the pertinent diagnostic signs of these life-threatening situations, their altered physiology, and the measures that can be employed from the most primitive to the more sophisticated.

In this presentation, we shall discuss as briefly as possible the diagnosis and treatment of chest injuries, from on-the-spot first aid to definitive hospital care. Those who desire a more comprehensive discussion of chest trauma are referred elsewhere.*

PRIORITIES OF TREATMENT

More often than not, injury to the chest is only part of the picture in a patient with multiple injuries. In many instances, injuries to other body areas may prove more serious than those involving the thorax. Obviously then, the priorities of treatment will vary from case to case.

A severely bleeding scalp wound, that can be controlled by digital pressure, should certainly receive early attention. However, one must bear in mind that a patient in shock from bleeding may survive for hours, even though his pulse is barely perceptible and his blood pressure cannot be obtained. On the other hand, a person who cannot breathe will be dead within minutes. Therefore, the first thing to look for, and treat if necessary, is:

---

*__Chest Injuries:__ *Physiologic Principles and Emergency Management.* Naclerio, E. A., Grune & Stratton, Inc., New York (In Press, April 1971).

75

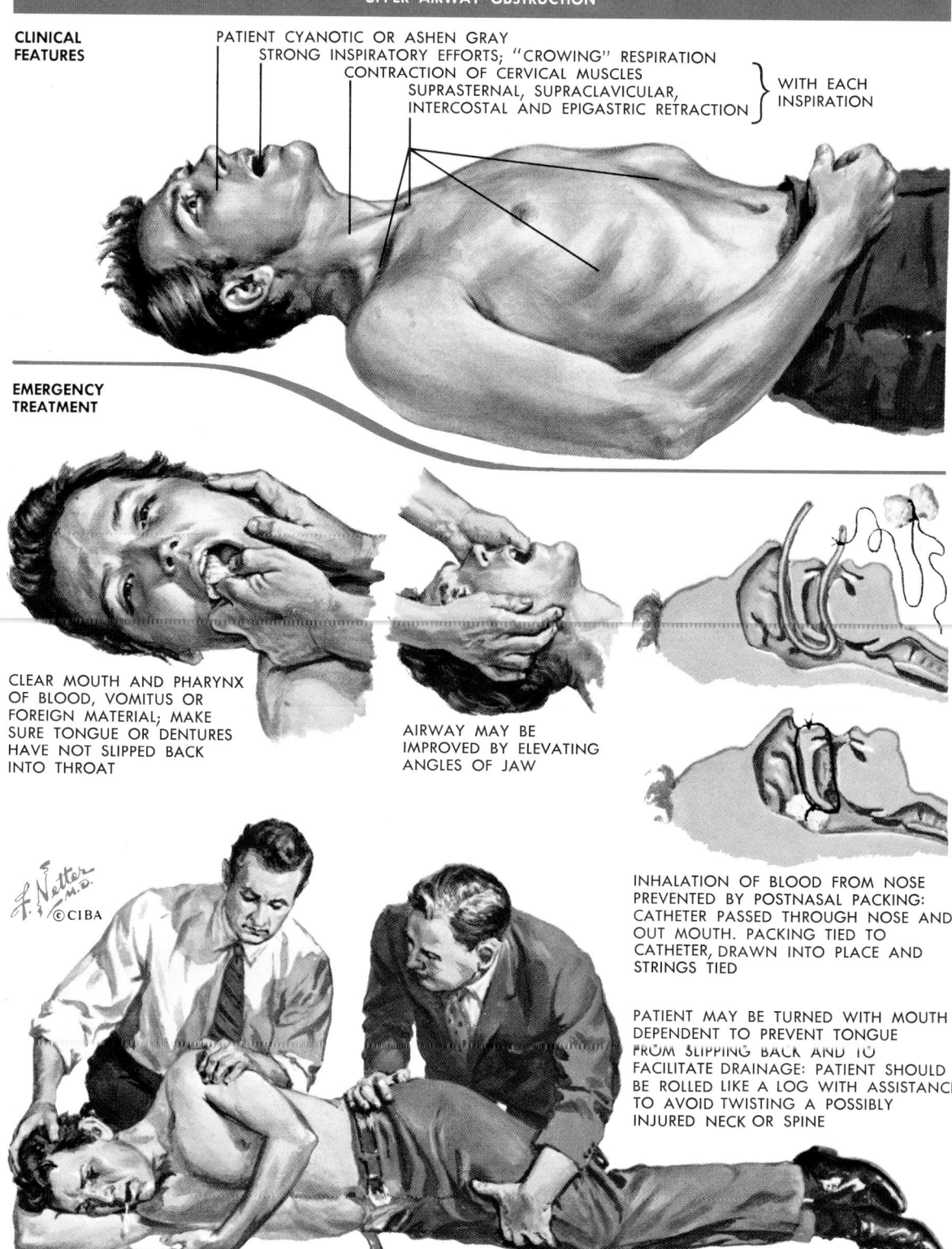

CLINICAL FEATURES

PATIENT CYANOTIC OR ASHEN GRAY
STRONG INSPIRATORY EFFORTS; "CROWING" RESPIRATION
CONTRACTION OF CERVICAL MUSCLES
SUPRASTERNAL, SUPRACLAVICULAR,
INTERCOSTAL AND EPIGASTRIC RETRACTION } WITH EACH INSPIRATION

EMERGENCY TREATMENT

CLEAR MOUTH AND PHARYNX OF BLOOD, VOMITUS OR FOREIGN MATERIAL; MAKE SURE TONGUE OR DENTURES HAVE NOT SLIPPED BACK INTO THROAT

AIRWAY MAY BE IMPROVED BY ELEVATING ANGLES OF JAW

INHALATION OF BLOOD FROM NOSE PREVENTED BY POSTNASAL PACKING: CATHETER PASSED THROUGH NOSE AND OUT MOUTH. PACKING TIED TO CATHETER, DRAWN INTO PLACE AND STRINGS TIED

PATIENT MAY BE TURNED WITH MOUTH DEPENDENT TO PREVENT TONGUE FROM SLIPPING BACK AND TO FACILITATE DRAINAGE: PATIENT SHOULD BE ROLLED LIKE A LOG WITH ASSISTANCE TO AVOID TWISTING A POSSIBLY INJURED NECK OR SPINE

PLATE I

UPPER AIRWAY OBSTRUCTION

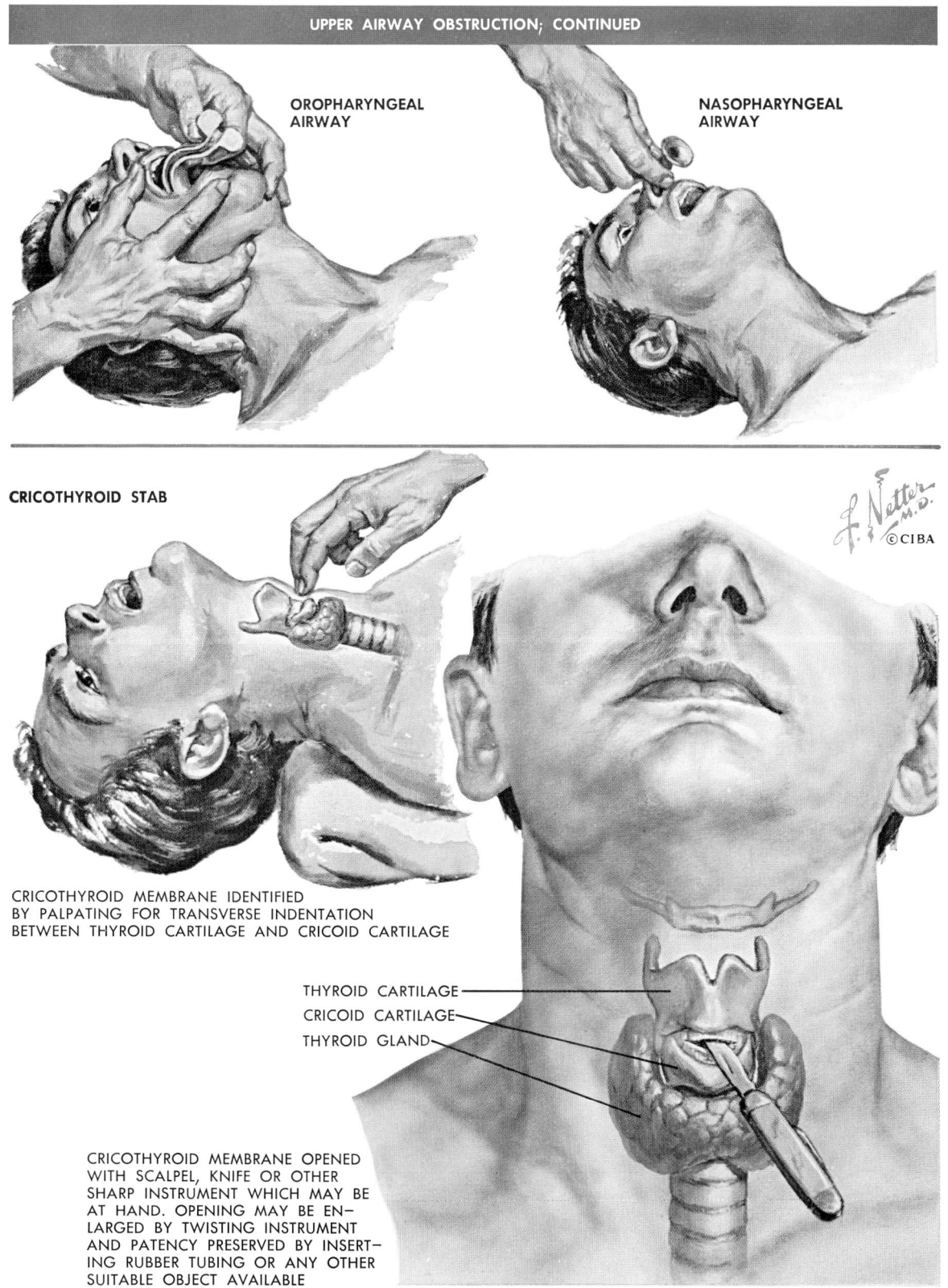

OROPHARYNGEAL AIRWAY

NASOPHARYNGEAL AIRWAY

CRICOTHYROID STAB

CRICOTHYROID MEMBRANE IDENTIFIED BY PALPATING FOR TRANSVERSE INDENTATION BETWEEN THYROID CARTILAGE AND CRICOID CARTILAGE

THYROID CARTILAGE
CRICOID CARTILAGE
THYROID GLAND

CRICOTHYROID MEMBRANE OPENED WITH SCALPEL, KNIFE OR OTHER SHARP INSTRUMENT WHICH MAY BE AT HAND. OPENING MAY BE EN-LARGED BY TWISTING INSTRUMENT AND PATENCY PRESERVED BY INSERT-ING RUBBER TUBING OR ANY OTHER SUITABLE OBJECT AVAILABLE

DIAGNOSIS

The patient will be making strong inspiratory efforts. A cursory look at the neck will reveal contraction of the cervical muscles with *retraction of the suprasternal notch and supraclavicular fossae* coincident with each inspiration. The intercostal spaces and epigastrium will also retract on inspiration. The patient's color may be cyanotic or ashen gray.

TREATMENT

Make sure that the tongue or loose dentures have not slipped back to occlude the throat. Clear the mouth and pharynx of blood, mucus, vomitus, and all foreign material with a finger, a gauze sponge, or by catheter suction. Aspiration of blood from the posterior nose and nasopharynx can be prevented by postnasal packing.

The possibility of the tongue slipping back into the throat can be eliminated by rolling the patient over so that his mouth is dependent. When assistance is available, the patient should be rolled like a log in one piece to avoid twisting a possibly injured neck or spine. Any rough or careless handling of these patients may lead to rapid fatality secondary to cervical cord injury or may convert a minor cord compression into one resulting in quadriplegia.

If the mouth and throat are clear, or have been cleared, the airway may be improved by simply elevating the posterior angles of the jaw.

If respiration is still labored, with retraction of the suprasternal notch, or if signs of laryngeal stridor are present, the next step will depend on the equipment at hand.

Oropharyngeal Airway

In the unconscious or comatose patient, a quick and easy way to provide a clear pathway for air is by the introduction of a plastic oropharyngeal airway. While this device will insure ample air flow, it will not prevent aspiration of blood, mucus, or vomitus.

Nasopharyngeal Airway

If a nasopharyngeal airway tube is available, it can be passed through the nose and down into the oropharynx. This will prevent complete blockage of the pharynx by the tongue, but like the oropharyngeal airway, it will not prevent aspiration.

Cricothyroid Stab

In desperate situations of complete or near complete upper airway obstruction secondary to extensive injuries to the face, mandible, or throat, or entrapped foreign bodies in the larynx, any measure short of an emergency cricothyroid stab may prove fatal. In these situations (if none of the previously described measures can be used), the cricothyroid membrane must be opened at once using any relatively sharp instrument, a penknife, scissors, or even a nail file.

The cricothyroid membrane can be identified by feeling for the transverse indentation which is located about ½ inch (1.5 cm) below the Adam's apple. This area is avascular so that serious bleeding cannot occur. The instrument should be inserted transversely so as to obtain a sufficient opening. Once the trachea has been entered, a piece of rubber tubing, if available, should be inserted into the airway to keep the edges of the aperture apart.

The insertion of intravenous needles in the cricothyroid membrane has been recommended, but even those of large bore will improve the airway very little.

Endotracheal Intubation (Plate III)

The quickest and easiest way to insure a clear upper airway in patients who cannot be treated adequately by the use of an oropharyngeal airway is by direct endotracheal intubation. Moreover, this measure allows a tube to be directed through the larynx, eliminating obstruction by vocal cord spasm. If a cuff-type endotracheal tube is used, inflation of the cuff will prevent aspiration by sealing off the trachea from the digestive tract. It will also permit positive-pressure ventilation.

In most cases, endotracheal intubation will provide an entirely adequate airway for hours or days, if necessary. A tracheostomy, if required, can be carried out later on an elective basis. In an emergency situation, endotracheal intubation can be accomplished by anyone who has a moderate degree of familiarity with the technique, which is illustrated in Plate III.

Most important is to properly position the patient, so as to bring the opening of the mouth into direct line with the trachea.

To do this, the neck is slightly flexed on the trunk. The head, which is supported by a pillow or its equivalent, is hyperextended. (Extension of the head without some neck flexion will not provide a straight line of approach to the larynx.)

In the absence of a mouth-spreader, a block of wood or some other solid object can be wedged between the teeth to keep the jaws apart.

Advantages of Endotracheal Intubation: Once in place, a cuffed endotracheal tube confers on the patient many advantages:

1. A clear upper airway is insured.

2. Aspiration of blood, mucus, and vomitus is prevented.

3. Resistance to air flow, and thus the oxygen-consuming work of breathing is reduced.

4. An Ambu bag or a positive-pressure respirator may be employed to assist ventilation.

5. The excessive secretions causing lower airway obstruction can be easily removed by direct aspiration.

6. Inhalation anesthesia can also be given easily, if required.

7. Upper airway patency having been

secured, the physician can concentrate on other urgent problems.

Tracheostomy

This procedure may be lifesaving in chest-injured patients. However, in an acute emergency, tracheostomy is far inferior to endotracheal intubation. In the first place, it will take 10 to 15 minutes, as compared to the few seconds required to insert an endotracheal tube. Furthermore, a hastily done tracheostomy with inadequate assistance, poor lighting, and improper instruments in a patient who is rapidly expiring, often leads to troublesome bleeding which may significantly increase the airway difficulty.

Tracheostomy, therefore, should be deferred until it can be carried out carefully under suitable conditions, preferably in the operating room. The endotracheal tube should not be withdrawn until the tracheostomy has been completed.

LOWER AIRWAY OBSTRUCTION

(PLATES IV AND V)

Blockage or impedance of air flow in the lower airways is brought about by one or more of the following:

1. Aspirated blood, vomitus, or other foreign material.

2. Bleeding from lacerated or contused lung tissue.

3. Bronchospasm.

4. Inhibition of cough by chest pain and/or narcotic drugs.

5. Mechanical and/or reflex cessation of ciliary movement and bronchial peristaltic action.

6. An abnormal outpouring of mucus and transudates characteristic of "traumatic wet lung."

In severe blunt trauma, the lung becomes edematous, like a thumb hit with a hammer. However, factors other than simple contusion must be involved, because pulmonary edema can result

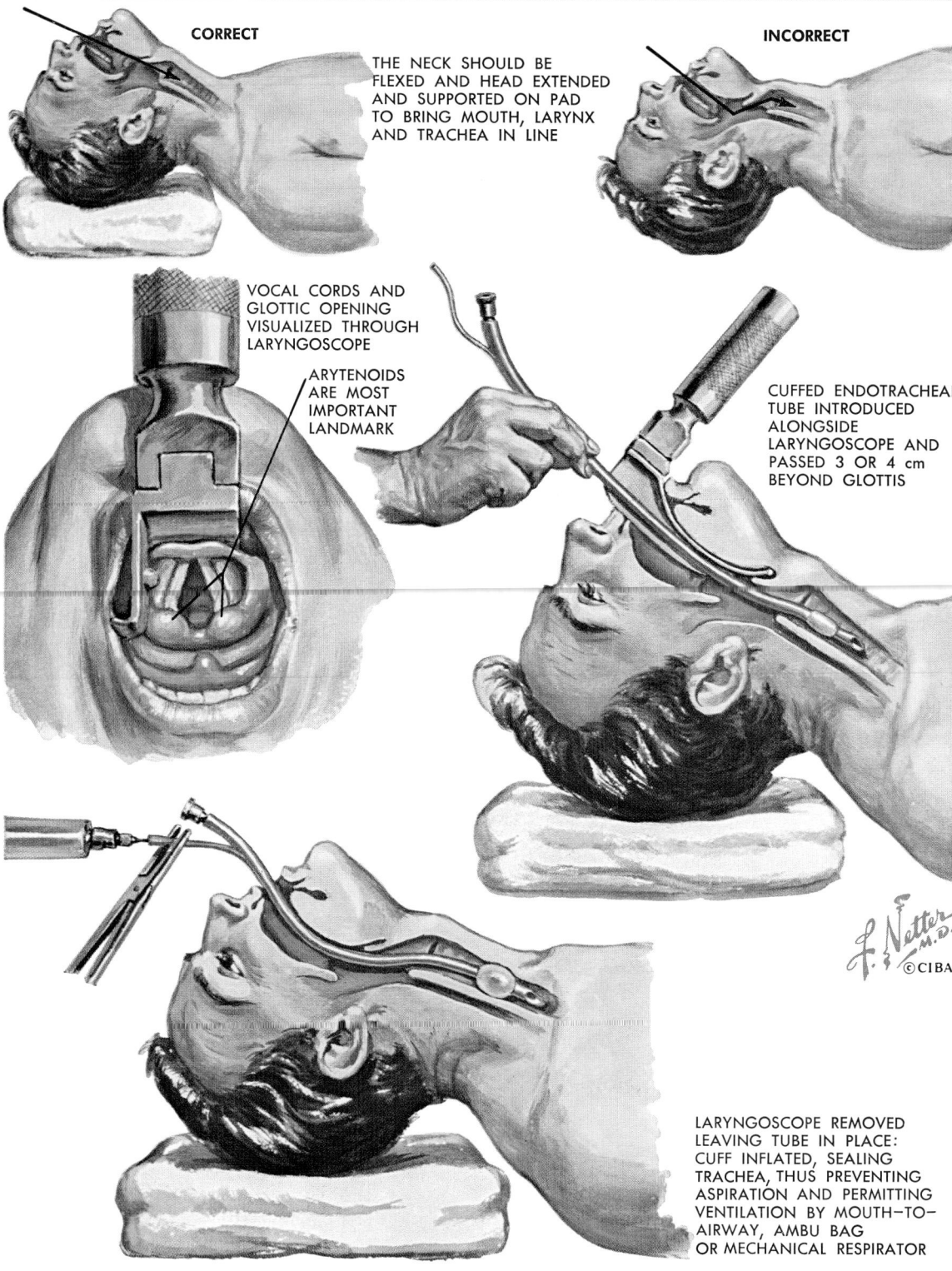

ENDOTRACHEAL INTUBATION
THE MOST RAPID AND EFFECTIVE WAY OF ESTABLISHING AND MAINTAINING A CLEAR AIRWAY

CORRECT

INCORRECT

THE NECK SHOULD BE FLEXED AND HEAD EXTENDED AND SUPPORTED ON PAD TO BRING MOUTH, LARYNX AND TRACHEA IN LINE

VOCAL CORDS AND GLOTTIC OPENING VISUALIZED THROUGH LARYNGOSCOPE

ARYTENOIDS ARE MOST IMPORTANT LANDMARK

CUFFED ENDOTRACHEAL TUBE INTRODUCED ALONGSIDE LARYNGOSCOPE AND PASSED 3 OR 4 cm BEYOND GLOTTIS

LARYNGOSCOPE REMOVED LEAVING TUBE IN PLACE: CUFF INFLATED, SEALING TRACHEA, THUS PREVENTING ASPIRATION AND PERMITTING VENTILATION BY MOUTH-TO-AIRWAY, AMBU BAG OR MECHANICAL RESPIRATOR

CLINICAL FEATURES

CYANOSIS

DYSPNEA

INEFFECTIVE COUGH

RALES, WHEEZES, RHONCHI

X-RAY SIGNS OF ATELECTASIS AND/OR PNEUMONIA

P_aCO_2 INCREASED
P_aO_2 DECREASED
pH DECREASED

TREATMENT

EVACUATION OF SECRETIONS

MANUAL SUPPORT OF CHEST TO FACILITATE COUGH AND RID TRACHEOBRONCHIAL TREE OF SECRETIONS (SEE ALSO PLATE V)

ANESTHESIA TO RELIEVE PAIN OF FRACTURED RIBS

INTERCOSTAL NERVE BLOCK AT ANGLE OF RIB; OPTIMUM POINT TO INJECT BECAUSE RIB IS HERE MOST SUPERFICIAL, MOST EASILY PALPABLE AND ACCESSIBLE

6 cm

10 cm

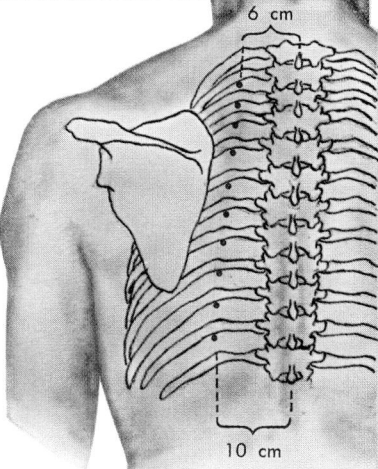

SITES FOR INJECTION TO RELIEVE PAIN OF FRACTURED RIBS:
1: PARAVERTEBRAL BLOCK
2: INTERCOSTAL BLOCK AT ANGLE OF RIB
3: INTERCOSTAL BLOCK AT POST. AXILLARY LINE
4: INTERCOSTAL BLOCK AT ANT. AXILLARY LINE
5: LOCAL INFILTRATION AT FRACTURE SITE
6: PARASTERNAL BLOCK

SKIN IMMOBILIZED BY INDEX FINGER; NEEDLE INTRODUCED THROUGH CUTANEOUS WHEAL PERPENDICULAR TO SKIN TO CONTACT LOWER BORDER OF RIB (1), WITHDRAWN SLIGHTLY, DIRECTED CAUDAD AND AD-VANCED 1/8 INCH TO SLIP UNDER RIB AND ENTER INTERCOSTAL SPACE (2): ASPIRATION ATTEMPTED PRIOR TO INJECTION OF 5 ml ANESTHETIC

PLATE IV

LOWER AIRWAY OBSTRUCTION
INTERCOSTAL NERVE BLOCK

from shock due to injury as far away as the leg. Pulmonary edema also occurs following brain injury, including cerebrovascular accidents, as well as in drug poisoning, and burns involving the head, neck, and chest. In these circumstances, neurogenic reflexes or humoral factors must be involved.

Regardless of the cause or causes in the individual patient, resistance to air flow is markedly increased. The elasticity of the lung, or lung compliance, is reduced ("the stiff-lung syndrome"). In these situations, more respiratory work is needed to move the necessary amount of air in and out of the lungs. At the same time, there is interference with the exchange of oxygen and carbon dioxide because of the increased fluid interface in the alveoli.

If these factors are severe and persist, the inevitable result is hypoxia and acidosis. These biochemical derangements can be particularly lethal in patients with associated respiratory disability due to asthma, chronic bronchitis, or emphysema.

SIGNS AND SYMPTOMS

Symptoms usually develop insidiously. The early clinical appearance of the patient is often deceptively reassuring. Although often hypoxemic, the $PaCO_2$ level may be normal or even reduced, due to reflex hyperpnea, and treatment may be deferred until it is too late.

In other patients in whom the lung is irritated by the aspiration of blood or gastric contents, or in those in whom there is bleeding from the pulmonary parenchyma, asphyxia develops far more rapidly. In the rare patient, in whom there is a communication between a bronchus and a blood-filled pleural cavity (see Hemothorax, Page 99), death may occur rapidly as a result of massive inundation of the tracheobronchial tree.

Rales, wheezes, or rhonchi are usually present in patients with secretional obstruction of lower airways. The findings are accentuated by deep or rapid breathing. They are not necessarily eliminated by cough, particularly in the presence of bronchospasm.

Cough is frequent and relatively nonproductive, but may yield mucoid, serosanguineous or frothy secretions, or blood. With progression of the secretional obstruction, cyanosis, which may not respond to the administration of oxygen, may develop rapidly.

Arterial blood gas studies at this time will show an increase in $PaCO_2$. Also PaO_2 will be decreased, as will the pH. These laboratory findings in association with the clinical signs and symptoms may be erroneously attributed to other conditions. For example: The respiratory distress and cyanosis may be thought to be due to pneumonia, heart failure, pulmonary embolus, or shock. Apprehension, boisterousness, and combativeness, which are really due to hypoxia, may be mistakenly assessed as a reaction to head injury or chest wall pain. Also, the development of shock or manifestations of impending shock secondary to the hypoxia may be attributed to the severe pain and/or internal hemorrhage.

Unfortunately, x-ray examinations are of little help in the early stages of lower airway blockage, usually being negative until atelectasis or pneumonia develops. In the presence of interstitial pulmonary edema, x-ray films may show patchy or diffuse "ground-glass" opacification.

TREATMENT

This depends upon the stage of the condition and the facilities at hand. The best way to clear the airways is by voluntary cough. If the patient is conscious, and rales are present, he should be made to cough every fifteen minutes or more, depending upon the amount of secretions. Cough should be encouraged while manual support is given the chest to decrease pain.

In the presence of a fractured rib or ribs, the cough-inhibiting pain can be eliminated by intercostal nerve block (see Page 87) and pain-relieving drugs (see Page 86).

In the unconscious patient, aspiration of secretions must be carried out by mechanical means. Here again the method used will depend upon the equipment at hand. The method requiring the least in the way of specialized equipment is:

Nasotracheal Suction (Plate V)

The equipment consists of a small rubber tube or a French catheter (preferably #14 or #16), an electric suction machine, tubing, several pieces of gauze, water-soluble lubricating jelly, and a connecting Y tube.

The technique consists of passing the lubricated catheter through a nostril down through the pharynx. The patient, if conscious, is asked to open his mouth wide and protrude his tongue, and the location of the catheter tip is checked with the aid of a tongue blade and bright light. The tongue is then held firmly in an extended position by the patient or an assistant. At this point, the patient is instructed to take several deep breaths. The catheter is then quickly advanced into the trachea. As the catheter passes through the larynx, the patient practically always coughs, and he can no longer phonate.

The catheter is advanced to a maximal depth. Suction is applied by occluding the open Y tube with the finger. Suction is terminated by removing the finger.

When suction is applied, it is very important that it be interrupted to allow the patient to inhale. Suction should be applied for *not more than* 3 or 4 seconds at one time. If longer than this, the patient may panic, because he cannot inhale during suction. Also, any patient with borderline respiratory reserve may be thrown into a state of severe hypoxia, and if suction is continued, prompt cardiac arrest may follow.

To introduce the catheter into the right main bronchus, the head is turned sharply to the left, and the chin is elevated. To enter the left stem bronchus, the head is turned to the right, and the chin is again elevated. In all patients, the catheter is gradually withdrawn while suction is applied, stopping temporarily wherever secretions are heard being aspirated.

Nasotracheal suction properly performed will eliminate the need for bronchoscopy and tracheostomy in many instances.

Bronchoscopy (Plate V)

Bronchoscopy has the advantage over nasotracheal aspiration in that foreign material can be extracted under direct vision. It also helps rule out a suspected injury to the trachea or a major bronchus and to identify a bleeding source in the lower respiratory tract. Also, with a ventilating bronchoscope, the patient can be continuously oxygenated.

Bronchoscopic aspiration is particularly indicated where gastric contents have been aspirated or when atelectasis has involved one or more lobes. In the severely dyspneic or cyanotic patient, the procedure is best carried out in the semi-upright position to improve ventilation. Anesthesia is frequently unnecessary in these patients.

Tracheostomy (Plate VI)

As we have pointed out previously (Page 79), tracheostomy is inferior to endotracheal intubation when a clear airway is needed with great urgency. However, all patients with multiple rib fractures, flail chest and/or contusion pneumonitis, complicated by severe chest wall pain and retained bronchial secretions, and those with associated head trauma should be subjected to tracheostomy as soon as possible. To wait until blood gases have become abnormal may be to have waited too long.

In these circumstances, tracheostomy in

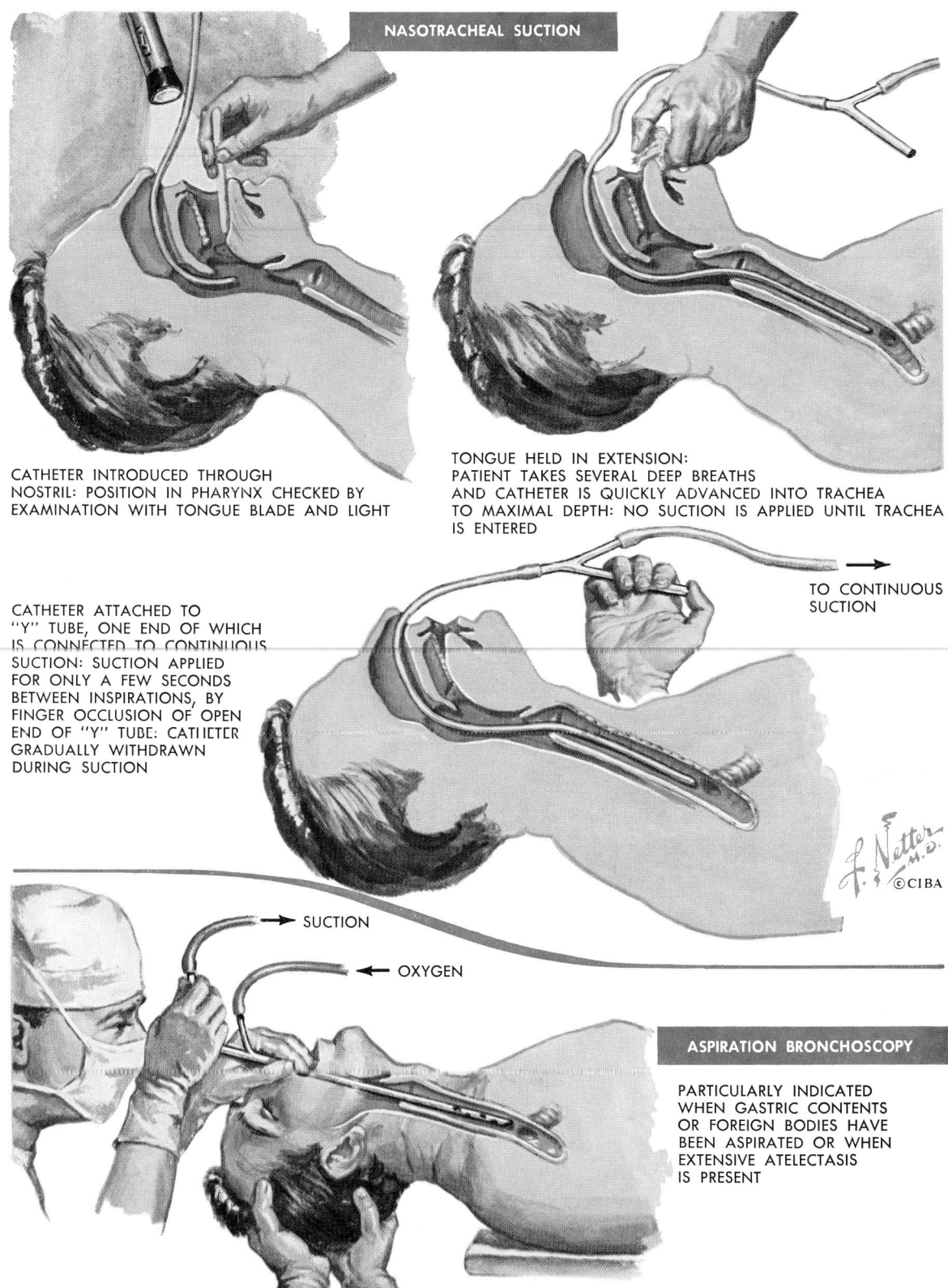

NASOTRACHEAL SUCTION

CATHETER INTRODUCED THROUGH
NOSTRIL: POSITION IN PHARYNX CHECKED BY
EXAMINATION WITH TONGUE BLADE AND LIGHT

TONGUE HELD IN EXTENSION:
PATIENT TAKES SEVERAL DEEP BREATHS
AND CATHETER IS QUICKLY ADVANCED INTO TRACHEA
TO MAXIMAL DEPTH: NO SUCTION IS APPLIED UNTIL TRACHEA
IS ENTERED

CATHETER ATTACHED TO
"Y" TUBE, ONE END OF WHICH
IS CONNECTED TO CONTINUOUS
SUCTION: SUCTION APPLIED
FOR ONLY A FEW SECONDS
BETWEEN INSPIRATIONS, BY
FINGER OCCLUSION OF OPEN
END OF "Y" TUBE: CATHETER
GRADUALLY WITHDRAWN
DURING SUCTION

TO CONTINUOUS
SUCTION

SUCTION

OXYGEN

ASPIRATION BRONCHOSCOPY

PARTICULARLY INDICATED
WHEN GASTRIC CONTENTS
OR FOREIGN BODIES HAVE
BEEN ASPIRATED OR WHEN
EXTENSIVE ATELECTASIS
IS PRESENT

PLATE V

NASOTRACHEAL SUCTION
BRONCHOSCOPIC ASPIRATION

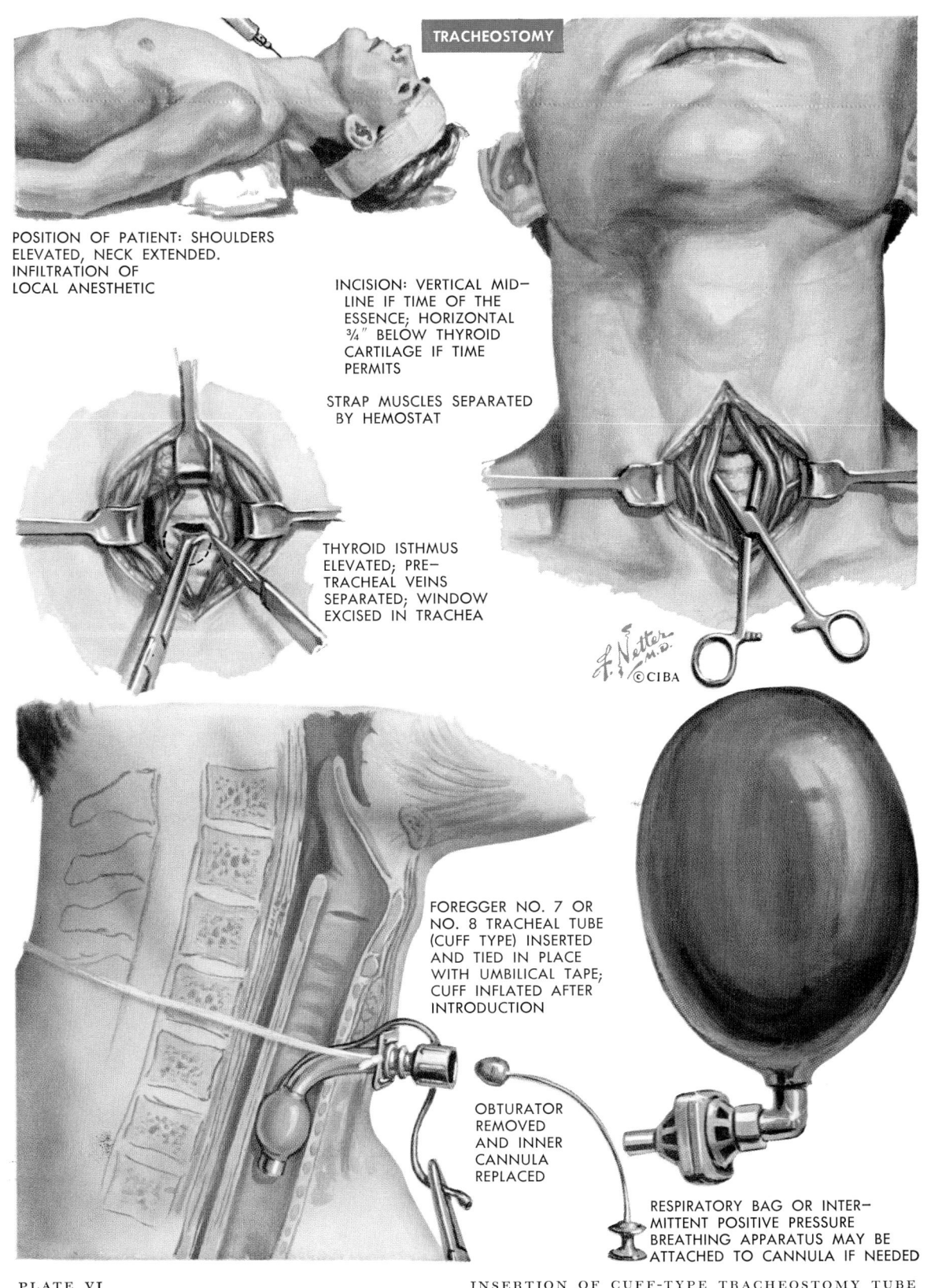

TRACHEOSTOMY

POSITION OF PATIENT: SHOULDERS ELEVATED, NECK EXTENDED. INFILTRATION OF LOCAL ANESTHETIC

INCISION: VERTICAL MID-LINE IF TIME OF THE ESSENCE; HORIZONTAL ¾″ BELOW THYROID CARTILAGE IF TIME PERMITS

STRAP MUSCLES SEPARATED BY HEMOSTAT

THYROID ISTHMUS ELEVATED; PRE-TRACHEAL VEINS SEPARATED; WINDOW EXCISED IN TRACHEA

FOREGGER NO. 7 OR NO. 8 TRACHEAL TUBE (CUFF TYPE) INSERTED AND TIED IN PLACE WITH UMBILICAL TAPE; CUFF INFLATED AFTER INTRODUCTION

OBTURATOR REMOVED AND INNER CANNULA REPLACED

RESPIRATORY BAG OR INTER-MITTENT POSITIVE PRESSURE BREATHING APPARATUS MAY BE ATTACHED TO CANNULA IF NEEDED

PLATE VI

INSERTION OF CUFF-TYPE TRACHEOSTOMY TUBE

itself often turns the tide. In addition to the advantages previously given for endotracheal intubation (Page 79), tracheostomy significantly decreases airway resistance and reduces the respiratory dead space of the adult airway by as much as 150 ml. These factors greatly reduce the high oxygen-cost of breathing.

Positive-Pressure Breathing

Positive-pressure breathing helps overcome the increased turbulence and resistance to air flow in secretion-containing bronchi, bronchioles, and alveolar ducts. It also helps expand the alveoli of "stiff lungs" where the compliance has become reduced by injury. In this way, it improves oxygenation and reverses respiratory acidosis. Indeed, the use of 50 per cent oxygen with proper humidification may bring about dramatic results, particularly in improving oxygenation of the myocardium.

Drugs

Narcotic drugs to relieve pain should be used cautiously because of their propensity for cough suppression and respiratory depression. In the patient with cardiovascular instability, repeated small doses of morphine, 2.5 to 5 mg, given intravenously are much safer and more effective than larger doses administered by the intramuscular route. Demerol has the advantage of causing less respiratory depression.

Bronchodilating drugs, such as isoproterenol, given in suitable dilution intravenously or as an aerosol, may improve breathing by relieving bronchial spasm. Aminophylline or epinephrine may be given intravenously for the same purpose.

If these drugs prove ineffective, corticosteroids may be beneficial. Prednisolone, 100 to 200 mg, is given in the first 24 hours, 50 to 100 mg during the next 24 hours, and 25 to 50 mg over the following 24 hours.

Nebulization of 20 to 50 per cent ethyl alcohol may help the respiratory efficiency by reducing surface tension and breaking down the foam of pulmonary edema.

Since these patients often develop obstructive atelectasis and secondary pneumonia, appropriate antibiotics should be given without delay in the hope of preventing this dreaded complication.

THE CHEST CAGE AND RESPIRATORY FUNCTION

Normal respiratory function depends upon clear airways and normally elastic lungs, as previously discussed. It is also dependent upon an intact thorax that can produce the pressure changes necessary for inspiration and expiration.

On deep inspiration, the ribs are elevated anteriorly. As a result, the ribs, which had slanted obliquely downward, become more horizontal, and the internal capacity of the thorax is increased.

At the same time, muscular contraction lowers the dome of the diaphragm. This diaphragmatic contraction makes by far the greatest contribution to the expansion of chest volume during inspiration. For example: During quiet respiration, the descent of the diaphragm of only 1 cm will increase thoracic volume by 270 ml, or more than one half of the total tidal volume of 500 ml. A diaphragmatic descent of 3 cm would increase thoracic volume by more than 700 ml.

Thus, with muscle splinting, or fixation of the injured thoracic cage by tape or sandbags, the diaphragm alone can be depended upon to maintain adequate aeration *provided* the airways are open, the lungs have not become contused and stiffened, and the pleural spaces are intact.

This statement presupposes previously normal lungs. However, in patients whose vital capacity (normally about 4.8 liters) has been reduced to a low level of 1 liter or less, by such conditions as asthma, chronic bronchitis, pulmonary emphysema, or congestive heart failure, even a simple rib fracture may result in death from asphyxia, particularly if complicated by severe pain or pulmonary contusion.

RIB FRACTURES

This, the most common of all chest injuries, should not be taken lightly, especially in the middle-aged and elderly, whose vital capacity is often seriously reduced. Moreover, rib fractures are frequently complicated by underlying injuries. A significant number will have lung contusion. About one-third have an associated pneumohemothorax. About one-fourth have a pneumothorax, and approximately one-fifth will have hemothorax. This high frequency of underlying complications should be recalled whenever one treats a broken rib as a matter of little consequence.

TREATMENT OF UNCOMPLICATED RIB FRACTURES

Where no underlying complication can be found by repeated examinations, including x-ray, the main problem is relief of pain, since such fractures all heal satisfactorily.

Chest Strapping

This, the method usually employed, does not always relieve the pain. However, it can be tried, bearing in mind that it will limit ventilation, and thus predispose to atelectasis and pneumonia.

Intercostal Nerve Block (Plate IV)

The quickest and surest way to relieve pain is by nerve block, which also abolishes the muscle splinting that limits respiratory excursion. Usually only one or two blocks will be required.

The best place to inject the nerve is in the region of the angle of the rib. The locations of the angle of the ribs in relation to the spinous processes are shown in Plate IV.

Where injection cannot be made at the angle, because of bruised or traumatized overlying tissue, which would increase the risk of infection, the injection can be made at the posterior axillary line where the lateral cutaneous branch will also be affected, in the midaxillary line, or even in the region of the sternum. Since there is some overlap of cutaneous innervation, adjacent nerves above and below the involved rib or ribs had best also be injected.

The technique of injection, as illustrated in Plate IV, utilizes a 5 cm, 25-gauge needle, or for obese or heavily muscled individuals, an 8 cm, 22-gauge needle, to which is attached a 10 ml syringe.

After a cutaneous wheal has been raised at the selected site, the needle is introduced through the wheal, perpendicular to the skin, until the lower border of the rib is contacted. The needle is then withdrawn slightly and carried caudad, so as to slip beneath the rib margin where further advancement of only about ⅛ inch or 4 mm will bring the tip into the intercostal space. Aspiration is attempted, and if negative, 5 ml of the chosen anesthetic solution is injected.

Local Infiltration

Injection directly into the fracture site, while also effective, has several disadvantages. Pain relief is neither as complete nor as long lasting. Also, tissues over the fracture are often contused or macerated, thus predisposing to infection.

Paravertebral Block

This not only produces anesthesia, but also affects centripetal and autonomic fibers. It therefore relieves visceral pain, vasospasm, and other reflex phenomena of trauma. However, this additional anesthetic coverage has the disadvantage that it may cause a precipitous fall in blood pressure, which occasionally is irreversible. Therefore, if a number of segments are to be blocked, vasopressors should be close at hand.

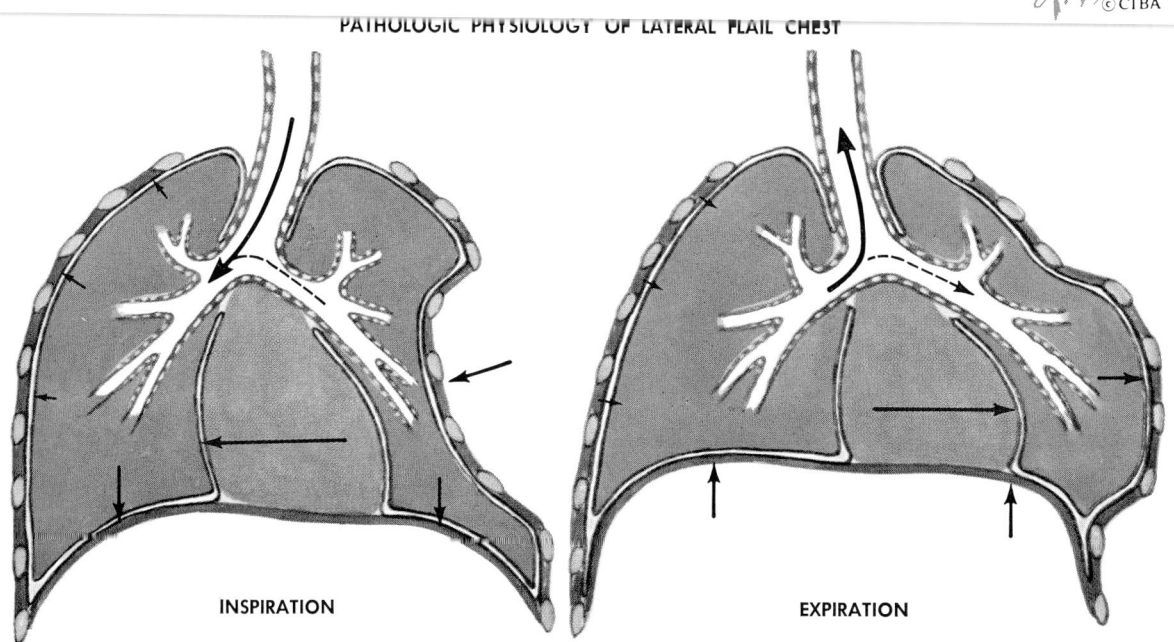

FLAIL CHEST

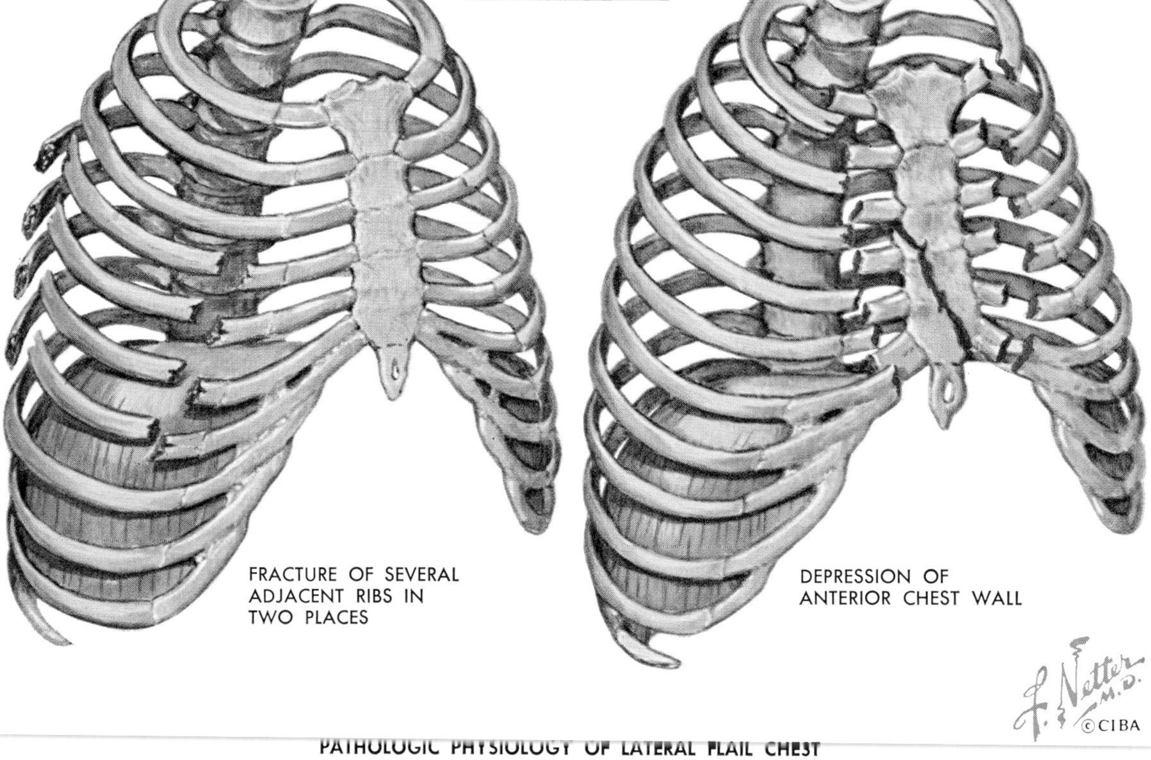

FRACTURE OF SEVERAL
ADJACENT RIBS IN
TWO PLACES

DEPRESSION OF
ANTERIOR CHEST WALL

PATHOLOGIC PHYSIOLOGY OF LATERAL FLAIL CHEST

INSPIRATION

EXPIRATION

ON INSPIRATION: AS CHEST EXPANDS, FLAIL SECTION SINKS IN, THUS IMPAIRING
ABILITY TO PRODUCE NEGATIVE INTRAPLEURAL PRESSURE TO DRAW IN AIR. MEDIA-
STINUM SHIFTS TO THE UNINJURED SIDE. ON EXPIRATION: THE FLAIL SEGMENT
BULGES OUTWARD, THUS IMPAIRING ABILITY TO EXHALE. MEDIASTINUM SHIFTS TO
INJURED SIDE. IN SEVERE FLAIL CHEST, AIR MAY SHIFT USELESSLY FROM SIDE
TO SIDE (PENDELLUFT) INDICATED BY BROKEN LINES

PLATE VII

FLAIL CHEST

MANAGEMENT OF FLAIL CHEST

COMPRESSION METHODS (FIRST AID)

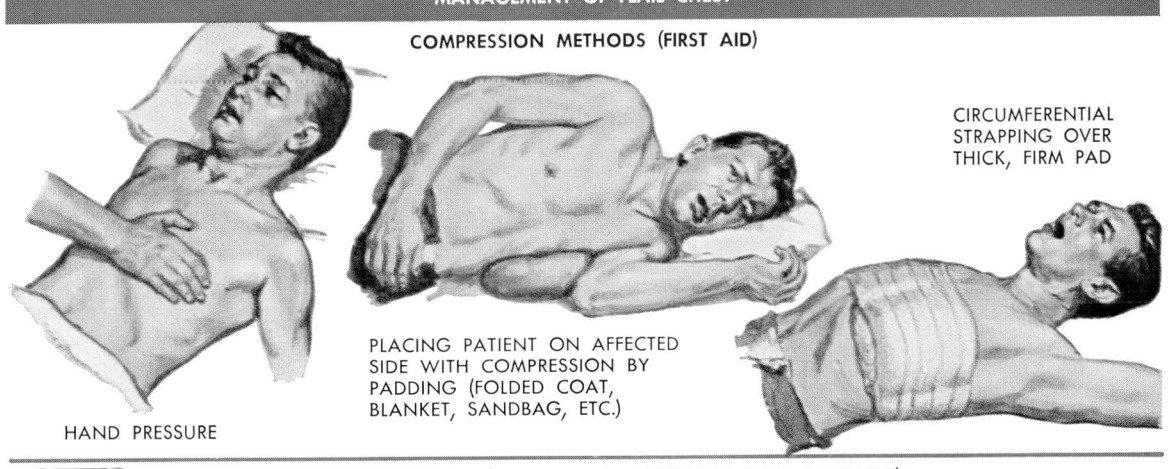

HAND PRESSURE
PLACING PATIENT ON AFFECTED SIDE WITH COMPRESSION BY PADDING (FOLDED COAT, BLANKET, SANDBAG, ETC.)
CIRCUMFERENTIAL STRAPPING OVER THICK, FIRM PAD

TRACTION METHODS (VALUABLE IF VENTILATOR NOT AVAILABLE)

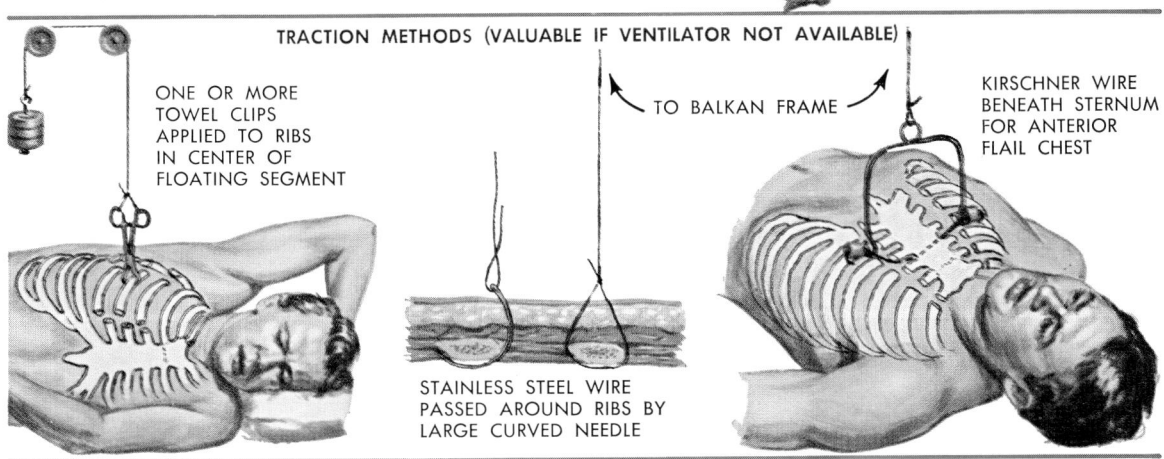

ONE OR MORE TOWEL CLIPS APPLIED TO RIBS IN CENTER OF FLOATING SEGMENT
TO BALKAN FRAME
STAINLESS STEEL WIRE PASSED AROUND RIBS BY LARGE CURVED NEEDLE
KIRSCHNER WIRE BENEATH STERNUM FOR ANTERIOR FLAIL CHEST

TRACHEOSTOMY AND MECHANICAL ASSISTED VENTILATION

FOR CRUSHED CHEST WITH MAJOR DEGREE OF FLAIL, ANY MEASURE SHORT OF TRACHEOSTOMY OR ENDOTRACHEAL INTUBATION PLUS MECHANICAL VENTILATION ALMOST ALWAYS PROVES FATAL

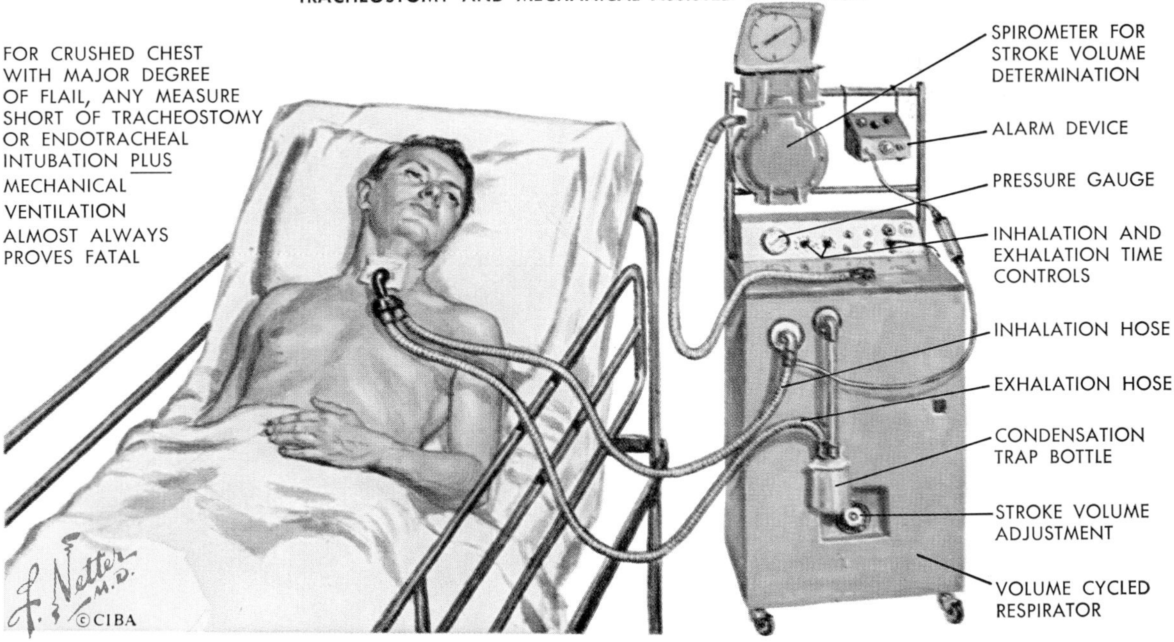

SPIROMETER FOR STROKE VOLUME DETERMINATION
ALARM DEVICE
PRESSURE GAUGE
INHALATION AND EXHALATION TIME CONTROLS
INHALATION HOSE
EXHALATION HOSE
CONDENSATION TRAP BOTTLE
STROKE VOLUME ADJUSTMENT
VOLUME CYCLED RESPIRATOR
F. Netter M.D.
©CIBA

MULTIPLE RIB FRACTURES —
FLAIL CHEST

(PLATE VII)

The term "flail chest" is used for a condition in which, because of double fractures of three or more adjacent ribs, or fractures of several ribs with costochondral separations, or sternal fractures, a portion of the chest wall loses its continuity with the rest of the rib cage and moves in a direction opposite to the rest of the thorax.

With inspiration, when the thorax is expanding, the portion that has lost its continuity sinks in, the outside atmospheric pressure forcing it inward against the negative intrathoracic pressure. On expiration, the reverse is true. As the rest of the chest cavity contracts, the isolated segment moves outward.

The result of these paradoxical movements is an inability to create the normal changes in intrathoracic pressure necessary to draw air in and to expel it from the lungs. Moreover, with severe degrees of flail, air may move to-and-fro within the bronchi (Plate VII).

In lateral flail chest, the abnormal pressure changes already described will cause the mediastinum to move from side to side during the respiratory cycle. This "mediastinal flutter" will tend to kink the great veins, thus reducing blood return to the heart.

The seriousness of the respiratory and circulatory handicap will depend upon the number of ribs involved, and whether the injury is unilateral or bilateral.

When three or more adjoining ribs or their cartilages are broken in more than one place, the paradoxical respiration of flail chest is often present from the start.

However, where a relatively small segment of the chest cage has lost its continuity, paradoxical respiration may not be evident. At least for a time, the position of the broken segment may be maintained by muscle splinting, particularly with the shallow breathing that is induced by pain.

However, with the passage of time (usually within a few hours, especially if there is lung contusion), secretions accumulate in the bronchi and bronchioles, and oxygen hunger overcomes both muscle splinting and voluntary inhibition of chest movement. Compliance of the underlying lung having been reduced, the patient must fight harder for each breath. Therefore, he must create a greater negative pressure during inspiration and positive pressure during expiration. The flail may then appear.

TREATMENT OF FLAIL CHEST

(PLATE VIII)

To delay or prevent the development of the "flail" where a relatively small segment of the chest wall is involved, efforts should be directed to relief of pain (preferably with intercostal nerve block). This is primarily to decrease the accumulation of secretions in the lower airways by improving ability to cough. Additional steps in this direction include chest strapping, placing the patient on the affected side, or simple manual support of the injured side while asking the patient to cough.

Where a detectable flail is already present, the first consideration is a clear airway and reduction of dead space. For major degrees of flail chest, tracheostomy and mechanical ventilation supersede all other methods.

In the meantime, other measures previously described for upper and lower airway obstruction must be instituted, and attention given to stabilizing the chest wall.

Stabilization of the Chest Wall

The methods whereby this may be accomplished include external compression, traction, surgical fixation, and mechanical assisted ventilation. Each of these methods has its specific indications, limitations, advantages, and disadvantages.

External Compression: The simplest and quickest way to stabilize the chest wall is by gentle but firm pressure of the palm of the hand against the floating segment. The mere turning of the patient on his injured side may prove effective in lateral injuries. When available, a sandbag can be placed against the involved portion.

As a first aid measure, firm, circumferential, adhesive strapping constitutes the method of choice, because the pressure can be adjusted easily to suit the patient's comfort. The adhesive tape should be applied over a thick, firmly rolled pad of cotton, wool, or folded towels to conform with the size and shape of the mobile area of the chest wall.

The Disadvantages of Compression include impairment of ventilation and interference with the cough mechanism, thus predisposing to lower airway obstruction, atelectasis, and pneumonia. Manual compression and the injured-side-down position are only temporary expedients. Circumferential strapping cannot be used for patients with anterior segment injuries or for those with multiple rib fractures that are bilateral.

Traction Methods: In an emergency, towel clips can be pushed through the skin to encompass one or more ribs, which can then be stabilized by manual traction. Where circumstances permit, the skin should be cleansed and draped, and the overlying tissues and periosteum infiltrated with an anesthetic agent before the towel clips are applied. Better than towel clips is stainless steel wire, which may be passed around the rib or ribs when swaged on a large, round, curved needle.

The sternum may be grasped for traction by using a uterine tenaculum inserted through small incisions on each side of the sternum, or a Kirschner wire passed behind the sternum. The latter procedure is an extremely effective method for stabilizing an anterior flail chest.

Traction on the skeletal attachments can be maintained by suitable pulleys, preferably with a Balkan frame, using 5 to 15 pounds of weight, depending on the individual case.

Costal traction has many disadvantages, which include difficulty in identifying the appropriate rib or ribs, inadequate control of paradox, infection, and necrosis when used for prolonged periods of time, iatrogenic pneumothorax, or hemothorax, and severe subsequent bony deformity. Therefore, this method should be used only in an emergency when a respirator is not available.

On the other hand, sternal traction with the use of Kirschner wire is not accompanied by any of these difficulties or complications.

Surgical Fixation: This method of handling may prove to be the treatment of choice in patients with flail chests complicated by intrathoracic injury requiring open thoracotomy, and in those who do not show evidence of decreased paradox after two weeks or more of assisted ventilation. Direct operative fixation may also constitute optimum therapy for flail chests of the anterolateral variety, especially when there is marked displacement of rib fragments. This type of injury lends itself to operative fixation, because the area involved permits rapid surgical exposure and rib fixation.

This method immediately eliminates severe chest wall pain, and thus minimizes the inhibition of cough and respiratory excursion. Also, because the integrity of the thoracic cage is immediately restored, the potential hazards of prolonged costal traction or positive-pressure breathing are completely eliminated.

Assisted Ventilation (Positive-Pressure Breathing)

For patients in marked respiratory distress, with severe paradoxical respiration, any measure short of immediate endotracheal intubation or tracheostomy *plus*

1: PENETRATION OF CHEST WALL

2: LACERATION OF LUNG

3: PERFORATION OF BRONCHUS OR TRACHEA

4: TEAR OF LUNG BY INDRIVEN RIB FRAGMENT

5: RUPTURE OF ALVEOLI SECONDARY TO BLUNT TRAUMA OR STRAINING

6: PULMONARY INTERSTITIAL EMPHYSEMA

7: MEDIASTINAL EMPHYSEMA

8: PNEUMO-THORAX

9: SUBCUTANEOUS EMPHYSEMA

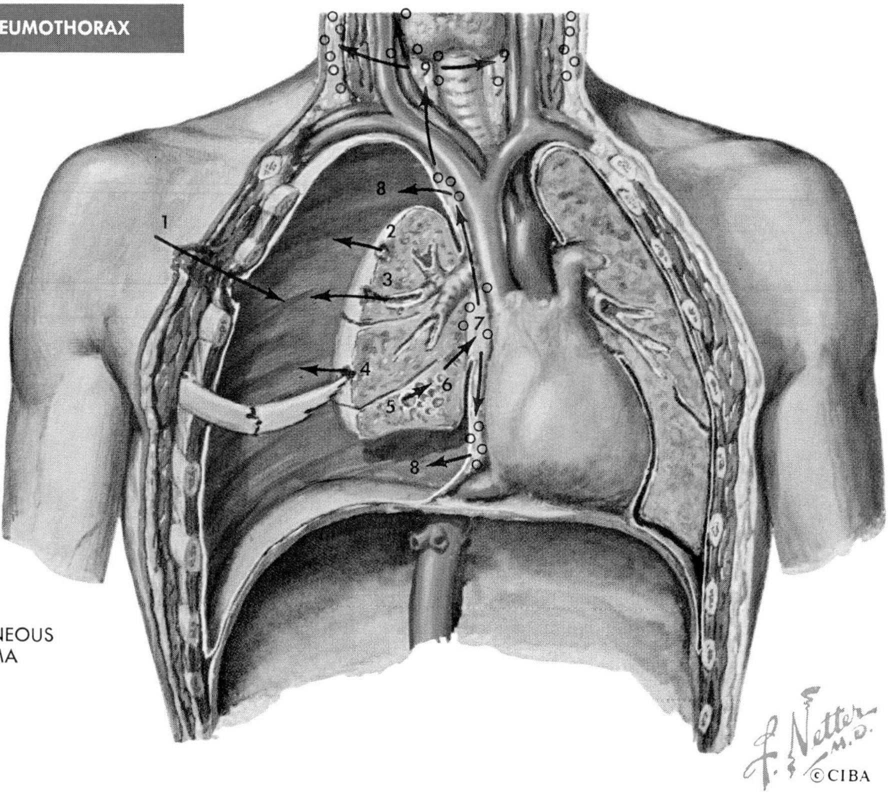

PATHOPHYSIOLOGY OF OPEN PNEUMOTHORAX

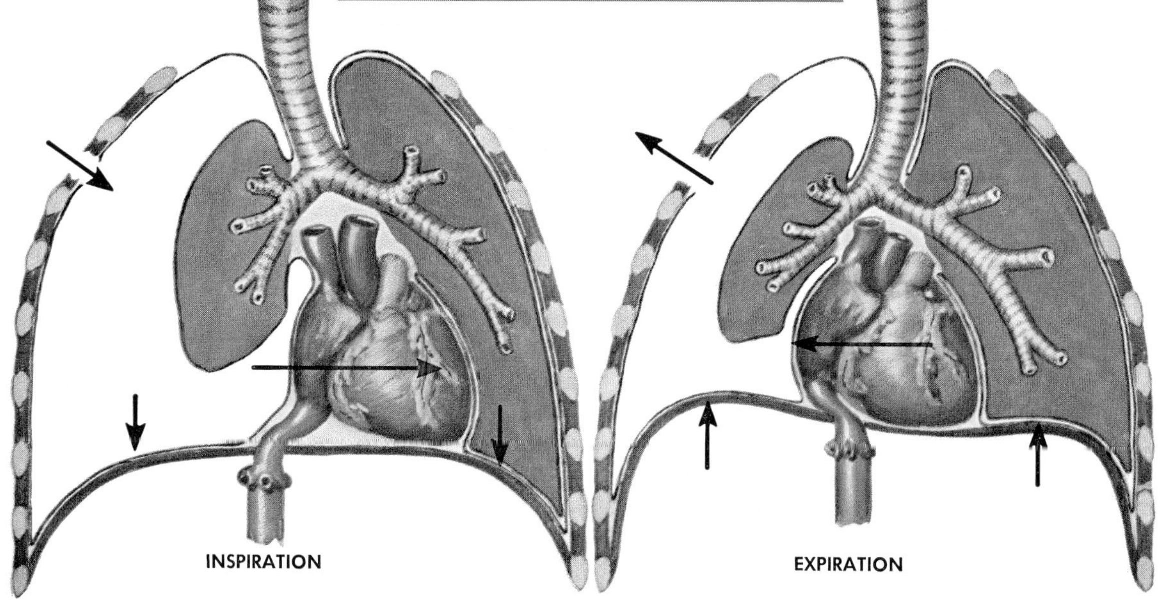

INSPIRATION

EXPIRATION

AIR ENTERS PLEURAL CAVITY. NEGATIVE PRESSURE IS DIMINISHED OR LOST, COLLAPSING IPSILATERAL LUNG AND REDUCING VENOUS RETURN. SHIFT OF MEDIASTINUM COMPRESSES OPPOSITE LUNG AND IMPAIRS ITS VENTILATION

AIR IS EXPELLED FROM PLEURAL CAVITY. MEDIASTINUM SHIFTS TO AFFECTED SIDE. SIDE-TO-SIDE SHIFT (FLUTTER) OF MEDIASTINUM FURTHER REDUCES VENOUS RETURN BY DISTORTING VENAE CAVAE

PLATE IX

PATHOPHYSIOLOGY OF PROGRESSIVE TENSION PNEUMOTHORAX

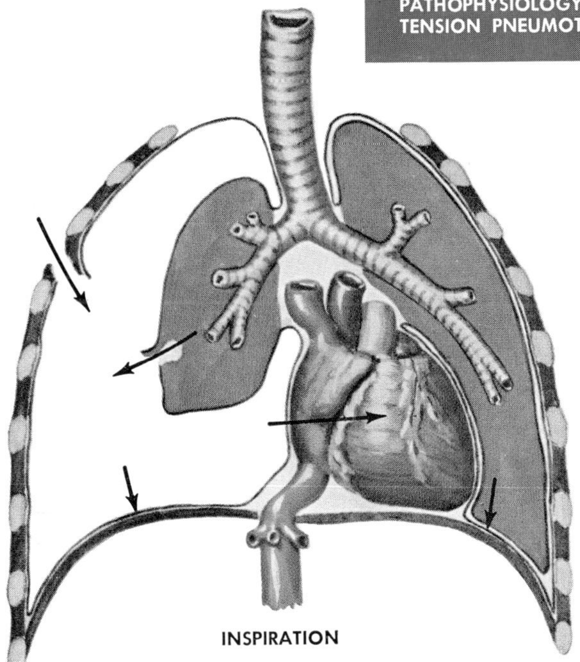

INSPIRATION

AIR ENTERS PLEURAL CAVITY FROM A LUNG PERFORATION (OR RARELY FROM AN EXTERNAL CHEST WOUND). LUNG COLLAPSES AND MEDIASTINUM SHIFTS TO OPPOSITE SIDE COMPRESSING CONTRA-LATERAL LUNG AND IMPAIRING ITS VENTILATING CAPACITY

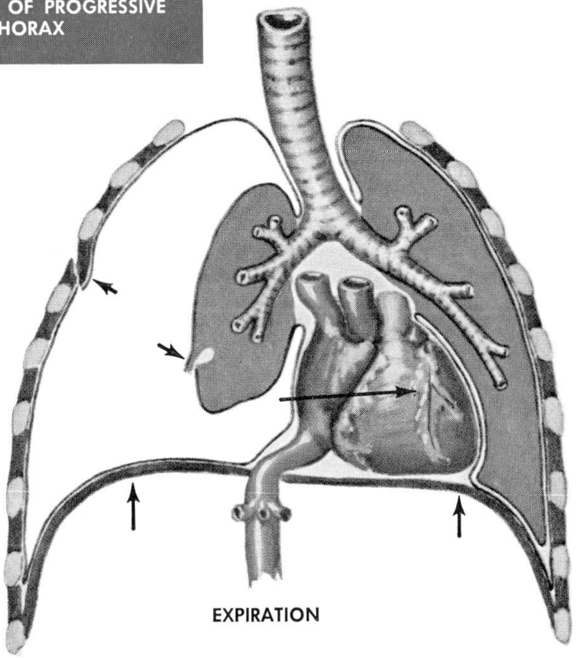

EXPIRATION

AS DIAPHRAGM RISES AND CHEST CONTRACTS, INTRAPLEURAL PRESSURE RISES AND VALVE-LIKE OPENING THROUGH WHICH AIR ENTERED CLOSES. PRESSURE IS THUS PROGRESSIVELY INCREASED AND MEDIASTINAL SHIFT AUGMENTED WITH EACH RESPIRATION. VENOUS RETURN IS IMPAIRED BY INCREASED INTRATHORACIC PRESSURE AND BY DISTORTION OF VENAE CAVAE

MANIFESTATIONS OF TENSION PNEUMOTHORAX

CYANOSIS

MARKED RESPIRATORY DISTRESS

TRACHEAL DEVIATION TO OPPOSITE SIDE

CHEST PAIN

HYPERRESONANCE

DIAGNOSTIC TAP; PLUNGER OF MOISTENED SYRINGE PUSHED OUT BY INTRA-THORACIC PRESSURE

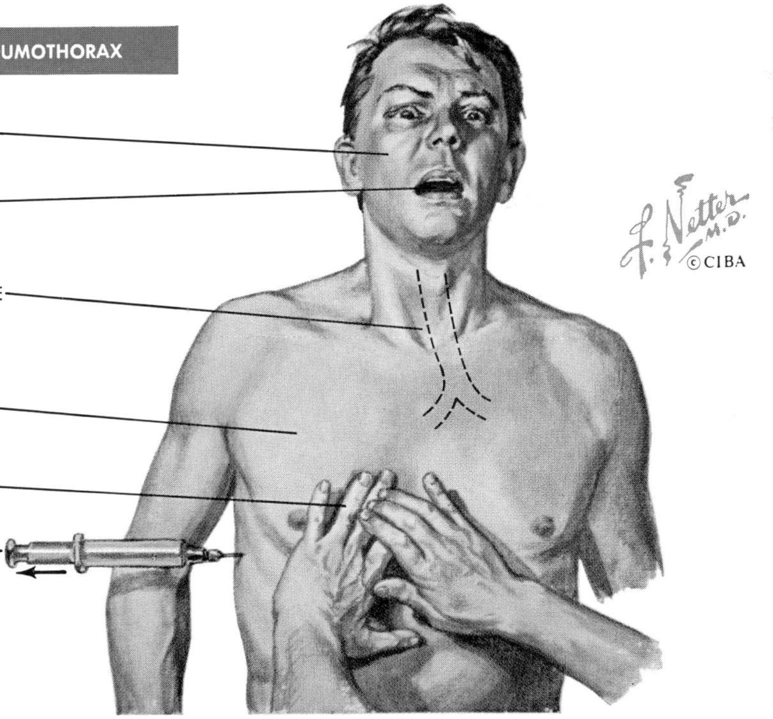

assisted mechanical ventilation almost always proves fatal.

Positive pressure should *not* be started until after a space-occupying pleural collection of blood or air has been ruled out, or if present, treated by intercostal tube drainage. (Air in the pleural cavity from a lacerated lung can quickly be converted into a tension pneumothorax by positive-pressure breathing.)

With mechanical respirators, room air or low percentages of added oxygen usually will be all that is required. Only exceptionally will mixtures of 60 per cent oxygen or higher be needed and these only for short periods. These machines are of two types, the volume controlled and pressure controlled. For patients with chest injuries, the volume-controlled type is far superior to those activated by pressure changes.

One of the potential disadvantages of the positive intrathoracic pressure produced by a respirator is a decrease in venous return and hence in cardiac output. This can usually be avoided if the pressure is set at the lowest level that produces adequate ventilation, usually between 15 and 20 cm of water.

BLOOD OR AIR IN THE PLEURAL SPACE

Effect on Respiratory and Circulatory Function (Plates IX and X)

Under normal conditions, the pleural space is not a space at all. Instead, the visceral and parietal layers are tightly adherent, due to the "hydraulic traction" of the moisture between them. (The power of this adhesive force, estimated to equal 3600 mm IIg, can be visualized by attempting to separate two wet glass slides or cover slips by simply pulling them apart.) This hydraulic traction, strong as it is, is quickly lost if air or blood is introduced between the layers, allowing them to shear away from each other. The deleterious effects of either air or blood between the layers of pleura are both respiratory and circulatory.

From the respiratory standpoint, the lung on the affected side, unless fixed by previously formed adhesions, will tend to collapse due to its inherent elasticity (Plate IX). Thus, depending on the volume of invading air or blood, the ipsilateral lung will become relatively useless from a ventilatory standpoint.

The mediastinum lying between the lungs, unless previously diseased, is not a rigid wall. Instead, it will move from side to side if there are differences in the pressure laterally.

With inspiration, the negative pressure on the unaffected side is greater than can be produced by the partially collapsed lung on the affected side. The mediastinum is thus displaced toward the *un*affected side, and the contralateral lung is also unable to expand fully.

With expiration, the negative pressure on the unaffected side is much reduced or may even become positive in labored breathing. As a result, the mediastinum is pushed back toward the affected side. This side-to-side movement, called mediastinal flutter, is increased as rate and depth of respiration increase, due to dyspnea.

Thus, the ventilatory efficiency of *both* lungs is impaired, even though to a much greater extent on the affected side. The seriousness of this reduction in alveolar ventilation will depend on the volume of the pleural space invasion and the pulmonary reserve of the patient.

From a circulatory standpoint, the effect is twofold. Blood is normally drawn cyclically into the thorax by the negative pressure of rhythmic inspiration. With accumulation of air or blood within the pleural space, this negative pressure is greatly reduced. This causes a concomitant reduction in venous return and in filling of the right atrium. In addition, the side-to-side swings of the mediastinum tend to kink the great veins, further

94

reducing venous return and cardiac filling.

As right heart filling is reduced, cardiac output is similarly reduced. Initially, this may be compensated by peripheral vaso-constriction, which tends to maintain a satisfactory blood pressure, despite a reduced circulating volume.

In addition to the effect on cardiac out put, there is a reduction in oxygen satura-tion of the circulating blood, predisposing to myocardial hypoxia and lactic acidosis. Where a portion of the alveolar bed has partially or completely lost its ventilatory capacity, the blood returning to the heart, fully saturated from normal alveoli, be-comes mixed with blood returning from the nonventilating or poorly ventilated areas.

Thus, even when 100 per cent oxygen is administered, the *arterial* oxygen tension of this *mixed* blood may be far below the *alveolar* oxygen tension that is derived only from functioning alveoli. This differ-ence between alveolar oxygen and blood oxygen tension ($A-aDo_2$) is a useful index of the seriousness of the deficiency of gas-eous exchange in all kinds of chest injury.

PNEUMOTHORAX

As illustrated in Plate IX, air may gain access to the pleural space from a number of different sources. Many of these are internal, which explains why pneumo-thorax is almost as frequent following blunt trauma as it is after stab wounds! In any event, the seriousness of the situa-tion from the standpoint of respiratory and circulatory function will depend upon the total volume of air that accumulates and whether or not it is under tension.

Small amounts of air may cause no symptoms and few if any physical signs. On the other hand, massive accumula-tions, particularly if under tension, may lead to rapid respiratory and/or circula-tory failure if not relieved promptly. The most serious forms of pneumothorax are the open and tension varieties. Later,

each of these will be discussed separately.

Diagnosis

The characteristic symptoms of dysp-nea and chest discomfort often tend to be overlooked because overshadowed by the severe pain of other thoracic complica-tions. On the affected side, chest wall movement is diminished, the percussion note may be hyperresonant, and breath sounds are distant. Quick, definitive diag-nosis can be made by thoracentesis.

Treatment

A minimal pneumothorax may be treat-ed expectantly if close observation is pro-vided, because the air will probably be absorbed over a period of several days.

For moderate or massive pneumothorax, repeated aspirations can be carried out. However, intercostal tube drainage (see Page 102 and Plate XIII) is by far the safest means of bringing about prompt and effective decompression of the pleural cavity. Therefore, this type of drainage should be instituted as soon as possible.

Rarely will exploratory thoracotomy be required. However, if the lung fails to expand following continuous, effective tube drainage, air is probably coming from a lacerated trachea or a main-stem bronchus. If confirmed by bronchoscopy, direct surgical repair should be under-taken without delay.

OPEN PNEUMOTHORAX

The seriousness of open pneumothorax, caused by a penetrating wound of the chest wall, will depend largely on the size of the opening. Where the wound is small, as from a knife blade, little air may enter the pleural space either from the lung or from the outside. On the other hand, depending on the location and direction, even the narrowest stab can cause an exsanguinating hemorrhage or a life-threatening tension pneumothorax.

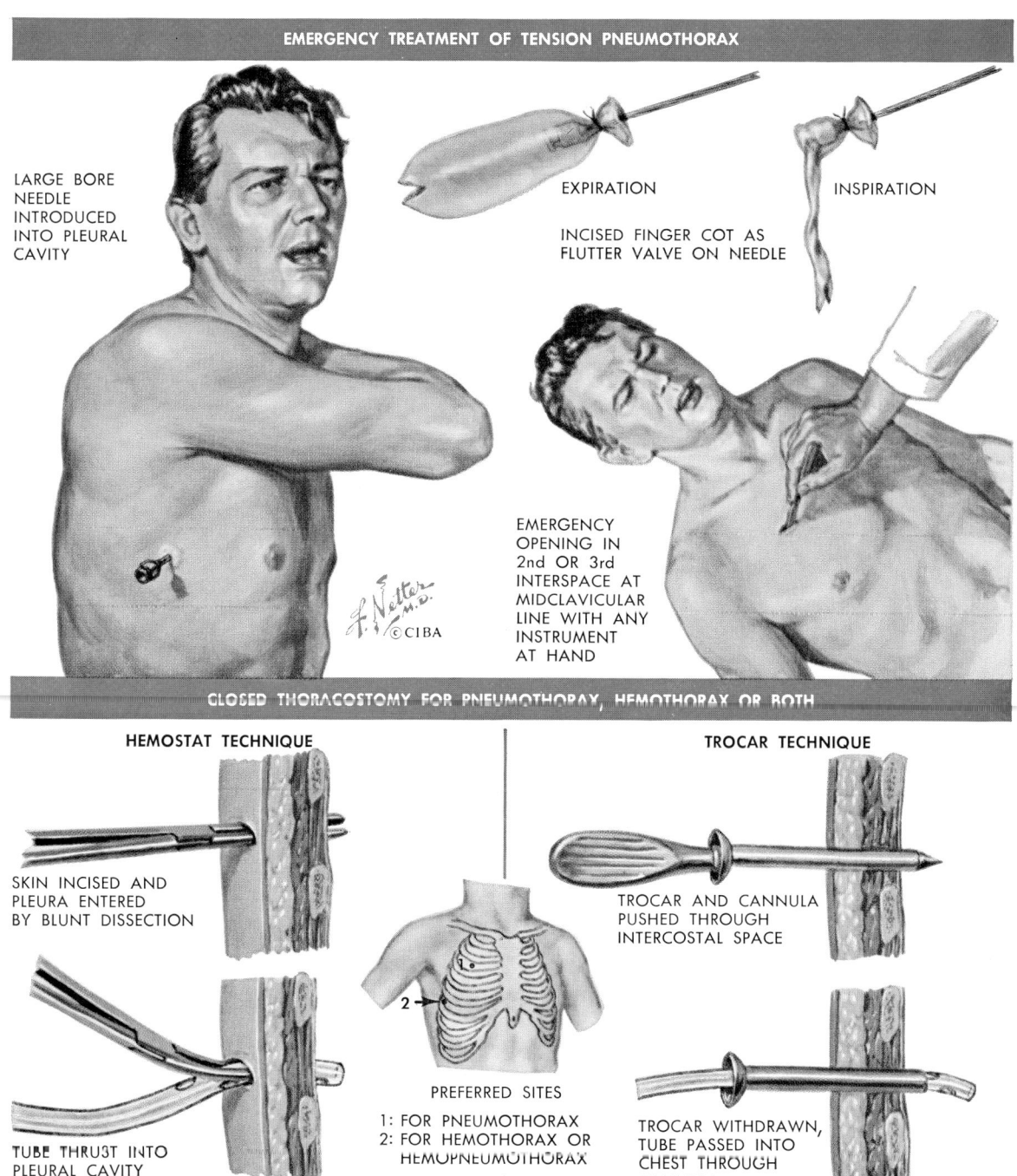

EMERGENCY TREATMENT OF TENSION PNEUMOTHORAX

LARGE BORE NEEDLE INTRODUCED INTO PLEURAL CAVITY

EXPIRATION

INSPIRATION

INCISED FINGER COT AS FLUTTER VALVE ON NEEDLE

EMERGENCY OPENING IN 2nd OR 3rd INTERSPACE AT MIDCLAVICULAR LINE WITH ANY INSTRUMENT AT HAND

CLOSED THORACOSTOMY FOR PNEUMOTHORAX, HEMOTHORAX OR BOTH

HEMOSTAT TECHNIQUE

SKIN INCISED AND PLEURA ENTERED BY BLUNT DISSECTION

TUBE THRUST INTO PLEURAL CAVITY

TUBE ATTACHED TO UNDER-WATER-SEAL SUCTION

PREFERRED SITES

1: FOR PNEUMOTHORAX
2: FOR HEMOTHORAX OR HEMOPNEUMOTHORAX

TROCAR TECHNIQUE

TROCAR AND CANNULA PUSHED THROUGH INTERCOSTAL SPACE

TROCAR WITHDRAWN, TUBE PASSED INTO CHEST THROUGH CANNULA

CANNULA WITHDRAWN, TUBE ATTACHED TO UNDER-WATER-SEAL SUCTION

PLATE XI

TREATMENT OF TENSION PNEUMOTHORAX
INSERTION OF DRAINAGE TUBES

1: LUNG

2: INTERCOSTAL VESSELS

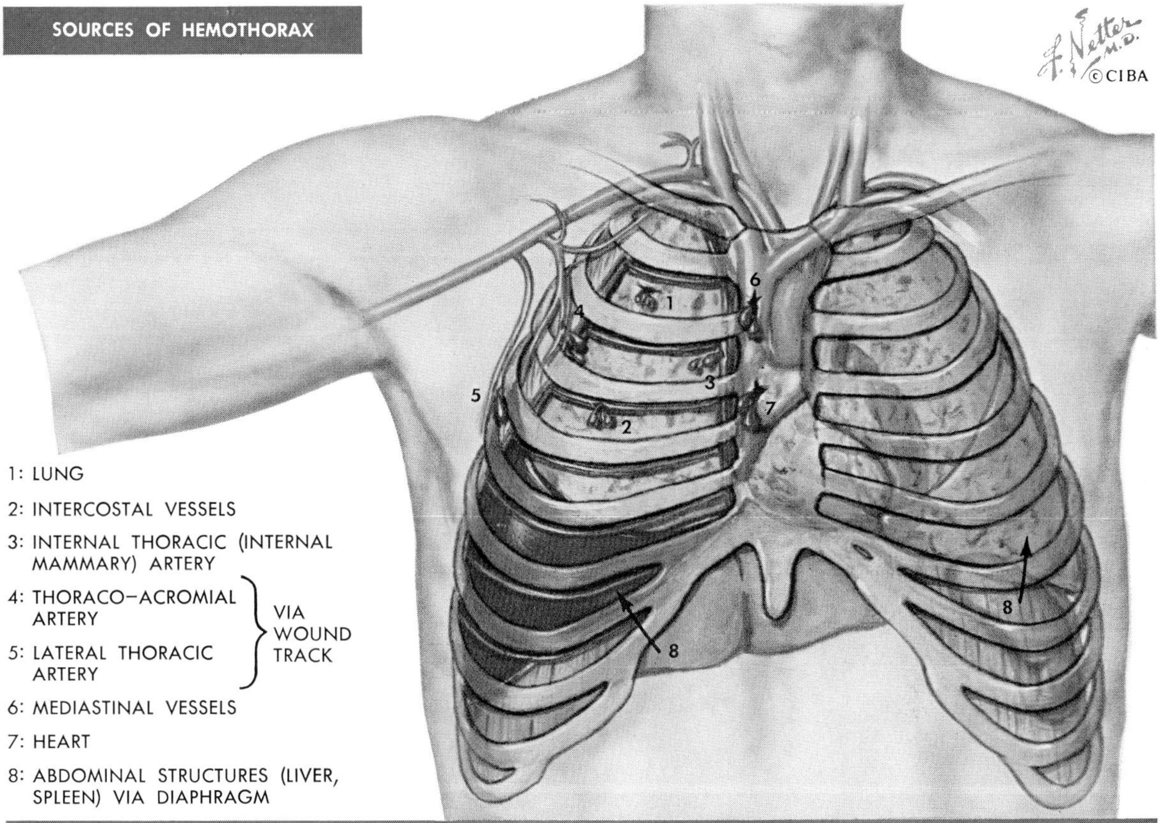

3: INTERNAL THORACIC (INTERNAL MAMMARY) ARTERY

4: THORACO–ACROMIAL ARTERY ⎱
5: LATERAL THORACIC ARTERY ⎰ VIA WOUND TRACK

6: MEDIASTINAL VESSELS

7: HEART

8: ABDOMINAL STRUCTURES (LIVER, SPLEEN) VIA DIAPHRAGM

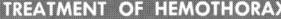

TREATMENT OF HEMOTHORAX

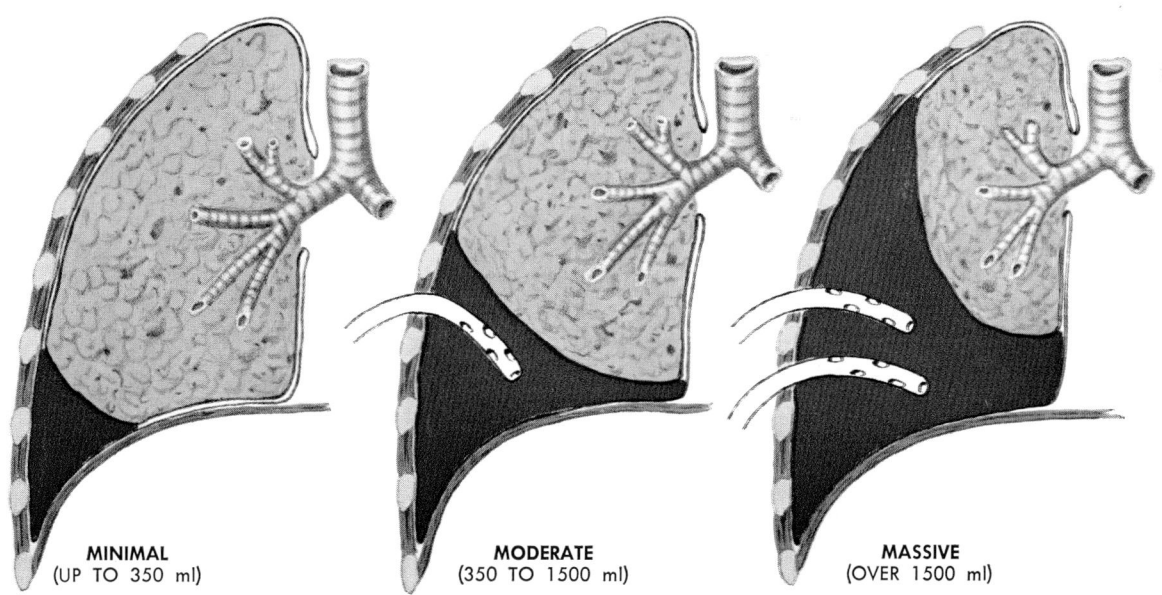

MINIMAL
(UP TO 350 ml)

MODERATE
(350 TO 1500 ml)

MASSIVE
(OVER 1500 ml)

BLOOD IS USUALLY RESORBED SPONTANEOUSLY: THORACENTESIS RARELY NECESSARY

THORACENTESIS AND/OR TUBE DRAINAGE USUALLY SUFFICES: THE LATTER IS PREFERRED TREATMENT

TWO DRAINAGE TUBES INSERTED SINCE ONE MAY CLOG: IMMEDIATE OR EARLY THORACOTOMY MAY BE NECESSARY

PLATE XII

HEMOTHORAX — SOURCES AND TREATMENT

Usually far more serious are the larger openings, such as those produced by gunshot at close range or forceful contact with some ragged object. These sucking wounds through which air moves in and out with a characteristic swishing sound will cause potentially lethal disturbances in cardiorespiratory dynamics (Plate IX).

Where the opening is larger than the glottis, air will enter through the chest wall in preference to the trachea, a situation incompatible with life. In addition, the foreign material frequently carried into these wounds poses the threat of serious pulmonary and pleural infection.

Treatment

Close the sucking wound immediately by any means available. Best is vaseline gauze, but as a temporary expedient, the open hand will do. Depending on the size of the hole, and the cooperation that can be obtained from the patient, he may be able to reexpand his own lung if a dressing is alternately removed and replaced. That is, the patient is asked to cough or strain, which will force air out of the pleural space. Then the dressing is slapped tightly in place to maintain whatever expansion has been accomplished. This can be repeated.

In extreme situations, the patient's arm may be fixed firmly to the chest. This will at least partially occlude the opening. As soon as possible, tube drainage of the thorax should be instituted (see Page 102 and Plates XI and XIII).

Emergency closure by sutures bringing the skin edges together without debridement should *not* be attempted. It will simply predispose to subcutaneous emphysema and infection. While small wounds may heal by secondary intention with just a sterile dressing, large wounds, particularly when contaminated, will require wide debridement and reconstructive surgery. This must be carried out as soon as the patient's condition permits.

In this variety of pneumothorax, the opening in the lung, bronchus, or chest wall acts as a valve to allow air to enter the pleural cavity on inspiration, but not to escape during expiration.

As a result, pressure is built up within the pleural space, particularly when the patient coughs. The elevated intrathoracic pressure collapses the ipsilateral lung, displaces the mediastinum, and significantly compresses the contralateral lung. Venous return to the heart is greatly diminished. Indeed, these effects are more pronounced and lethal in tension pneumothorax than in any other pleural involvement.

Diagnosis

These patients will be cyanotic, with extreme air hunger, and violent agitation due to the rapid development of severe hypoxia. The trachea will be deviated toward the opposite side. The affected side will be hyperresonant.

Diagnostic Aspiration: The quickest and surest way to reach a conclusive diagnosis of tension pneumothorax is by aspiration. All that is required is a 17- or 18-gauge needle attached to a moistened 10 ml syringe.

The needle is inserted into any interspace on the affected side. As soon as the thorax is entered, the high intrapleural pressure will suddenly push the plunger of the syringe outward.

Treatment

The increased intrapleural pressure must be relieved immediately. If nothing else is available, an opening should be made in the chest wall, preferably about the second interspace in the midclavicular line, using any semisharp tool, a screwdriver, or even a nail file. The possibility of producing an empyema is a small price to pay when death is threatening.

If a large-bore needle (14- to 16-gauge) is available, immediate relief may be accomplished by introducing it into the pleural cavity. If the patient is to be transported, pleural decompression can be maintained by attaching a flutter valve to the end of the needle. This can be improvised by tying a perforated finger cot or condom to the hub of the needle (Plate XI).

The treatment of choice is under-water-seal drainage of the pleural cavity (see Plates XI and XIII). If the air continues to leak into the pleural space, one must consider the possibility of injury to the trachea or a main stem bronchus. If this is confirmed by bronchoscopy, surgical repair is indicated.

HEMOTHORAX

The seriousness of hemothorax and the treatment indicated will depend on the volume of blood that invades the pleural cavity (Plate XII).

MINIMAL HEMOTHORAX

Where the accumulation is minimal, amounting to less than 350 ml, obliteration of the costophrenic angle on x-ray may be the only positive sign.

Treatment

No treatment is necessary. Since resorption is rapid, the chest film is usually clear within 10 to 14 days. However, all patients with minimal hemothorax should be observed closely, because occasionally, bleeding will continue and go on to a moderate or even a massive hemothorax after an elapse of hours or days.

MODERATE HEMOTHORAX

Total accumulations of up to 1500 ml will produce shortness of breath due to lung compression. At the upper levels of this accumulation, shock may be produced by the loss of circulatory blood volume. X-ray in the upright position will show a shadow curving upward laterally on the involved side. (In the supine position, only a diffuse light opacity may be observed.) Physical signs, including dullness and distant breath sounds, will depend on the amount of bleeding and the position of the patient. Diagnostic confirmation is obtained by aspiration.

Treatment

Thoracentesis, which may yield 500 ml of blood initially, should be repeated every six hours, or preferably tube drainage should be instituted (see Page 102 and Plate XIII). For either needle aspiration or tube drainage of hemothorax, the pleural cavity is entered in the 5th or 6th interspace in the midaxillary line (Plate XI). Insertion into a lower interspace may injure a high-lying diaphragm and underlying organs, such as the liver or spleen.

Since minimal and moderate degrees of hemothorax are usually caused by bleeding from the lung parenchyma, a hemopneumothorax is usually present, both air and blood being obtained from the pleural space. Since the bleeding is from low-pressure vessels, it will almost always cease spontaneously. Therefore, exploratory thoracotomy should not be considered unless rapid accumulation of blood continues.

MASSIVE HEMOTHORAX

Rapid and continuous bleeding into the pleural cavity usually comes from larger, high-pressure vessels, such as the intercostals and/or the internal thoracic (internal mammary). Less common sources are the liver and spleen in thoraco-abdominal wounds and the pectoral branches of the thoracoacromial artery, the blood entering the pleura through the penetrating wound after the external opening had been sutured.

AUTOTRANSFUSION USING PLEURAL BLOOD

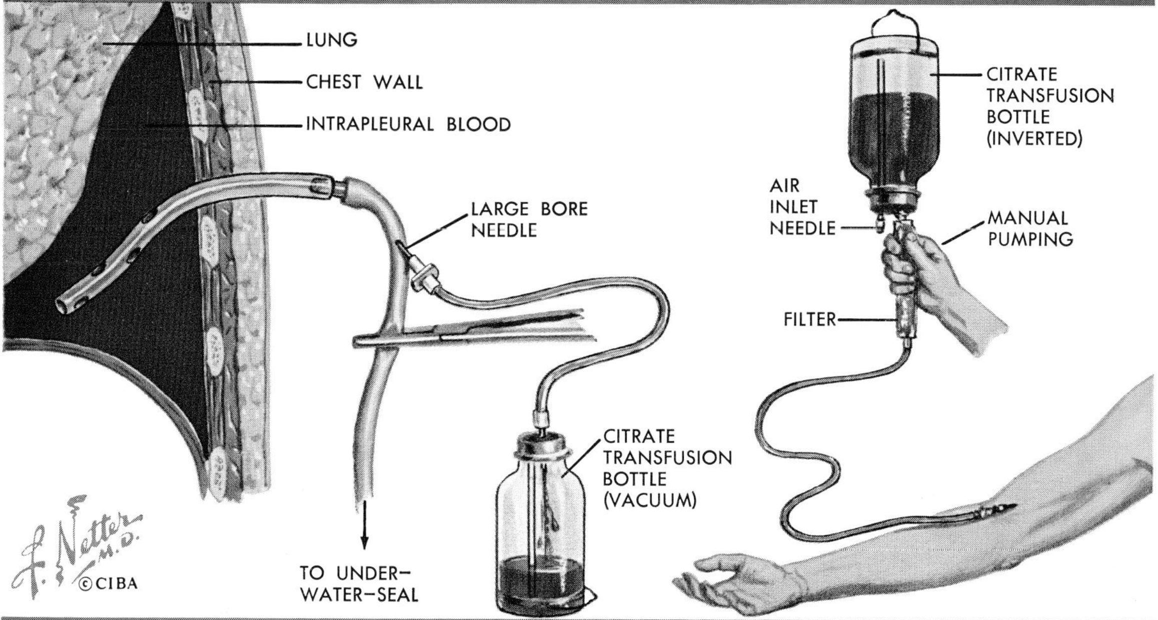
LUNG
CHEST WALL
INTRAPLEURAL BLOOD
LARGE BORE NEEDLE
CITRATE TRANSFUSION BOTTLE (VACUUM)
TO UNDER-WATER-SEAL
CITRATE TRANSFUSION BOTTLE (INVERTED)
AIR INLET NEEDLE
MANUAL PUMPING
FILTER
F. Netter M.D.
©CIBA

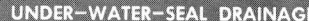

UNDER-WATER-SEAL DRAINAGE

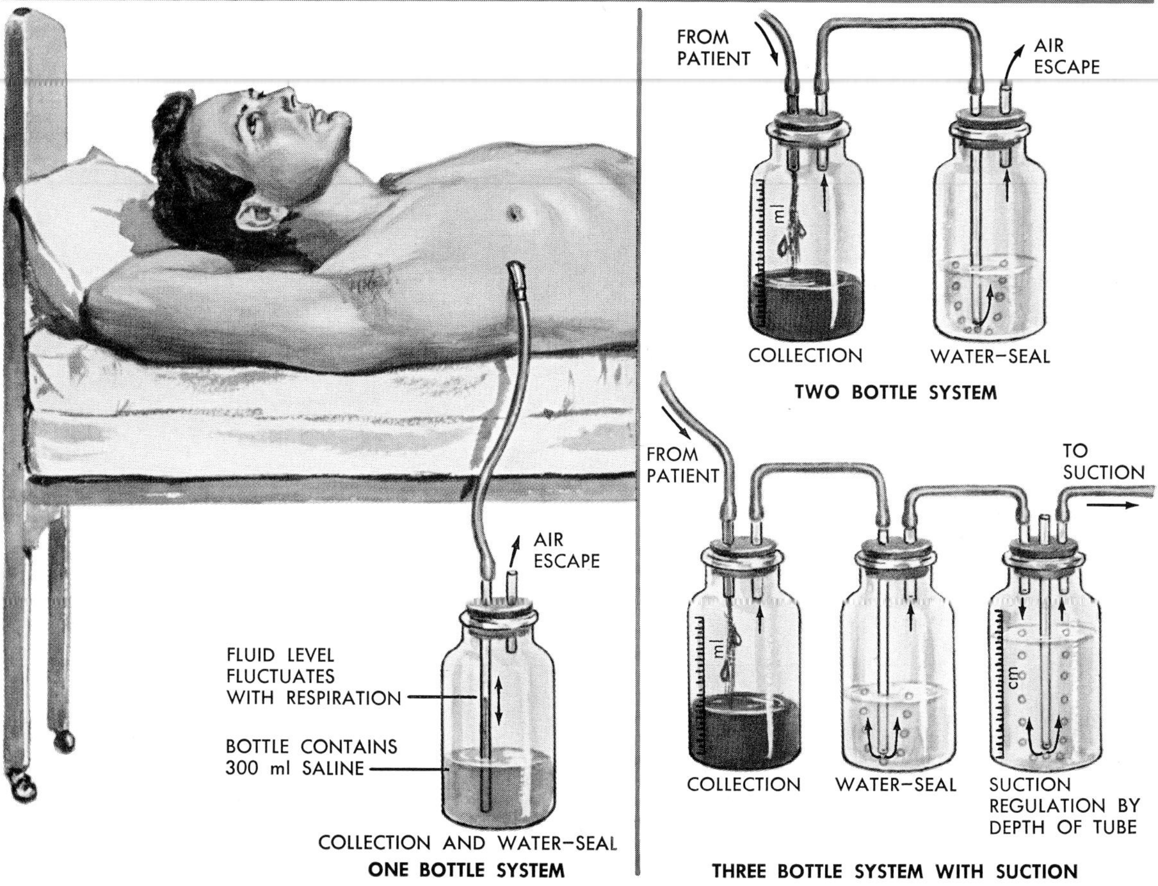
AIR ESCAPE
FLUID LEVEL FLUCTUATES WITH RESPIRATION
BOTTLE CONTAINS 300 ml SALINE
COLLECTION AND WATER-SEAL
ONE BOTTLE SYSTEM
FROM PATIENT
AIR ESCAPE
ml
COLLECTION
WATER-SEAL
TWO BOTTLE SYSTEM
FROM PATIENT
TO SUCTION
ml
cm
COLLECTION
WATER-SEAL
SUCTION REGULATION BY DEPTH OF TUBE
THREE BOTTLE SYSTEM WITH SUCTION

PLATE XIII

AUTOTRANSFUSION OF PLEURAL BLOOD
UNDER-WATER-SEAL DRAINAGE

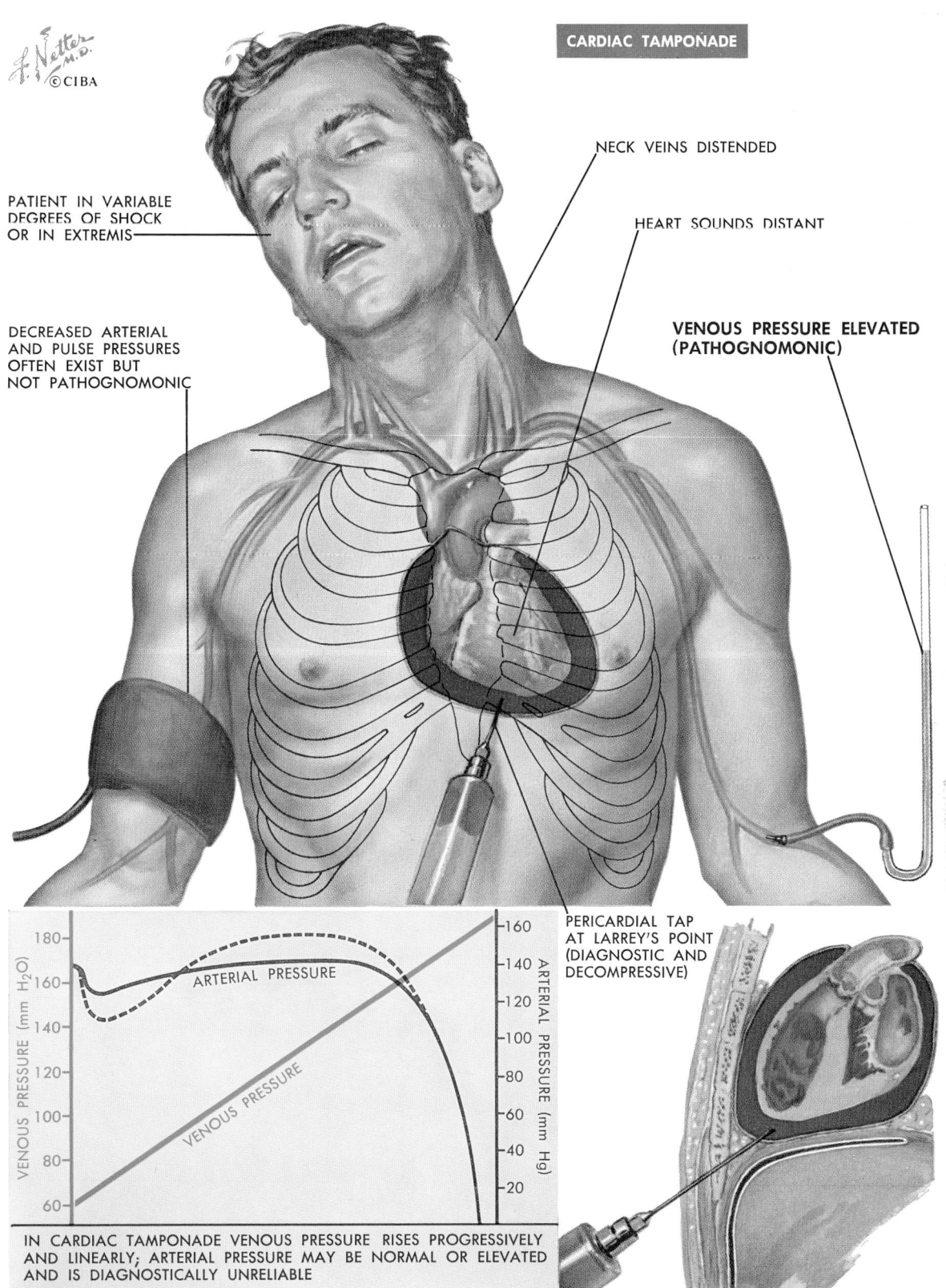

NECK VEINS DISTENDED

HEART SOUNDS DISTANT

PATIENT IN VARIABLE DEGREES OF SHOCK OR IN EXTREMIS

VENOUS PRESSURE ELEVATED (PATHOGNOMONIC)

DECREASED ARTERIAL AND PULSE PRESSURES OFTEN EXIST BUT NOT PATHOGNOMONIC

PERICARDIAL TAP AT LARREY'S POINT (DIAGNOSTIC AND DECOMPRESSIVE)

ARTERIAL PRESSURE

VENOUS PRESSURE

VENOUS PRESSURE (mm H_2O)

ARTERIAL PRESSURE (mm Hg)

IN CARDIAC TAMPONADE VENOUS PRESSURE RISES PROGRESSIVELY AND LINEARLY; ARTERIAL PRESSURE MAY BE NORMAL OR ELEVATED AND IS DIAGNOSTICALLY UNRELIABLE

PLATE XIV

Signs and Symptoms

Compression of the lungs and the great veins produces cyanosis, tightness or severe pain in the chest, and engorgement of the veins in the neck. The trachea may be felt displaced to the contralateral side in the suprasternal notch. The affected side will show dullness, absence of breath sounds, and limitation of respiratory excursion. Profound shock is produced by the loss of circulating blood.

Treatment

Blood volume must be restored and the pleural cavity emptied. Both of these prerequisites for the saving of life must be undertaken immediately. If feasible, autotransfusion can be carried out, the blood removed from the pleural cavity being citrated and injected intravenously (Plate XIII). However, a coexisting laceration of the trachea, major bronchus, stomach, colon, or liver is a contraindication to autotransfusion because of the possibility of contamination and infection.

Blood may be removed from the pleural cavity by needle and syringe, as a temporary expedient. But as soon as possible, a large-bore tube, size 34 or 36, should be inserted, as shown in Plate XI, and connected with a continuous suction, underwater-seal drainage system illustrated in Plate XIII. Two tubes should be used, since clotting in a single tube will eliminate an important means of estimating the rate and volume of blood loss which, if undetected, may lead to disastrous results.

In addition, the necessity for prompt exploratory surgery should always be considered in these patients. Decision in the individual case will depend on the location of the wound, the amount and rapidity of blood accumulation as shown by serial x-ray films, and particularly by observation of the drainage bottles at intervals of 10 or 20 minutes. With these considerations in mind, a decision on the necessity for operation can usually be reached within one hour.

Profound or increasing shock, despite active treatment with intravenous fluid and blood, calls for prompt thoracic exploration.

CONTINUOUS WATER-SEAL DRAINAGE
(PLATE XIII)

The most effective way of emptying the pleural space and keeping it clear is by water-seal drainage.

This can be carried out without suction. The chest drainage tube is attached to a bottle partially filled with water that stands on the floor, well below the patient's chest. The chest is sealed off from the contamination of the outside air by the water in the bottle. A negative pressure greater than the 15 cm H_2O negative pressure within the chest is produced by the column of water in the tube.

Such a system has several disadvantages, not least of which is the tendency of thoughtless personnel to lift the bottle in order to empty it. If this is done without first clamping the drainage tube, fluid will siphon back into the chest.

The disadvantages of a single bottle can be partially overcome by the use of two bottles. However, best is a three-bottle system, connected to suction. Here the first bottle does the collecting, the second provides the underwater seal, and the third bottle maintains the chest suction at the level of the water in the bottle, without the use of gauges.

Sterile, compact, disposable units containing the equivalent of a three-bottle system are commercially available.

CARDIOCIRCULATORY DYNAMICS OF BLOOD IN THE PERICARDIAL CAVITY

Acute hemopericardium with cardiac tamponade is caused by small penetrating wounds of the heart wall or the intrapericardial portions of aorta, pulmonary artery, or venae cavae. The trapping of blood in the pericardial sac results in three major physiologic alterations:

1. *On the venous side,* the increased intrapericardial pressure causes compression of the venae cavae and the auricles. It thereby impedes venous return to the heart and elevates venous pressure.

2. *On the arterial side,* cardiac compression lowers the cardiac output. This reduces coronary filling, predisposing to myocardial hypoxia and failure.

3. *On the systemic side,* the reduced cardiac output is initially compensated by a generalized vasoconstriction. Blood pressure is thus temporarily maintained at near-normal or even higher-than-normal levels. Eventually, the blood pressure will suddenly fall.

CARDIAC TAMPONADE
(PLATE XIV)

Extensive lacerations or large caliber gunshot wounds of the heart are quickly fatal due to sudden and voluminous blood loss. However, small wounds, as from a penknife or even a small caliber bullet, should rarely cause death, because the blood becomes trapped within the pericardium (cardiac tamponade), thus tending to arrest the hemorrhage.

This trapping of blood in the pericardial sac, while temporarily lifesaving, often offers only a transient reprieve, lasting several minutes to several hours.

The pericardium is inelastic. Therefore, while a small amount of blood within the sac is of little consequence, when the volume reaches 150 to 200 ml, the patient may suddenly go into shock or die.

Diagnosis

A small puncture wound in the vicinity of the heart, in the upper abdomen, the axilla, or even in the back should immediately arouse suspicion.

The characteristic features include muffled and distant heart sounds, a falling or absent blood pressure, and a progressively rising venous pressure. The presence of deep shock, that seems out of proportion to the severity of the wound and the amount of blood loss, weighs heavily in favor of tamponade. Aspiration of blood from the pericardial sac confirms the diagnosis.

Treatment

Immediate aspiration of the pericardial sac is mandatory if life is to be saved. The removal of as little as 15 to 20 ml of blood may be sufficient to revive an apparently moribund patient.

The aspiration is carried out by placing the patient in a semi-Fowler position, so that accumulated blood will be dependent. A three-inch, 16- to 18-gauge, short-bevel needle is attached to a 50 ml syringe inserted slightly to the left of the xyphoid cartilage. The needle is then pushed upward as shown in Plate XIV until blood can be aspirated or the heart wall is encountered, as evidenced by a scraping sensation against the needle tip, produced by the beating heart. The depth of insertion will usually be about 1½ inches or 4 centimeters.

Unless there is great urgency, pericardiocentesis should be performed in the operating room with electrocardiographic monitoring. Oscilloscopic electrocardiography will be helpful in determining whether or not the myocardium has been penetrated or abrupt change in cardiac action has occurred.

Once aspiration has been carried out, the relief must be considered temporary and the patient observed continuously, because bleeding, which may prove rapidly fatal, may recur within minutes or days. For this and other rather compelling reasons, we believe it is safer to do an immediate or early thoracotomy with cardiac repair in all patients with penetrat-

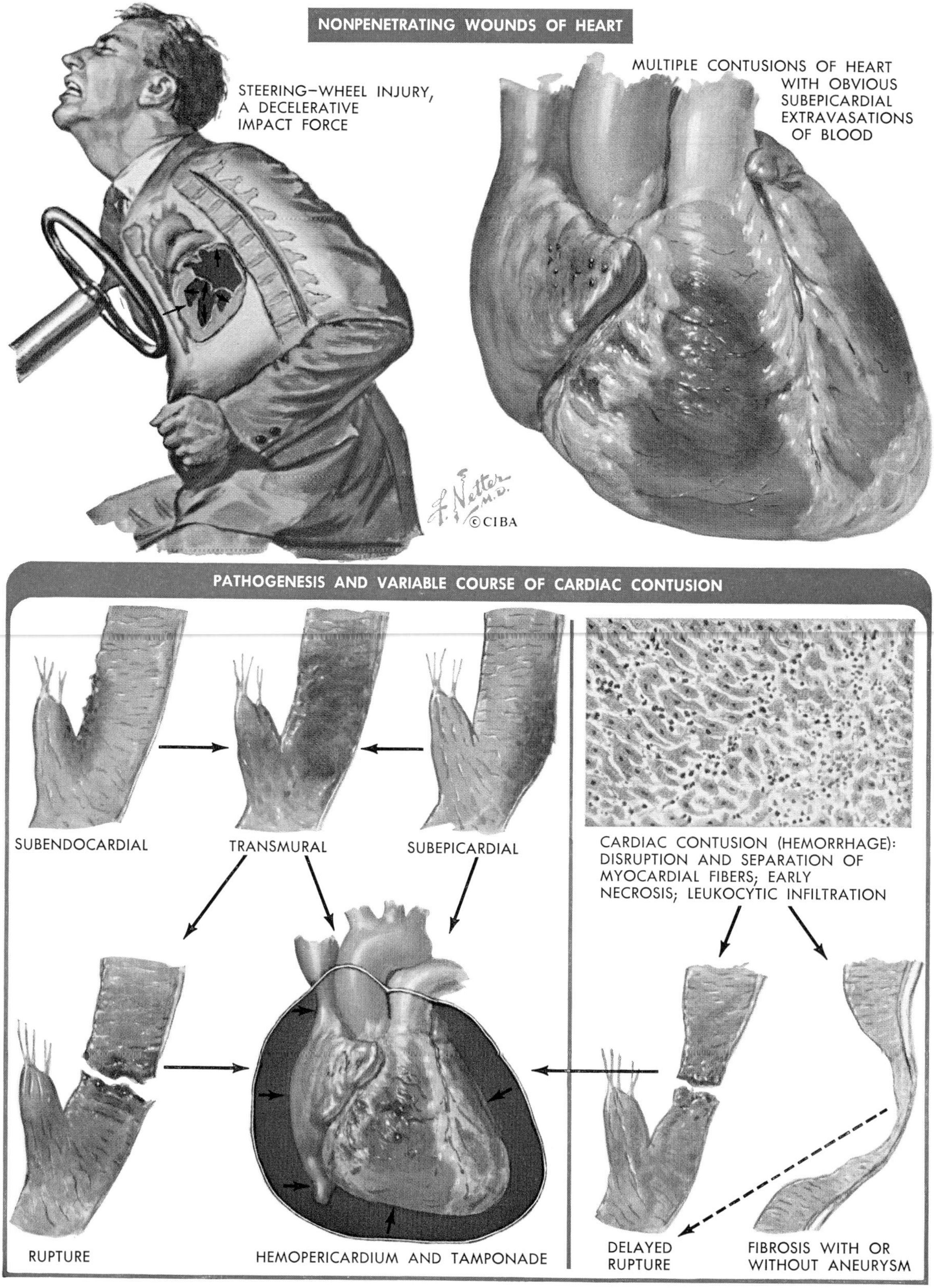
NONPENETRATING WOUNDS OF HEART
STEERING–WHEEL INJURY, A DECELERATIVE IMPACT FORCE
MULTIPLE CONTUSIONS OF HEART WITH OBVIOUS SUBEPICARDIAL EXTRAVASATIONS OF BLOOD
F. Netter M.D.
©CIBA
PATHOGENESIS AND VARIABLE COURSE OF CARDIAC CONTUSION
SUBENDOCARDIAL
TRANSMURAL
SUBEPICARDIAL
CARDIAC CONTUSION (HEMORRHAGE): DISRUPTION AND SEPARATION OF MYOCARDIAL FIBERS; EARLY NECROSIS; LEUKOCYTIC INFILTRATION
RUPTURE
HEMOPERICARDIUM AND TAMPONADE
DELAYED RUPTURE
FIBROSIS WITH OR WITHOUT ANEURYSM

PLATE XV

CARDIAC CONTUSION

ing wounds of the heart complicated by acute hemopericardium and tamponade.

CARDIAC CONTUSION
(PLATE XV)

Depending upon the degree of blunt force, the cardiac injury sustained may vary from simple contusion, with or without the electrocardiographic signs of infarction, to rupture of the atria with rapidly developing hemopericardium and tamponade occasionally salvageable by prompt pericardiocentesis and immediate operation, or complete ventricular rupture, which is invariably fatal.

Simple cardiac contusion, although often associated with minor degrees of hemorrhage into the pericardial cavity, rarely causes death and, when uncomplicated, the prognosis is usually excellent.

Probably the most frequent cause of contusion is the steering wheel injury of sudden automobile deceleration. Frequently, cardiac contusion is present without any disruption of the bony thorax. Also, this condition can be caused by indirect violence, such as falls from heights, blast explosions, and even sudden force transmitted hemodynamically from the abdomen or an extremity.

As in contusion elsewhere, the primary lesion is capillary hemorrhage, which may vary in size from petechial to hemorrhagic involvement of the full thickness of the myocardium. The coronary vessels, except when they are atheromatous, are rarely involved in the hemorrhage.

Diagnosis

The clinical symptoms and signs consist of:

1. Pain, which may be immediate or delayed (even days later). The pain is retrosternal or anginal in character, refractory to nitroglycerin, and responsive to oxygen.

2. Conduction disturbances, which include ectopic beats, paroxysmal tachycardia, or atrial flutter or fibrillation.

3. ECG alterations, which will depend on the severity and location of the lesion. A severe contusion may result in progressive degeneration and necrosis of the heart muscle, which will terminate either in delayed rupture, fibrous healing, or aneurysm formation.

Treatment

Patients in whom the history suggests the possibility of cardiac contusion, particularly those with severe steering wheel accidents, should be followed by serial ECG studies and treated like coronary thrombosis if tracings suggestive of an infarct are obtained (see CLINICAL SYMPOSIA, Volume 20, Number 4). Acute hemopericardium, of a degree to produce tamponade, requires immediate aspiration of the pericardial sac.

CARDIAC ARREST

Cardiac arrest is to be presumed on the absence of arterial pulsation and detectable blood pressure. Often the presence or absence of a peripheral pulse is difficult to determine with certainty. However, since the brain can survive the lack of oxygen-carrying hemoglobin for only 3 to 4 minutes, active, energetic support of both ventilation and circulation must be started immediately, even though some doubt exists.

Ventilatory Support

If help is available, attention should be given to both ventilation and circulation at the same time. However, the first priority must be given to ventilatory support.

An adequate airway must be established by one of the methods previously outlined. In an emergency, once the mouth and pharynx have been cleared of blood, secretions, and other foreign material, mouth-to-mouth ventilation is started. To do this, the patient's head is hyperextended, the jaw pulled forward, and the nostrils occluded with the fingers.

The resuscitator then covers the patient's open mouth with his own lips and exhales with a force and depth that will noticeably expand the patient's chest. The mouth is then withdrawn, allowing the patient's chest to contract. This is repeated intermittently and regularly at a rate of about 20 times per minute. A self-expanding Ambu bag, if available, is far superior to the mouth-to-mouth method.

A volume-cycled respirator should be employed when available. However, a pressure-cycled respirator should not be used to assist ventilation because these devices are often cycled by the act of closed-chest compression. For this reason, the Ambu bag technique should be used whenever a volume-cycled respirator is unavailable.

Closed-Chest Cardiac Compression

In order for closed-chest compression to be effective, the patient must be placed supine on a firm, level surface. The shoulders of the person applying the compression should be high enough so that force can be applied with the arms straight and the elbows stiff. The heel of one hand, with the other hand superimposed, is placed on the lower third of the sternum. Sharp, downward force is then applied with the weight of the torso, sufficient to depress the sternum by an inch or two (2.5 to 5 cm). Pressure is then promptly released.

These short, sharp compressions are repeated rhythmically at a rate of 60 to 80 per minute. After each three compressions, the resuscitator should pause momentarily to permit maximum lung expansion.

If this technique is properly applied and successful, a carotid or femoral pulse should return, and a blood pressure of at least 60 to 70 mm Hg should be obtained.

Contraindications to Closed-Chest Compression

Compression is contraindicated by certain injuries of the chest, the presence of which can often be surmised by the history (for example, stab or gunshot wounds *vs* blunt trauma) and a rapid diagnostic evaluation.

In the patient with a *wound of the heart or a great vessel*, bleeding and/or tamponade will be increased, and the patient's life will quickly become irretrievable. (The diagnosis of tamponade has already been discussed. Diagnosis of traumatic rupture of the thoracic aorta is established by a widening of the superior mediastinum on x-ray.)

The condition of the patient whose cardiac arrest is secondary to hypoxia caused by pulmonary compression of *tension pneumothorax* (the diagnosis of which was already discussed) or *extensive traumatic diaphragmatic herniation* (as evidenced by mediastinal shift, distant or absent breath sounds, and frequently the auscultation of borborygmi in the thorax) will also be rapidly worsened by closed-chest compression. Also, depending on location and extensiveness, *fractured ribs* may be forced to penetrate a vital intrathoracic and/or intra-abdominal organ during compression.

These conditions all contraindicate closed-chest compression. They demand immediate thoracotomy, and *internal* cardiac massage, along with means to establish and maintain ventilation, and simultaneous efforts to control hemorrhage and/or any other underlying causative factor.

Open Cardiac Massage

In the presence of one of the conditions just mentioned, or when external compression proves ineffective within a few minutes, an incision should be made quickly in the left fourth or fifth intercostal space (preferably in the fifth), without regard for sterility. The ribs are rapidly separated manually by an assistant, or if available, with a rib spreader. The operator then thrusts his hand into the chest, grasps the heart, and rhythmically compresses it through the intact pericardium against the sternum.

If this is not immediately effective, the pericardial sac should be opened longitudinally, anterior to the phrenic nerve. The heart is then grasped by placing the fingers behind and the thumb anterior, Plate XVI. It is now compressed at a rate of about 70 per minute using a gliding motion from its apex to its base. Complete relaxation must be permitted between each compression to allow for adequate cardiac filling.

If on entering the chest it becomes obvious that tamponade is present, the pericardium must be incised immediately, clots and fluid blood evacuated from the sac, and bleeding from the myocardial wound controlled by digital pressure. The myocardial wound can then be sutured in accordance with circumstances.

If it appears that major bleeding is emanating from a lacerated aorta or a hilar pulmonary vessel, cardiac massage must be performed at once and continued, the patient being turned to the semisupine or lateral position so that the incision can be extended laterally, and the chest opened adequately to permit the bleeding source to be identified and controlled.

For small wounds of the aorta, control of bleeding can often be accomplished temporarily by digital pressure or a partially occluding, noncrushing vascular clamp. Patients with large penetrating wounds of the aorta approaching transection may require immediate cross clamping above and below the site of injury to permit perfusion of the brain and coronary arteries. Such complete occlusion however cannot be tolerated for longer than 15 minutes. Thus, unless extracorporeal circulation is quickly available, such cases are practically hopeless.

Pulmonary hilar bleeding can often be controlled quickly by manual compression. As a temporary measure, cross clamping can be done. Or a ligature or two can be thrown around the hilum for control.

Sometimes myocardial damage secondary to hypoxia will be irreversible, and spontaneous electrical and mechanical activity cannot be induced. If the heart fails to resume activity within 45 minutes to the resuscitative measures mentioned, all hope must be abandoned.

Other Important Therapeutic Measures: If the heart fails to beat despite adequate cardiac massage, 0.5 to 1 ml of 1:1000 epinephrine should be injected directly into the heart to trigger cardiac action (Plate XVI). Cardiac massage is continued. If myocardial contractions are restored but are feeble, 5 to 10 ml of a 10 per cent solution of calcium chloride, or 1 to 2 ml of isoproterenol, should be injected directly into the heart, or into a vein, to improve both myocardial tone and contractile force.

Intravenous sodium bicarbonate is mandatory to combat metabolic acidosis. Acidosis not only depresses myocardial contractile force but also renders the heart refractory to the action of epinephrine and isoproterenol. Immediate correction of acidosis is therefore essential. In general, 44.6 mEq (one ampul) of sodium bicarbonate is given by the intravenous route for each estimated minute of arrest. After injection of the first ampul, the sodium bicarbonate is preferably given by continuous intravenous drip.

If ventricular fibrillation is present, countershock should be used (electrical defibrillation). The dose range of direct current countershock is from 20 to 100 watt-seconds. A single shock often proves effective. If not, a series of 2 or 3 shocks in rapid succession should be given. For electrical defibrillation to be effective, the heart must be maximally oxygenated and in good tone.

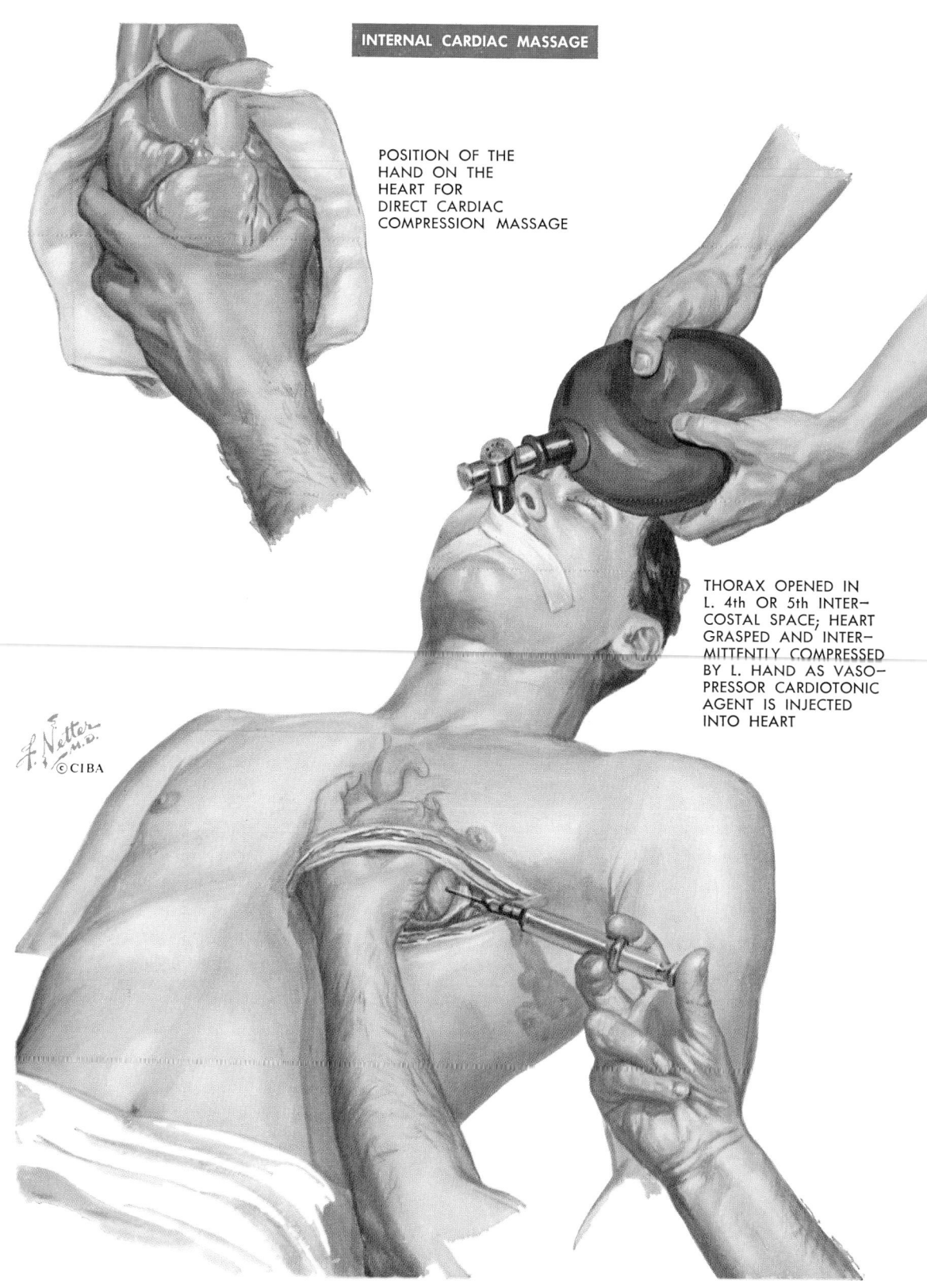

POSITION OF THE
HAND ON THE
HEART FOR
DIRECT CARDIAC
COMPRESSION MASSAGE

THORAX OPENED IN
L. 4th OR 5th INTER-
COSTAL SPACE; HEART
GRASPED AND INTER-
MITTENTLY COMPRESSED
BY L. HAND AS VASO-
PRESSOR CARDIOTONIC
AGENT IS INJECTED
INTO HEART

PLATE XVI

INTERNAL CARDIAC MASSAGE
INJECTION OF VASOPRESSOR

OTHER CONDITIONS DEMANDING IMMEDIATE OR EARLY THORACOTOMY

Most of the conditions demanding immediate or early thoracotomy have been discussed earlier in this presentation. One other condition, not previously mentioned, that requires either immediate or early thoracotomy is *rupture or perforation of the esophagus*. This injury is suggested by the presence of subcutaneous emphysema, or mediastinal emphysema as shown by x-ray. It is confirmed by a roentgenogram showing extravasation after a water-soluble contrast medium is swallowed.

Also, *large diaphragmatic herniations* require prompt surgical intervention in order to correct or prevent strangulation of portions of the gastrointestinal tract, as well as the potentially lethal cardio-respiratory embarrassment that such herniations will produce.

Penetrating thoraco-abdominal wounds on the left side are far more demanding of surgical exploration than those on the right. On the right side the liver affords some protection to intra-abdominal organs. On the left, however, injuries to the spleen, stomach, colon, and small bowel are very common complications.

Except for cardiac arrest, uncontrollable massive intrathoracic bleeding, or continuing shock when there is no response to rapid blood replacement, surgery should not be performed until after all resuscitative measures have been applied, and at a time when response to therapy is optimum.

CONDITIONS CONTRAINDICATING THORACOTOMY

Certain conditions contraindicate an opening into the chest. These include: 1. lacerations and/or contusions of the lung, 2. blast injuries of the lung, and 3. myocardial contusion.

INDICATIONS FOR LATE THORACOTOMY

Days, weeks, or even months after a chest injury, thoracotomy may be necessitated by one of the following: 1. retained foreign bodies, 2. clotted hemothoraces, 3. tracheobronchial tears, 4. valvular and septal injuries of the heart, 5. diaphragmatic herniations, and 6. traumatic aneurysms of the thoracic aorta.

Thus the importance of careful and prolonged follow-up of every chest-injured patient.

SECTION F

C I B A

OTOLOGIC DIAGNOSIS
AND THE TREATMENT OF DEAFNESS

David Myers, M.D., Woodrow D. Schlosser, M.D.,
Robert J. Wolfson, M.D., Richard A. Winchester, Ph.D.,
and Norman H. Carmel, M.A.

OTOLOGIC DIAGNOSIS AND THE TREATMENT OF DEAFNESS*

DAVID MYERS, M.D., WOODROW D. SCHLOSSER, M.D., ROBERT J. WOLFSON, M.D., RICHARD A. WINCHESTER, PH.D., AND NORMAN H. CARMEL, M.A.

EDITOR'S NOTE: Such was the popularity of *Otologic Diagnosis and The Treatment of Deafness*, which originally appeared in CLINICAL SYMPOSIA in 1962, that it has been impossible to maintain an adequate supply despite several reprintings. In the interim certain newer microsurgical techniques have been developed. These will be found in the following pages along with basic physiology and other sections that have been found so useful.

INTRODUCTION

To be deaf or "hard of hearing" is probably one of the most emotionally disabling conditions suffered by the human race. The baby who is deaf at birth learns to speak only with the most intensive training and remains six to eight years behind his fellows, regardless of the amount of effort devoted to his training and education.

The person who later becomes deaf or "hard of hearing" lives in a world of subdued or distorted sound, or even of silence. Thus deprived of his primary means of communication, he tends to withdraw from the world and live within himself.

If these consequences of hearing loss are to be avoided, early diagnosis is essential — before, rather than after, the infant is treated as though feeble-minded, the child fails in school work, or the older patient loses his job or becomes a partial recluse.

It will be the purpose of this article to review briefly the physiology of hearing, the various tests of acuity that can be applied, and a few of the modern techniques of treating this emotionally disabling condition.

PHYSIOLOGY OF HEARING

The function of the ear is to transmit to the brain an accurate pattern of all sound vibrations received from the environment, their relative intensity, and the directions from which they may emanate. Although much remains to be learned, and some aspects of the mechanism are conjectural or even controversial, the following summary should help in understanding the various causes of hearing impairment and the steps that can be taken in diagnosis and treatment.

Nature of Sound

The sounds that we hear are actually vibrations of the air moving away from the source in all directions, like the ripples produced by throwing a stone into a pool of water. These ripples, or waves of sound, have two main characteristics, both determined by the source.

---

* From the Presbyterian-University of Pennsylvania Medical Center, and Women's Medical College Hospital of Pennsylvania.

The first is *frequency* or wave length. Since sound travels at a uniform speed in a given conducting medium, the closer the waves are together (shorter wave length), the more frequently the waves will strike the ear drum. From the top of one wave to the top of the next is a single cycle of the wave. Thus, the frequency or number of vibrations per second is more often referred to as the cycles per second (abbreviated to cps and later to *Hertz* or Hz). The greater the frequency (and shorter the wave length), the higher the pitch. For example, middle C is produced by 256 vibrations or cycles per second (Hz), while the same note one octave above will have a vibration rate of 512 Hz.

The human ear can perceive sounds over a very wide range of frequencies (from as low as 16 Hz to as high as 30,000 Hz). However, there is a great deal of individual variation. As a general rule, perception of high frequencies is best in early childhood, with a gradual decrease throughout life, so that a normal adult may have difficulty with anything over 10,000 or 12,000 Hz.

In advanced years a condition known as presbycusis develops, in which perception of sound both by air and bone conduction grows progressively poorer as frequencies increase (Figure 1 on page 41).

The intensity of sound (or height of the waves) is customarily expressed in decibels (dB), where zero decibels is the intensity that we can barely hear. Each increase of 10 dB indicates a tenfold increase of sound intensity. Thus a sound of 10 dB is ten times as intense as that which is barely audible. Twenty dB indicates a sound 10 times 10, or 100 times as intense, while a sound of 60 dB is 1 million times as intense. At a distance of about 4 feet, an average whisper produces a level of 20 dB and ordinary conversation about 60 dB. A riveter about 35 feet away produces a sound, the intensity of which is 100 dB, or 10 billion times the intensity that is barely audible. Such is the tremendous range of intensity that we are able to hear.

The Auricles

Even though fixed in position and lying close to the head, the external ear tends to concentrate sound waves, especially those of high frequency, and conduct them into the external auditory meatus. Just as the two eyes give us stereoscopic vision, enabling us to judge distance, the two ears provide us with stereophonic hearing so that we can accurately judge the direction of a sound. This is accomplished because of the difference in the phase of the vibration as it arrives at the two ears and also by differences in intensity and quality or timbre, since in the far ear the sound must go around the corner. Probably the shape of the auricles helps us to differentiate between the sound coming directly from behind and that located directly in front.

The External Auditory Meatus

This canal shelters the ear drum and maintains the relatively constant conditions of temperature and humidity necessary to preserve its elasticity. In addition, it acts as a tubal resonator so that the vibrations of sound at the drum have a considerably higher intensity of "pressure" than at the external ear. This is particularly true in the range between 2,000 and 5,500 Hz, where the pressure amplification is between 5 and 10 dB.

The Ear Drum

This structure, composed of both circular and radial fibers, is kept tense for better reception of vibrations, particularly those of higher frequencies, by the tensor tympani muscle.

Here the pressure changes of the sound waves are transformed into mechanical vibrations of incredible minuteness, during ordinary conversation displacement of the drum being only the diameter of a molecule of hydrogen!

The drum not only acts as the receptor of vibrations, but also serves as a barrier to shelter the delicate contents of the middle ear. It also provides an acoustic dead space so that air vibrations in the middle ear will be broken up and dissipated by the irregular walls, epitympanic recess, and mastoid cells, and thus will not exert pressure against the round window in competition with vibrations coming through the cochlea in the other direction from the oval window.

The Ossicles

The anatomic relationships of these three small bones are shown in Plate I. Acting as a unit above 800 Hz, they conduct vibrations from the drum (to which the long and lateral processes of the malleus are attached) to the oval window, over which lies the footplate of the stapes.

These delicately suspended bones not only transmit vibrations almost completely without distortion, but they provide part of the increased power that is essential when going from a lighter conducting medium (air) to a heavier medium, the perilymph. This is partly accomplished by leverage. The incus being shorter than the long process of the malleus, vibrations at the oval window are reduced in amplitude but increased in power by a ratio of about 2 to 1.

An even more important factor in increasing the power of vibrations transmitted to the inner ear is the difference in the relative areas of drum and oval window. The pressure of vibrations received by the much larger drum is increased by a ratio of about 10 to 1 when transmitted to the much smaller area of the oval window.

The Inner Ear

Vibrations transmitted into the oval window by the footplate of the stapes set up vibrations in the perilymph, which surrounds and bathes the membranous labyrinth containing the end-organs of hearing and balance. Grossly viewed, the membranous labyrinth has two parts: the sacculocochlear section and the utriculovestibular portion. These two parts are joined by the ductus reuniens, which provides for physiologic continuity in all parts of the membranous labyrinth.

The cochlea itself is shaped like a snail shell; a cross section is shown in Plate II. The inside of this spiral contains a horizontal partition, producing two parallel circular stairways (scalae), an upper *scala vestibuli* and a lower *scala tympani*, both of which contain perilymph.

The partition is formed by three structures: Extending from the inside of the spiral is a bony ridge (the spiral lamina), while from the outside extends a thick ligament known as the spiral ligament. These two structures are connected by the relatively thin basilar membrane, on which is superimposed the organ of Corti.

A third wedge-shaped compartment lying between the scalae is known as the cochlear duct. This is separated from the scala vestibuli by Reissner's membrane and from the scala tympani by the basilar membrane. The cochlear duct contains a fluid called endolymph which resembles intracellular fluid (the perilymph resembles extracellular or cerebrospinal fluid). The function of the endolymph is probably the nourishment of the organ of Corti, freeing it of any vibrations or noise that its own intrinsic blood supply would produce. The cochlear duct being closed at the helicotrema, there is no direct communication between endolymph and perilymph. However, it is continuous via the ductus reuniens with the semicircular canals, a fact that explains the combination of symptoms present in Meniere's disease.

The organ of Corti, previously mentioned as lying upon the basilar membrane, is composed of a complex assortment of supporting cells, interspersed between and lying upon which are the hair cells, which are the sensory end-

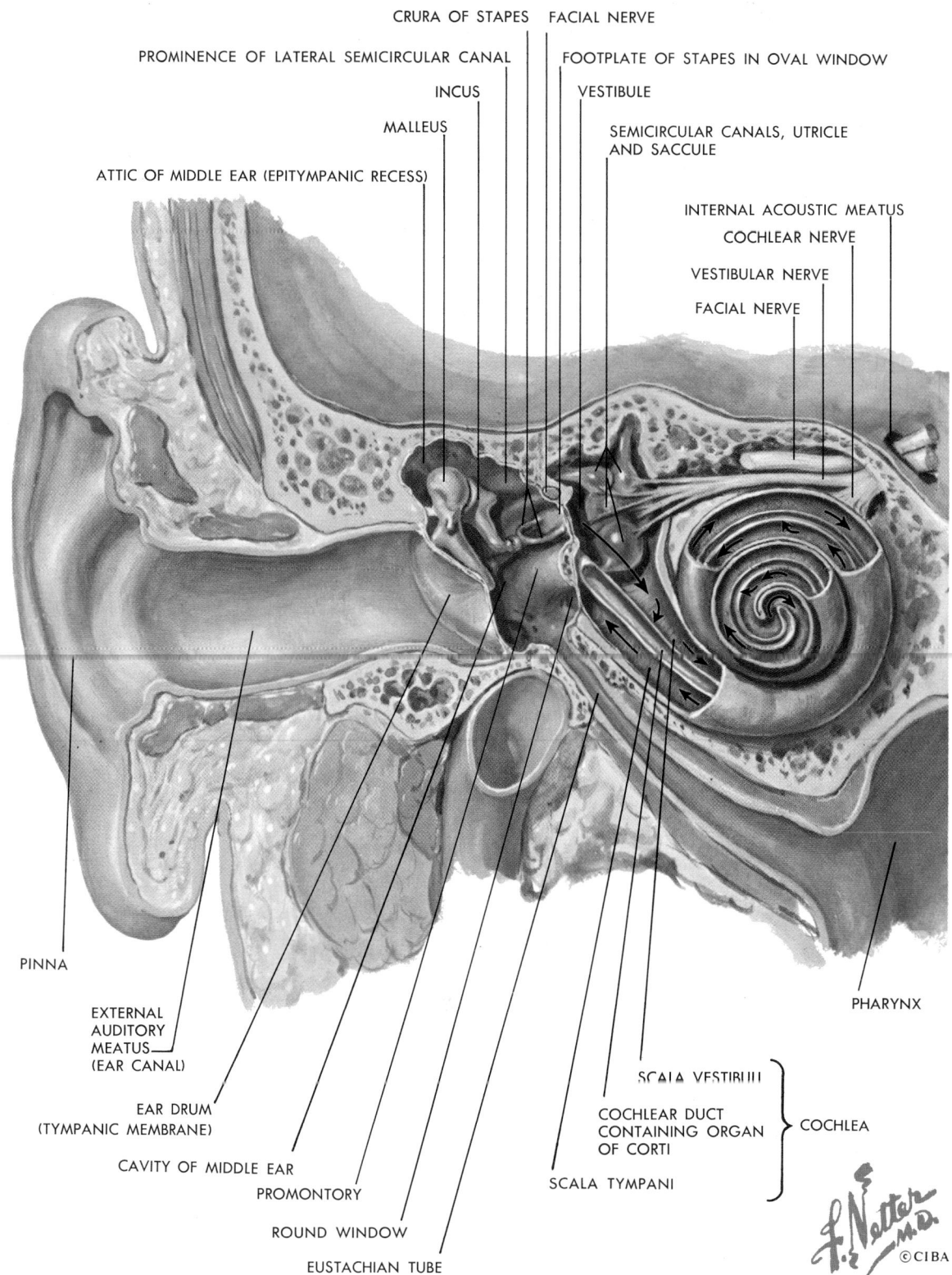

CRURA OF STAPES FACIAL NERVE

PROMINENCE OF LATERAL SEMICIRCULAR CANAL FOOTPLATE OF STAPES IN OVAL WINDOW

INCUS VESTIBULE

MALLEUS SEMICIRCULAR CANALS, UTRICLE AND SACCULE

ATTIC OF MIDDLE EAR (EPITYMPANIC RECESS)

INTERNAL ACOUSTIC MEATUS
COCHLEAR NERVE

VESTIBULAR NERVE

FACIAL NERVE

PINNA

EXTERNAL
AUDITORY
MEATUS
(EAR CANAL)

EAR DRUM
(TYMPANIC MEMBRANE)

CAVITY OF MIDDLE EAR

PROMONTORY

ROUND WINDOW

EUSTACHIAN TUBE

PHARYNX

SCALA VESTIBULI

COCHLEAR DUCT
CONTAINING ORGAN
OF CORTI

SCALA TYMPANI

COCHLEA

F. Netter M.D.
©CIBA

PLATE I

PATHWAY OF SOUND RECEPTION

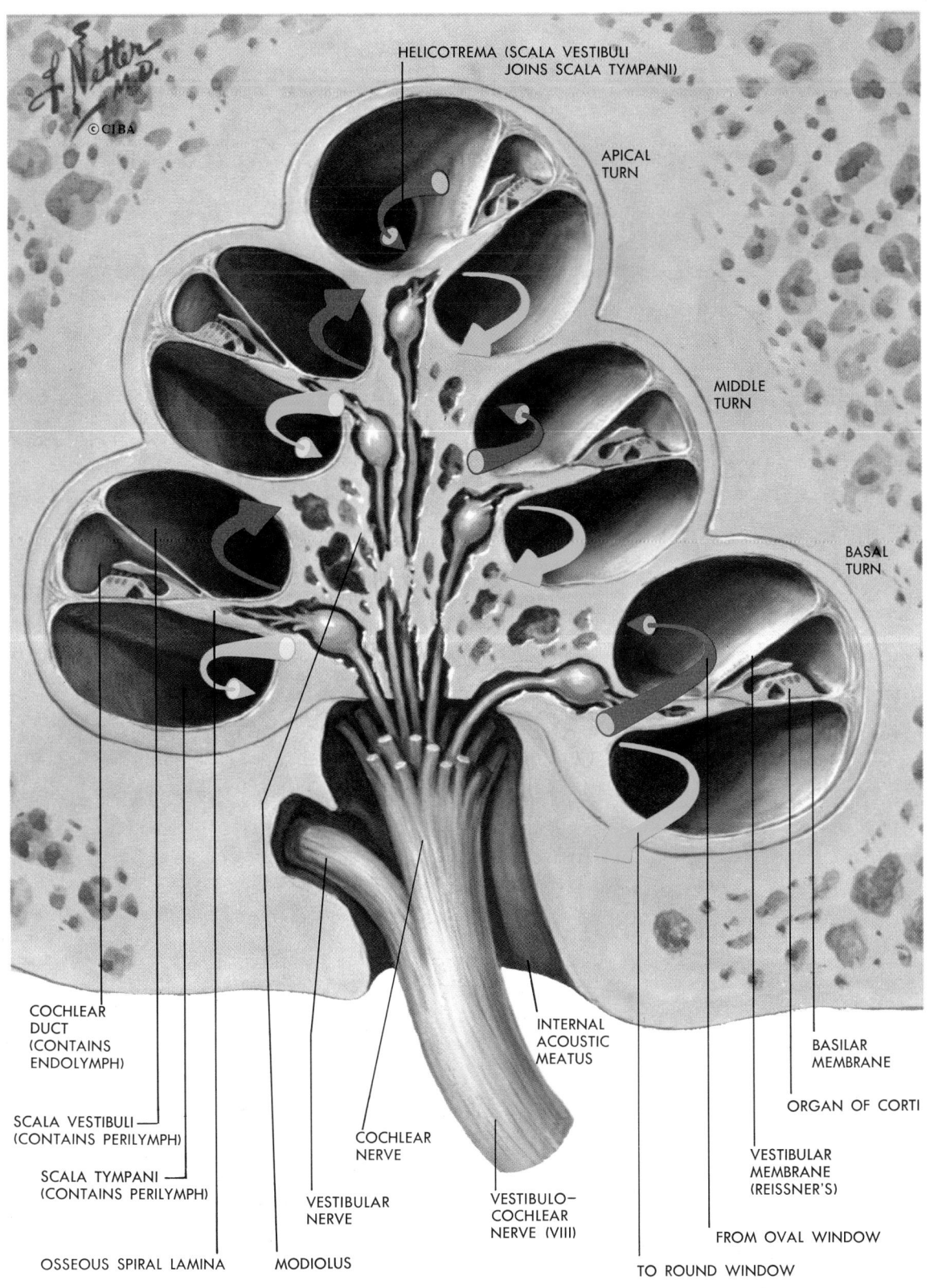

HELICOTREMA (SCALA VESTIBULI JOINS SCALA TYMPANI)

APICAL TURN

MIDDLE TURN

BASAL TURN

COCHLEAR DUCT (CONTAINS ENDOLYMPH)

SCALA VESTIBULI (CONTAINS PERILYMPH)

SCALA TYMPANI (CONTAINS PERILYMPH)

OSSEOUS SPIRAL LAMINA

MODIOLUS

VESTIBULAR NERVE

COCHLEAR NERVE

VESTIBULO-COCHLEAR NERVE (VIII)

INTERNAL ACOUSTIC MEATUS

TO ROUND WINDOW

FROM OVAL WINDOW

VESTIBULAR MEMBRANE (REISSNER'S)

ORGAN OF CORTI

BASILAR MEMBRANE

©CIBA

PLATE II

CROSS SECTION OF COCHLEA

organs. These hair cells are arranged segmentally in well-defined rows, a single row of inner hair cells and several rows of outer hair cells (three rows in the lowermost turn, four rows in the middle turn, and five rows in the apical turn). The total number of inner hair cells is about 3,500, of outer hair cells about 12,000.

Each hair cell terminates on its free surface in a clump of hairs like a small bristle, 40 per cell in the lower turn, as many as 100 per cell at the apex. Overhanging the hair cells is a gelatinous structure known as the tectorial membrane, in which the hair ends are imbedded.

Transmission of Vibrations in the Inner Ear

The vibrations of the stapes at the oval window are transmitted in the perilymph upward in the scala vestibuli (Plates II and III). These vibrations are transmitted through Reissner's membrane to the endolymph and thence through the basilar membrane to the scala tympani, where they pass downward to the round window. The vibrations of the round window thus coincide with those at the oval window, although a fraction of a second later and in opposite phase (when the oval window is forced inward, the round window "gives" outward).

Transformation of Mechanical Energy to Electrical Potential

As can be seen from Plate IV, vibrations of the basilar membrane will cause a pull, or a shearing force, on the hair cells which are attached to the tectorial membrane. It is this action which transforms the energy, which thus far has been mechanical, into electrical impulses that stimulate the fibers of the eighth nerve to the brain, thus giving rise to the action potentials responsible for nerve transmission.

It is generally agreed that hair cells transmitting different frequencies are arranged segmentally, those mainly responsible for transmitting the higher tones being located at the lower end of the cochlea, those transmitting lower tones being located near the apex (Plate III). It is now generally accepted that this segmental activation is caused by "standing waves in the endolymph," the specific actions of which are beyond the scope of this discussion.

Transmission of Impulses to the Brain

Each hair cell is supplied by a nerve fiber, some by more than one. Also each nerve fiber contacts one hair cell; some will contact several. In general, the inner hair cells are each served by only one neuron, the outer hair cells by many. The exact reason for this overlapping of nerve connections is unknown, but it may be to supply a flexibility of function and a capacity to compensate for damage to single hair cells or certain neurons.

The auditory nerve consists of 30,000 individual neurons. The nerve cells are located in the spiral ganglia shown in Plates II and IV, from which axons pass via the cochlear nerve to the dorsal and ventral cochlear nuclei located in the pons.

From these way stations, fibers pass to the superior olive on the same side, or some may decussate to the opposite side. Or they may pass upward to the medial geniculate body with or without intermediate synapses, with neurons located in the lateral lemnisci and the inferior colliculi. Between the latter nuclei located in the midbrain, a second though smaller pathway of decussation exists so that stimuli received in the two ears may be "synchronized" at either one of two levels, or both. On reaching the cortex, it is believed that tones of various pitch are perceived as indicated in Plate V. Generally speaking, as the nerve impulses ascend the auditory pathways, there is increasing interaction and synchronization between the two ears. For this reason, lesions above the level of the lower brain stem require very complicated methods of audiologic diagnosis, which as yet have

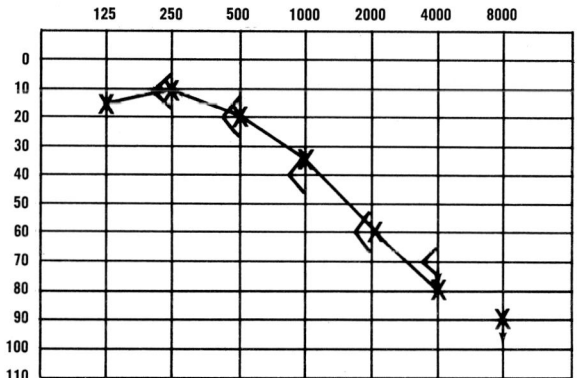

CONVENTIONAL AUDIOGRAMS
ISO—1964

FIGURE 1. Audiogram typical of presbycusis (hearing loss due to age). Air and bone conduction are equally affected, and loss is mainly in higher tones. No improvement can be expected from surgery.

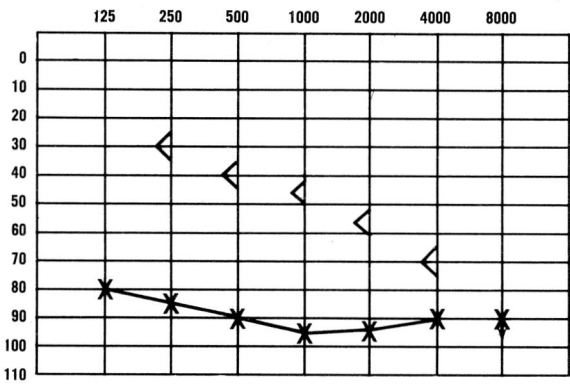

FIGURE 2. Severe mixed hearing loss. Although a great differential exists between air conduction and bone conduction, considerable high-tone deafness is inescapable, regardless of the results of surgery.

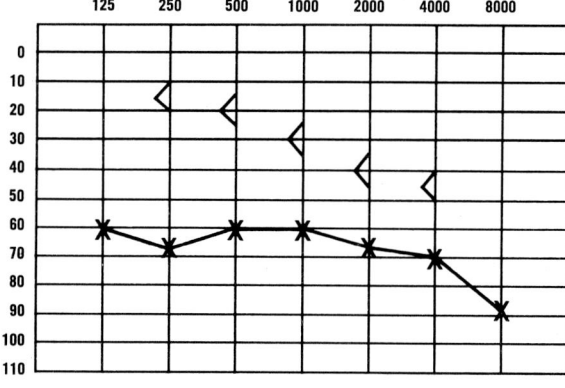

FIGURE 3. Moderately severe mixed hearing loss. Hearing may be considerably improved by surgery, but perception of the higher frequencies may be inadequate.

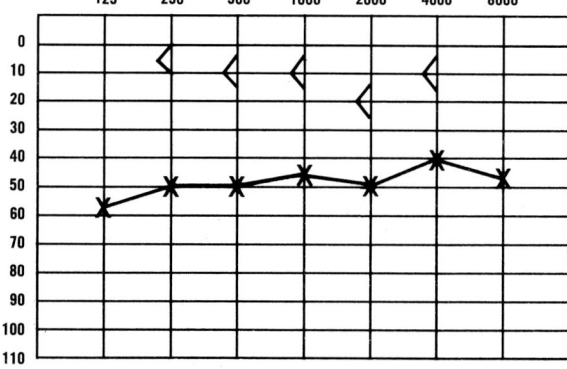

FIGURE 4. This audiogram illustrates a pure conduction loss because of uncomplicated otosclerosis. In such a case, surgery should give excellent results.

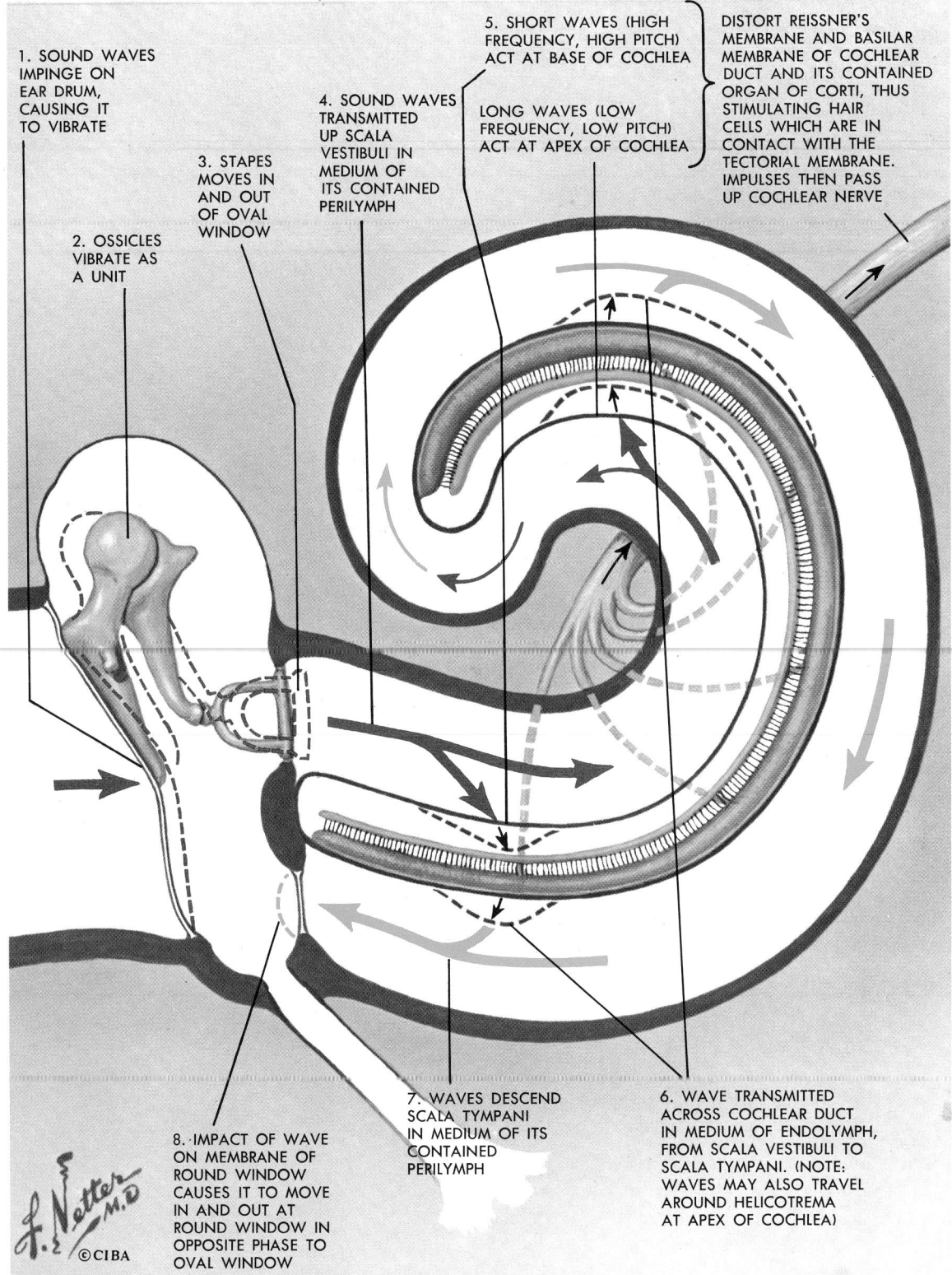

1. SOUND WAVES IMPINGE ON EAR DRUM, CAUSING IT TO VIBRATE

2. OSSICLES VIBRATE AS A UNIT

3. STAPES MOVES IN AND OUT OF OVAL WINDOW

4. SOUND WAVES TRANSMITTED UP SCALA VESTIBULI IN MEDIUM OF ITS CONTAINED PERILYMPH

5. SHORT WAVES (HIGH FREQUENCY, HIGH PITCH) ACT AT BASE OF COCHLEA

LONG WAVES (LOW FREQUENCY, LOW PITCH) ACT AT APEX OF COCHLEA

DISTORT REISSNER'S MEMBRANE AND BASILAR MEMBRANE OF COCHLEAR DUCT AND ITS CONTAINED ORGAN OF CORTI, THUS STIMULATING HAIR CELLS WHICH ARE IN CONTACT WITH THE TECTORIAL MEMBRANE. IMPULSES THEN PASS UP COCHLEAR NERVE

8. IMPACT OF WAVE ON MEMBRANE OF ROUND WINDOW CAUSES IT TO MOVE IN AND OUT AT ROUND WINDOW IN OPPOSITE PHASE TO OVAL WINDOW

7. WAVES DESCEND SCALA TYMPANI IN MEDIUM OF ITS CONTAINED PERILYMPH

6. WAVE TRANSMITTED ACROSS COCHLEAR DUCT IN MEDIUM OF ENDOLYMPH, FROM SCALA VESTIBULI TO SCALA TYMPANI. (NOTE: WAVES MAY ALSO TRAVEL AROUND HELICOTREMA AT APEX OF COCHLEA)

F. Netter M.D. ©CIBA

PLATE III   TRANSMISSION OF VIBRATIONS FROM DRUM THROUGH THE COCHLEA

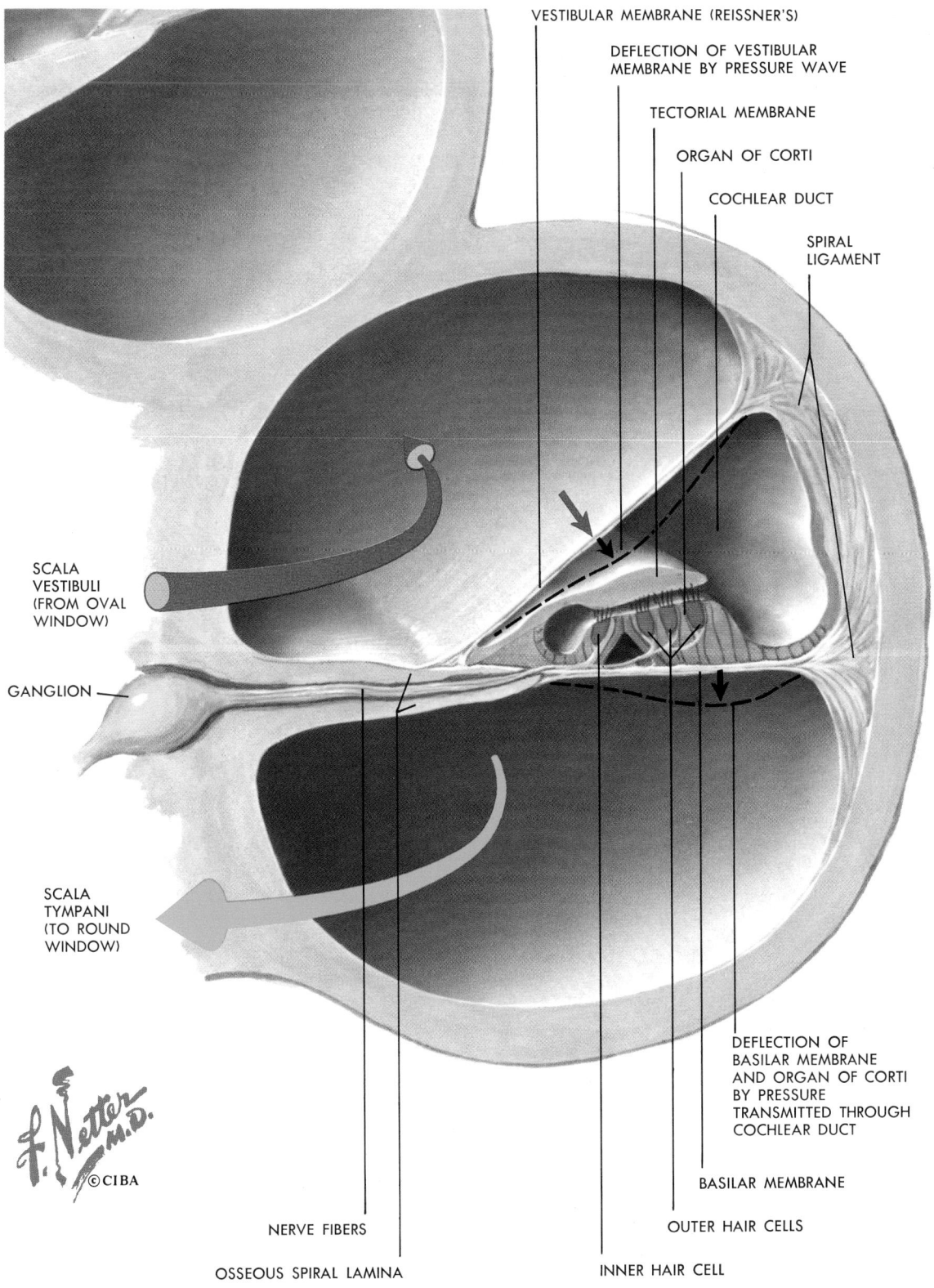

VESTIBULAR MEMBRANE (REISSNER'S)

DEFLECTION OF VESTIBULAR
MEMBRANE BY PRESSURE WAVE

TECTORIAL MEMBRANE

ORGAN OF CORTI

COCHLEAR DUCT

SPIRAL
LIGAMENT

SCALA
VESTIBULI
(FROM OVAL
WINDOW)

GANGLION

SCALA
TYMPANI
(TO ROUND
WINDOW)

DEFLECTION OF
BASILAR MEMBRANE
AND ORGAN OF CORTI
BY PRESSURE
TRANSMITTED THROUGH
COCHLEAR DUCT

BASILAR MEMBRANE

OUTER HAIR CELLS

INNER HAIR CELL

NERVE FIBERS

OSSEOUS SPIRAL LAMINA

PLATE IV TRANSMISSION OF SOUND ACROSS COCHLEAR DUCT STIMULATING HAIR CELLS

not been standardized, as well as comprehensive radiologic study.

A tuning fork is inexpensive. Its use takes less than a minute. It differentiates between conductive and perceptive deafness, which the whispered voice or the watch tick will not do. Therefore, considering the importance of early diagnosis of a hearing defect to the emotional and economic well-being of the patient, tuning fork tests should be a part of every physical examination of both children and adults.

If only a single fork is used, one should be selected that has a frequency of 500 Hz because this will be less influenced by the usual noises of office or examining room than one pitched lower. If a second fork is used, it should be of 2,000 Hz because this is the frequency area in which sensorineural loss is most important in the perception of speech. The fork is best activated with a rubber reflex hammer.

The Weber Test

Here the fork is placed on the forehead as shown in Plate VI. If the patient has normal hearing or if he has deafness equal on both sides, he will say, "I hear it in the middle of my head." If he has nerve deafness which is worse in one ear than the other, the tone will be heard best in the better ear. The tone will be heard in the poorer ear if he has asymmetric conductive deafness. This test furnishes only a comparison of the two ears. The next step will then be:

The Rinne Test

In this test, after striking the tuning fork, the handle is first placed against the mastoid process. Then the tines are held beside the ear as shown in Plate VI. Now the question is, "Where did you hear it better or longer?" If it was heard the same in both places, he may have a mixed loss. If it was louder in front, hearing is normal or there is a sensorineural loss. If louder in back, there is a conductive component. If much louder in back, there is probably a pure conductive loss.

Thus, these two simple tests give a comparison of the two ears and indicate when a conductive component is present. They do not, however, give quantitative information throughout the entire hearing range, which is an important thing to know before selecting a hearing aid or deciding on surgery. This can be determined only by audiologic study.

The Audiologic Analysis

Pure Tone Audiogram: Examples of the information obtained from an audiogram will be found in Figures 1 through 4 on page 41. By this method of analysis, one can determine whether hearing is normal for pure tones of different frequencies by both bone and air conduction or just how much deficit, if any, exists.

Speech Discrimination: People with sensorineural deafness who tend to have loss in the higher frequencies, with or without recruitment, have difficulty in understanding speech for two reasons: The consonants are higher pitched, and they are pronounced less loudly than the vowels. Therefore, such a patient hears the voice but has difficulty in understanding what is being said.

Because the understanding of speech is really more important than any other aspect of hearing, and since the audiometric curve may not indicate accurately just how well speech will be comprehended, it is customary to give tests for speech discrimination. This is carried out by giving the patient a list of fifty phonetically balanced words, such as "deck" and "peck," at about 30 dB above the *speech reception threshold.* (This is obtained by presenting words specially selected on the basis of the perception of vowel components rather than consonants.) In this way a speech discrimination ability is determined. This reading generally agrees quite well with the audiometric curve for pure tones, except in the case of a retrocochlear lesion, where speech discrimination scores will be noticeably poorer than expected.

von Békésy Test: In this test, the patient controls the test signal. The test tone becomes louder and louder until the patient presses a switch to indicate he hears it. Then the tone gets weaker and weaker, until a release of the switch indicates it is no longer being heard. Then the process is repeated with progressively higher tones. This results in a continuous tracing as shown on page 48. First a tracing has been made using a tone that is interrupted every 2.5 seconds, thus producing short beeps; then the same process is repeated with a sustained tone. With this apparatus it is possible to compare the patient's hearing for both the continuous and interrupted tones, and thus distinguish between the sensorineural deafness confined to the cochlea and that in which the difficulty is in the eighth nerve (usually a cerebellopontile angle tumor).

The von Békésy audiograms may be classified into five distinct types, in all of which the tracing for the interrupted tone will follow the standard audiometric curve for pure tones. In Type I, the continuous and interrupted tones are superimposed on one another. This type indicates either normal hearing or a conductive deafness with intact sensorineural functions. In the Type II curve, the two tracings are superimposed up to about 1,000 Hz. Above this frequency, however, the continuous tone tracing falls below the interrupted tone. Also, as shown on page 48, the swings in response to the continuous tone becomes smaller. This type is characteristic of cochlear deafness.

In the Type III von Békésy audiogram, the interrupted tone follows the conventional audiogram, but the hearing for the continuous tone falls away sharply as frequency increases. This is characteristic of retrocochlear deafness, usually an eighth nerve tumor, and is often present long before any other neurological signs can be elicited. In Type IV audiograms, the continuous tone falls below the interrupted tone at all frequencies. This type is usually indicative of more severe cochlear lesions as well as very early retrocochlear deficits. Type V is the only one in which the interrupted tone tracing falls below the continuous. This is indicative of a "functional" hearing loss. It is found in the malingerer or in one who is exaggerating an existing loss.

Retrocochlear versus Cochlear Deafness

The terms "nerve deafness," "perceptive deafness," and "sensorineural deafness" are applied to hearing deficits, the cause of which is central to the conducting mechanisms of the middle ear. Often it is important to localize the difficulty more precisely.

In addition to the typical von Békésy audiograms just mentioned, other findings serve to distinguish between damage in these two locations. In eighth nerve damage, high frequencies are lost first. Indeed, only a few fibers of the eighth nerve need to be preserved to conduct frequencies up to about 125 Hz. In contrast to cochlear deafness, loud sounds are well tolerated. Speech discrimination is poor however, and amplification of speech is of little help.

In cochlear deafness the first tones affected are usually between 4,000 and 6,000 Hz. In addition, there is recruitment which will be referred to later under "Meniere's Disease." With this characteristic of damage to the hair cells, the sensation of loudness will increase from say 10 to 40 dB, while intensity of the sound is increasing only from 10 to 20 dB. Patients with this condition find loud noises painful. A simple office test is to try both the whispered and spoken voice (the index vocalis test). The whisper may not be heard at all, whereas the spoken voice,

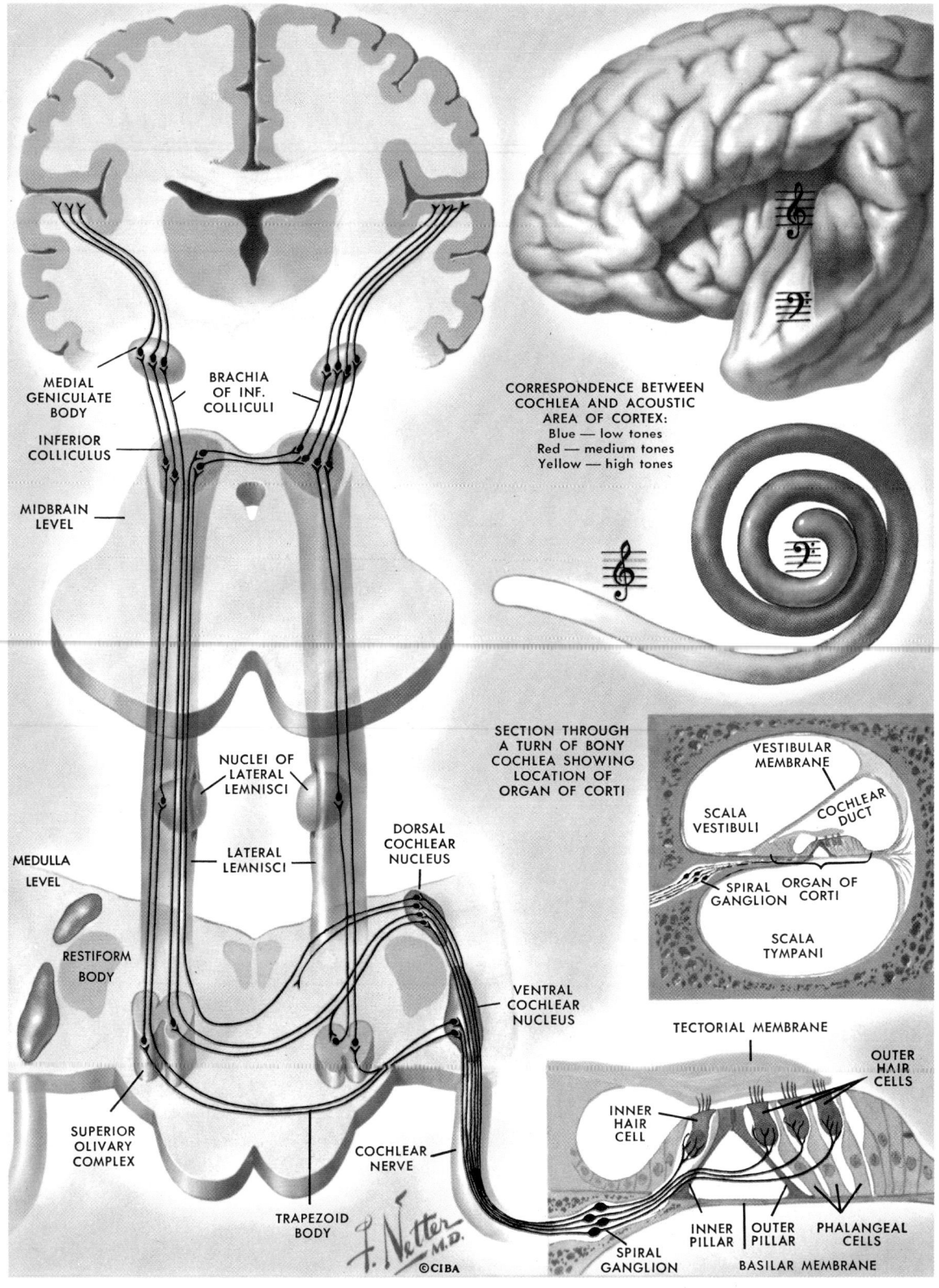

MEDIAL GENICULATE BODY

BRACHIA OF INF. COLLICULI

INFERIOR COLLICULUS

MIDBRAIN LEVEL

CORRESPONDENCE BETWEEN COCHLEA AND ACOUSTIC AREA OF CORTEX:
Blue — low tones
Red — medium tones
Yellow — high tones

NUCLEI OF LATERAL LEMNISCI

LATERAL LEMNISCI

DORSAL COCHLEAR NUCLEUS

MEDULLA LEVEL

RESTIFORM BODY

VENTRAL COCHLEAR NUCLEUS

SUPERIOR OLIVARY COMPLEX

COCHLEAR NERVE

TRAPEZOID BODY

SECTION THROUGH A TURN OF BONY COCHLEA SHOWING LOCATION OF ORGAN OF CORTI

VESTIBULAR MEMBRANE

SCALA VESTIBULI

COCHLEAR DUCT

SPIRAL GANGLION

ORGAN OF CORTI

SCALA TYMPANI

TECTORIAL MEMBRANE

OUTER HAIR CELLS

INNER HAIR CELL

INNER PILLAR

OUTER PILLAR

PHALANGEAL CELLS

SPIRAL GANGLION

BASILAR MEMBRANE

F. Netter M.D.

©CIBA

PLATE V

CENTRAL PATHWAYS OF HEARING

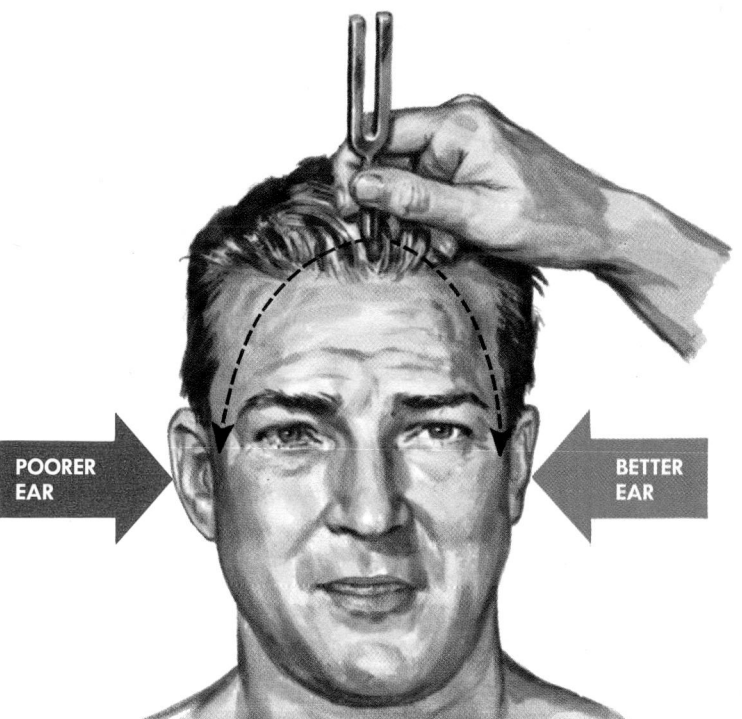

WEBER TEST

TONE REFERRED TO POORER EAR INDICATES CONDUCTIVE IMPAIRMENT

POORER EAR

BETTER EAR

TONE REFERRED TO BETTER EAR INDICATES PERCEPTIVE IMPAIRMENT

RINNE TEST

STAGE 1

STAGE 2

TONE HEARD LONGER BY AIR CONDUCTION = RINNE POSITIVE: INDICATES PERCEPTIVE LOSS

TONE HEARD LONGER BY BONE CONDUCTION = RINNE NEGATIVE: INDICATES CONDUCTIVE LOSS

PLATE VI   SIMPLE TESTS OF HEARING

VON BÉKÉSY AUDIOGRAMS

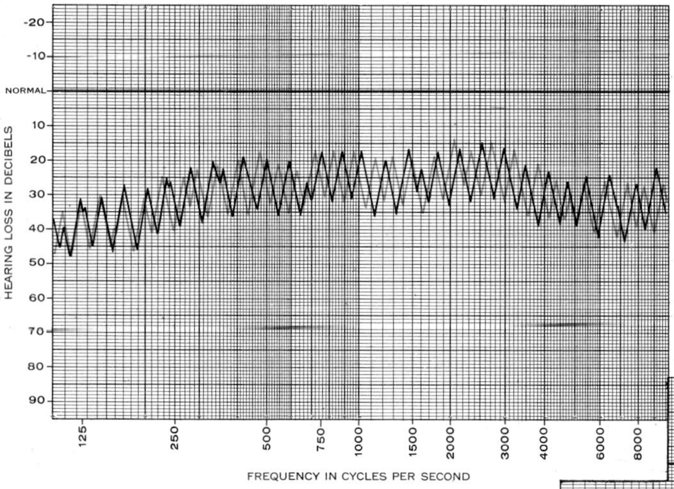

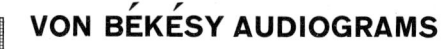

TYPE I: The tracings for the continuous and interrupted tones (shown by blue and black lines respectively) are superimposed. These tracings are found with normal hearing or a conduction deafness with normal sensorineural function.

TYPE II: Tracings are superimposed to 1,000 Hz. Above this frequency, tracing of continuous tone drops below the interrupted tone and the swings are reduced in amplitude. This is characteristic of cochlear deafness such as is found in Meniere's disease.

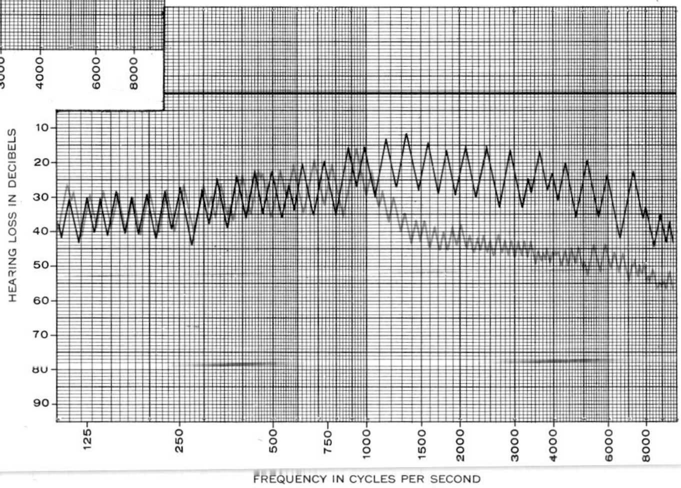

TYPE III: Tracing of the interrupted tone follows conventional audiogram for the same patient, but the continuous tone falls away sharply toward zero as frequencies increase. Characteristic of retrocochlear deafness, usually a cerebellopontile angle tumor.

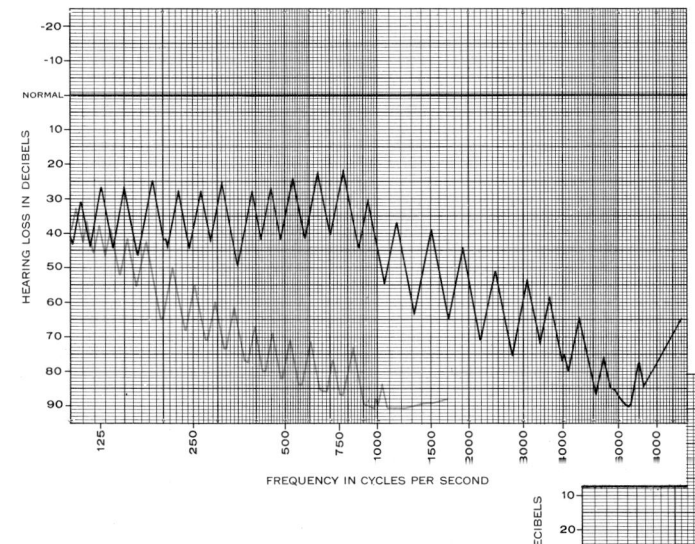

TYPE IV: The continuous tone curve falls below the interrupted tone at all frequencies. This is indicative of a severe cochlear lesion (occurs during and immediately after an acute attack of Meniere's disease) or of early retrocochlear deficits.

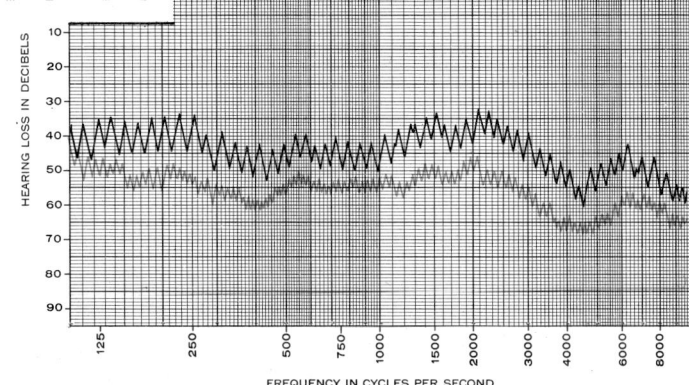

because of recruitment, is heard easily.

Special Tests

It will be impossible to mention here all the special methods available to determine the presence and location of a hearing loss. However, since it is so important to diagnose, not only the presence of a hearing loss, but also the exact site of pathology, we must mention tests that will identify lesions in the central nervous system.

Speech can be divided on two tapes, the one registering frequencies above 750 Hz, the other registering frequencies below this level. Fed into separate ears, the sounds are normally synthesized and the speech understood. Where there is a lesion in the central auditory pathways, no synthesis occurs and the result is gibberish.

Another test which may be of interest is the feeding into the right and left ears of sounds having a different phase. For example, the phase of the sound wave transmitted to one ear may lead that delivered to the other ear by 90 degrees. Normally the brain will synthesize the two and lateralize the sound around the points of the compass. With a lesion in the brain stem or midbrain, sound localization ability is reduced or lost.

HEARING AIDS AND REHABILITATION

With a conductive hearing loss but a normal sensorineural mechanism, the most important thing that is required is adequate amplification. The sound merely needs to be made louder. Here the only difference between instruments is in their fidelity, which usually increases with price. (Whatever hearing aid is chosen, it is wise to select one produced by a well-known company, for obvious reasons.) Some hearing aids have what is known as a compression amplifier, which tends to suppress sounds as they get louder. This protects the ear from sudden loud noises

and is particularly desirable in a patient with recruitment.

In a patient having sensorineural damage, there is a greater problem. Here the loss of sensitivity is not "across the board"; rather reduction in acuity is confined to or more marked at certain frequencies. Therefore, there is distortion in the hearing loss, and if the distortion of a poorly selected hearing aid is added, the patient's ability to hear is worse rather than better.

This is one reason that so many hearing aids are found in the bureau drawer rather than on the person after purchase. Another reason is that a hearing aid is often obtained long after the patient has become deaf and has therefore forgotten what various sounds are really like. His hearing aid will then place him in a new world of noises that he finds difficulty in interpreting.

In patients with these difficulties, it is important to do several things:

1. Select a hearing aid, the amplification curve of which *compensates* for, rather than adds to, the hearing distortion already present.

2. Help the patient to interpret what he hears with the hearing aid. First, he must learn to recognize gross sounds such as bells, horns, etc. Then the audiologist goes on to the sounds of speech, first the vowels, then the consonants. Here particular attention must be given to consonants that usually cause the most trouble, such as the "p" and "t," the "d" and "b," the "m" and "n," etc.

3. Teach the patient to read lips and to correlate lipreading with the sounds he now hears with his hearing aid.

Some patients require only a few visits after a proper hearing aid has been selected. Others may require a more prolonged course before they can be conversationally "adequate." Although time-consuming, the extra time and expense are more than justified, for otherwise the hearing aid often lies unused in the bureau drawer, while the patient continues

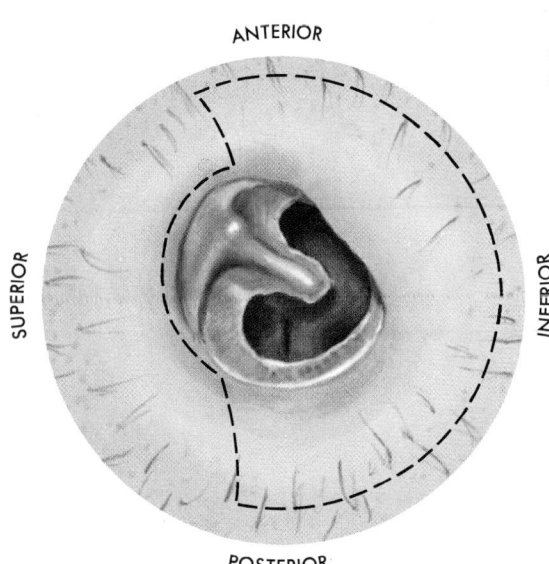

ANTERIOR

SUPERIOR

INFERIOR

POSTERIOR

1. INCISION IN SKIN
OF CANAL WALL
(RIGHT EAR)

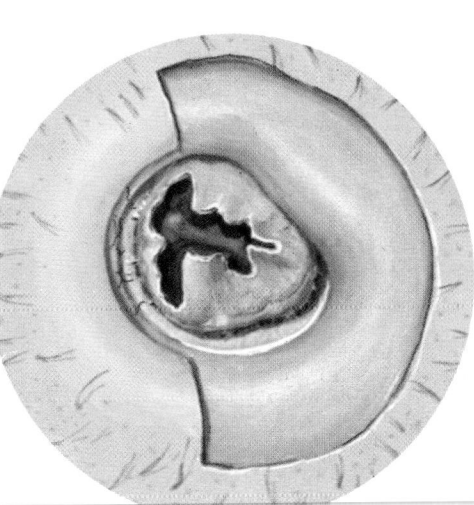

2. SKIN HAS BEEN
SEPARATED FROM
BONY CANAL WALL,
THE DISSECTION
BEING CARRIED
DOWN TO INCLUDE
EXTERNAL EPITHELIAL
LAYER OF DRUM

3. ANTERO–INFERIOR
BONY CANAL WALL
HAS BEEN BURRED AWAY,
EXPOSING ENTIRE
DRUM CIRCUMFERENCE

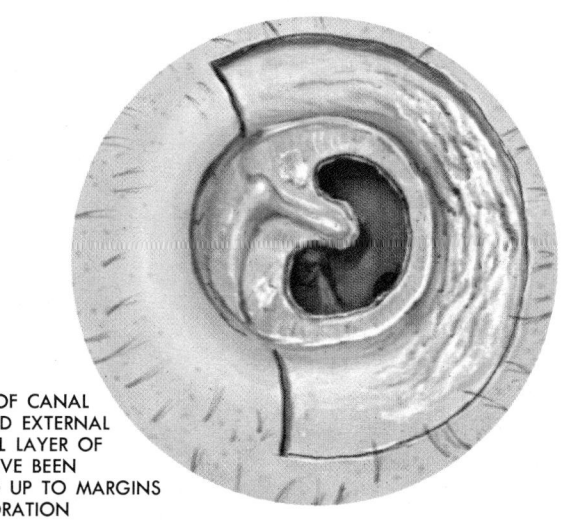

4. SKIN OF CANAL
WALL AND EXTERNAL
EPITHELIAL LAYER OF
DRUM HAVE BEEN
REMOVED UP TO MARGINS
OF PERFORATION

PLATE VII

EXPOSURE IN TRANSMEATAL TYMPANOPLASTY

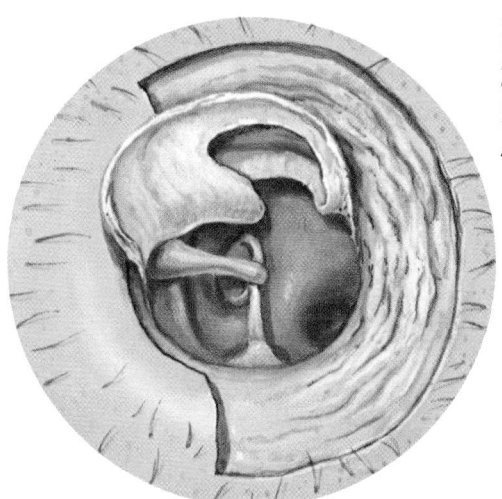

5. DRUM HAS BEEN FREED FROM
ITS ANNULUS ALONG POSTERO–INFERIOR
MARGIN AND REFLECTED ANTERIORLY
OVER MANUBRIUM OF MALLEUS, THUS
EXPOSING MIDDLE EAR AND OSSICLES
WHICH ARE NOW CLEANED AND TREATED
AS REQUIRED

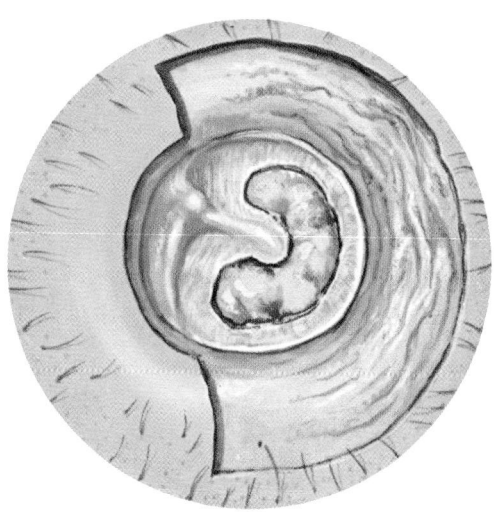

6. MIDDLE EAR
FILLED WITH
GELFOAM AND
DRUM REPLACED

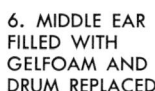

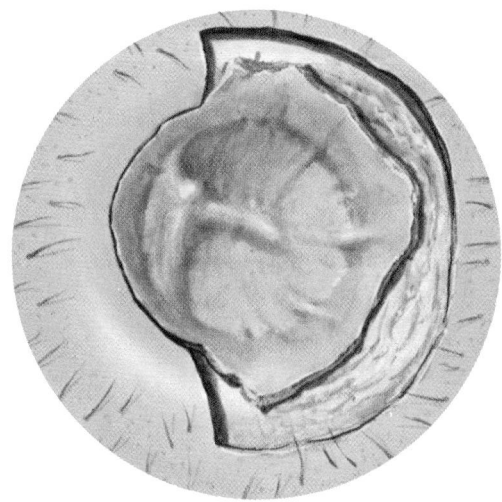

7. SKIN WHICH WAS
REMOVED FROM EAR CANAL
PLACED OVER DRUM
AS A GRAFT

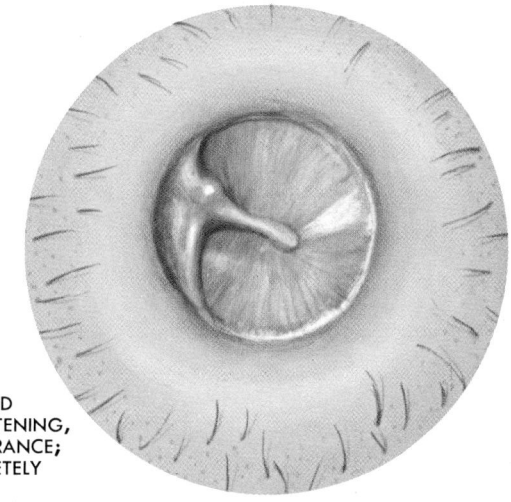

8. THREE MONTHS
POSTOPERATIVELY;
DRUM HAS REASSUMED
NORMAL GRAY, GLISTENING,
TRANSLUCENT APPEARANCE;
CANAL WALL COMPLETELY
EPITHELIALIZED

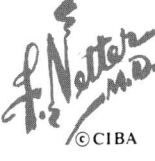

PLATE VIII

REPAIR AND CLOSURE IN TRANSMEATAL TYMPANOPLASTY

to live his life as a comparative recluse.

THE DEAF INFANT

In no field of medicine is an early, accurate diagnosis more important than in children who are congenitally deaf or acoustically handicapped due to hereditary or developmental defect. Training of a deaf child should begin as soon as the hearing loss is identified. If the condition is amenable to surgery or the use of a hearing aid, the child should have help immediately. Many hospitals have screening programs so that, where indicated, more elaborate audiologic testing can be carried out within the first year. Hearing aids have been used as early as the sixth month.

The two things most easily noticed in a deaf infant are that he does not become startled by a sudden noise like a hand clap, and that he does not develop speech normally.

The totally deaf child does not learn to talk because he cannot imitate what he cannot hear; he cannot even hear the "gooing" and babbling sounds that he makes himself. Therefore, he remains inarticulate.

Here it is important to remember that deafness is not the only cause of a child being inarticulate. In about 50 percent of cases it is, but in the remainder the fault is elsewhere. The child may have a receptive aphasia where the auditory center will not store words, or there may be a motor aphasia where the child can hear but cannot talk. The former is extremely difficult to train; the latter can be helped quite easily by training.

Then there is a type of childhood schizophrenia, infantile autism, in which the child is unable to communicate because of psychological factors. Still another group of nonverbal children is composed of the mentally retarded.

A careful history, coupled with shrewd observation, may serve to differentiate these groups. With his special techniques and equipment, the audiologist can more accurately distinguish the deaf or acoustically handicapped from those suffering from other conditions. He can also separate those having a conductive deafness that can be helped by medical or surgical treatment from those with sensorineural losses for whom amplification and special training are indicated.

DEAFNESS IN OLDER CHILDREN AND ADULTS

Deafness or defective hearing, acquired after birth, may arise from a variety of causes. These include diseases such as meningitis, virus infections, particularly measles or mumps, nonspecific high fevers, diabetes, syphilis, and myxedema, as well as ototoxic drugs such as streptomycin, kanamycin, salicylates, and quinine. Each of these drugs may affect the cochlea, and here it is important to consider the desirability of discontinuing any drug if the patient complains of tinnitus, the first indication that cochlear damage may be developing. Also included as causes of deafness or defective hearing are traumatic injuries such as skull fracture, injury to the drum from diving, and exposure to sudden loud noise. Sometimes overlooked is the effect of constant exposure to a noisy environment. This latter cause is an ever-increasing source of claims for compensation, now recognized in a number of states.

Advancing age of itself causes hearing to become less acute, usually beginning with high frequencies and progressing downward. A typical audiogram of this condition, known as presbycusis, is shown in Figure 1 on page 41.

The causes of acquired deafness thus far mentioned are not, as a rule, amenable to definitive therapy. However, certain conditions of the middle and inner ear can be favorably influenced by medical or surgical treatment. These will now be discussed in greater detail.

This is probably one of the *most* important causes of acquired deafness because it is most insidiously progressive and *very* often overlooked.

Pathology

Sterile fluid, which may be clear, mucoid, or purulent, is present in the middle ear. This collection of fluid is sometimes due to allergy. More often it follows a respiratory infection. Untreated, the continued presence of this fluid will produce metaplasia of the mucosa, formation of scar tissue, and a chronic adhesive form of deafness, often with the formation of cholesteatoma.

Symptoms

Usually serous otitis media follows a respiratory infection which was treated promptly with antibiotics, so that the symptoms of earache, fever, and drainage commonly associated with otitis media never appear. Or, if symptoms were present, they appeared to be completely controlled by the antibiotic. The child seems to make a complete recovery. Then a week or two later, the mother notices that she must speak more loudly to get the child's attention. All too often, even when the physician is consulted, appropriate treatment is not instituted because the drum looks relatively normal, and no hearing test is performed. The complaint of faulty hearing is attributed to "inattention," and the problem is dismissed with the advice that the child will "outgrow it."

Signs

The drum may appear normal. On closer inspection, however, it is seen to be opaque, a yellowish or bluish light reflex is present, and there is some fullness. On occasion a fluid level may be seen, or bubbles may be present in the fluid. Tuning fork examination will reveal a conductive deafness, except when carried out in a background of noise where a false positive Rinne may be encountered. Audiometric study shows conductive deafness largely limited to lower frequencies (below 2,000 Hz), with some impairment also in the higher tones (4,000 to 8,000 Hz).

Diagnosis

The discovery of a conductive hearing impairment not previously present, particularly in a patient with a history of allergy or respiratory infection (especially when treated with an antibiotic), calls for careful inspection of the drum and, if necessary, a diagnostic myringotomy.

Treatment

A postero-inferior quadrant myringotomy should be carried out. This may have to be repeated. If the fluid is not too viscid, mild suction through a fine 18-gauge needle, introduced in the postero-inferior quadrant of the drum, may be all that is needed.

For this procedure in adults, a local anesthetic is injected circumferentially beneath the skin of the external canal, particularly in the posterior portion. General anesthesia is recommended for children.

Ancillary measures include the instillation of nose drops, with the head inclined toward the affected side, in the hope of promoting patency of the eustachian tube. Hypertrophied adenoid tissue should be removed. Respiratory infections should be avoided as much as possible and treated aggressively when they occur. In children with repeated attacks, the possibility of allergy should be investigated.

Where the fluid tends to reaccumulate, a tiny plastic tube can be inserted through the drum and allowed to remain in place for several months. This does not act as a drainage tube, but instead acts as an auxiliary eustachian tube, allowing access of air to ventilate the middle ear. With this treatment the mucosa may eventually return to normal, and the patient's hearing will be saved.

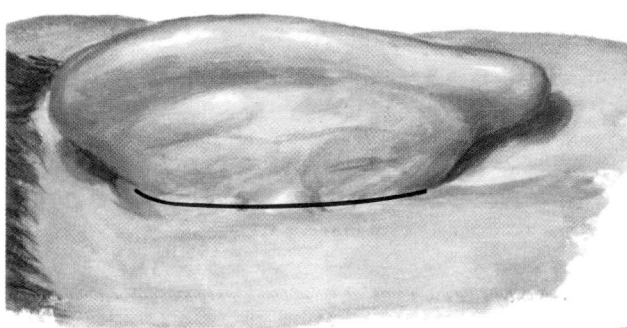

1. POSTAURICULAR INCISION

2. SKIN, FASCIA AND PERIOSTEUM RETRACTED; EAR CANAL OPENED FROM BEHIND EXPOSING DRUM WITH PERFORATION

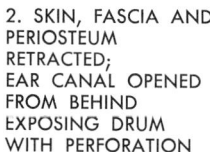

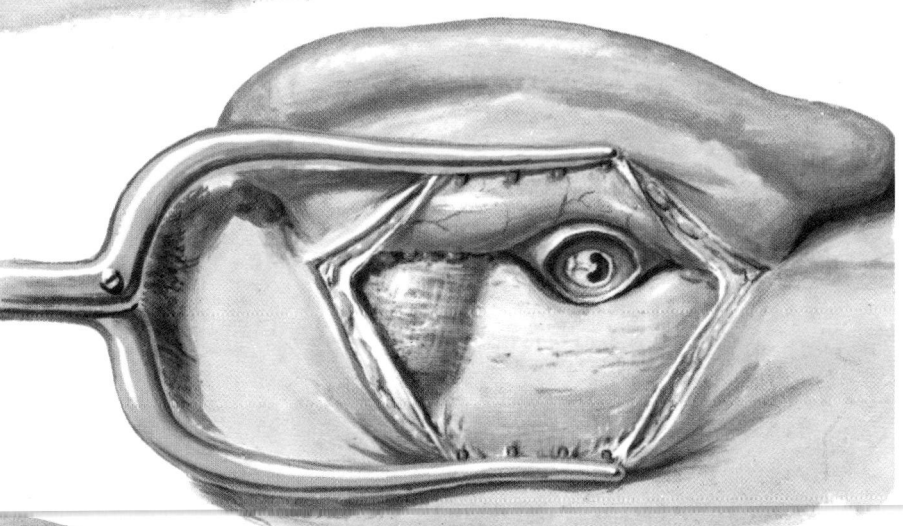

3. VIEW THROUGH OPERATING MICROSCOPE; BEGINNING REFLECTION OF SKIN OF POSTERIOR WALL OF EAR CANAL

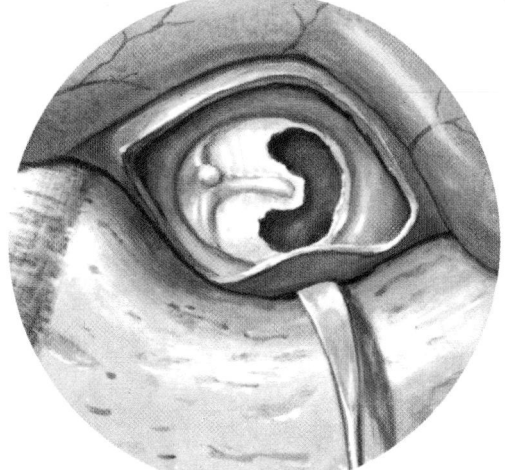

4. SKIN OF POSTERIOR WALL OF CANAL WALL AND EAR DRUM HAVE BEEN REFLECTED FORWARD OVER MANUBRIUM OF MALLEUS, EXPOSING MIDDLE EAR; POSTERIOR BONY WALL OF EAR CANAL HAS BEEN BURRED AWAY SOMEWHAT

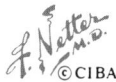

PLATE IX

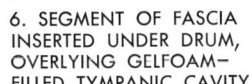
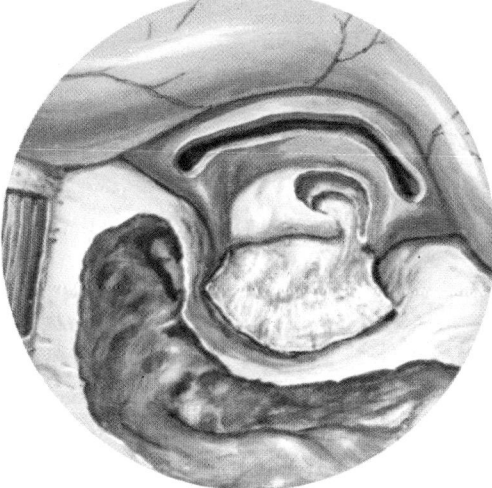
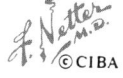
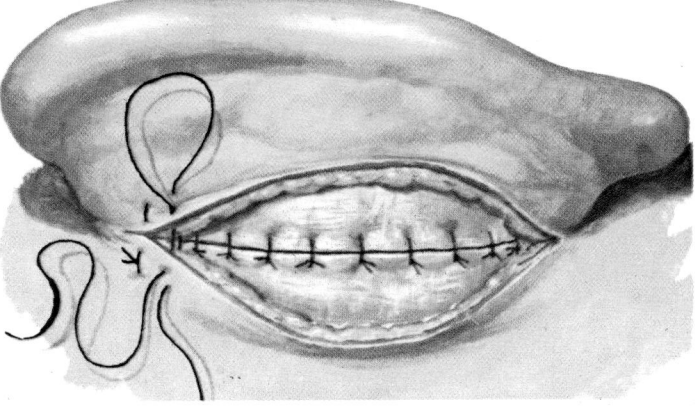

5. MASTOIDECTOMY COMPLETED, LEAVING BRIDGE OF BONE FOR POSTERIOR WALL OF EAR CANAL; TYMPANIC CAVITY PACKED WITH GELFOAM; SEGMENT OF TEMPORALIS FASCIA BEING EXCISED

6. SEGMENT OF FASCIA INSERTED UNDER DRUM, OVERLYING GELFOAM–FILLED TYMPANIC CAVITY

7. EAR DRUM AND SKIN OF POSTERIOR CANAL WALL REPLACED; FASCIAL POSITION ADJUSTED

8. POSTAURICULAR FASCIA AND PERIOSTEUM SUTURED TO FASCIA OF AURICLE; SKIN AND SUBCUTANEOUS TISSUE CLOSED WITH ON–END MATTRESS SUTURES

PLATE X   POSTAURICULAR TYMPANOPLASTY—CONTINUED

In patients not seen until after scar tissue has produced a chronic adhesive deafness, perhaps with cholesteatoma, the only hope of restoring hearing is tympanoplasty with removal of adventitious tissue. Because of the well-known tendency of scar tissue to re-form, relief obtained by this method often is not permanent, and a hearing aid may be required.

CHRONIC OTITIS MEDIA

In considering the question of chronic otitis media, its course, prognosis, and the desirability of surgical intervention, one must make a sharp distinction between three different forms of the disease, which we shall therefore discuss separately.

Chronic Otitis Media Simplex

This is the end result of an acute suppurative otitis media which has produced an unhealed perforation in the tense portion of the drum. Usually, with the passage of time the perforation increases in size until a large central or horseshoe-shaped opening is present, behind which one can see a red, edematous, and thickened mucosa.

An ear of this type rarely becomes involved with cholesteatoma. Therefore, it is not essentially a dangerous ear. Rather it is an annoyance because of persistent or periodically recurring discharge. In addition, with repeated flare-ups, a gradual loss of hearing can be expected. This is due not only to the edema and thickening of the lining mucosa, but ultimately to an actual necrosis of the ossicular chain, usually the incus.

To eliminate the discharge and the inevitable progression of hearing loss, several operative techniques are available. The simplest is transmeatal tympanoplasty where the perforation is covered by skin of the external auditory canal (see Plates VII and VIII). This procedure is applicable to uncomplicated cases having a perforation no larger than 30% of the drum area. The ear should also have been dry or free of drainage for several months.

Transmeatal Tympanoplasty: The lines of skin incision are shown in Plate VII. The first incision is carried from the drum outward in the anterosuperior portion of the canal, following the petrotympanic suture line into the cartilaginous part of the canal. The posterior incision follows similarly the petrosquamous suture line. These incisions are then joined distally, as indicated in Plate VII, and the skin is then elevated downward toward the drum.

In order to visualize the entire circumference of the tympanic membrane, it is necessary to burr away the bulge on the anterior canal wall. The epithelium is then removed from the annulus and carried from the periphery toward the edge of the perforation.

In the superior part of the canal, known as the vascular strip, the skin is incised close to the annulus as shown, and the skin and epithelium of annulus and drum are elevated from the periphery toward the edge of the perforation. In this way a patch of skin is obtained which is already accustomed to the bacterial flora of the region, and at the same time the drum has been completely freed of epithelial covering.

As shown in Plate VIII, the drum is then freed from the annulus and reflected anteriorly so that the ossicular chain may be inspected for disease, necessity for surgical repair, or replacement by a prosthesis. The middle ear is then packed with Gelfoam. This forms a bed on which the drum can lie, and prevents the graft from being displaced through the perforation. This Gelfoam is absorbed in about three weeks. Then the graft, which has been thinned out a little in the cartilaginous portion, is repositioned. The thicker part is placed against the vascular strip so as to cover Shrapnell's area. The ear canal is then packed with Gelfoam, which protects the graft and allows the still denuded bony area to re-epithelialize, a process that is usually complete in three to four weeks.

Postoperative Course: Since this is systemically a minor procedure, usually carried out under local anesthesia, the patient is out of bed the next day and discharged in a few days. The Gelfoam in the external canal remains in place for three weeks.

Postauricular Tympanoplasty and Mastoidectomy

Where there is evidence that the mastoid cells are involved and must be cleaned out, postauricular tympanoplasty with mastoidectomy should be carried out.

As shown in Plate IX, the postauricular incision is carried down through the periosteum of the mastoid. The ear canal, which has been elevated forward, is opened from behind at the osseous-cartilaginous junction, exposing the drum and its perforation.

The skin of the ear canal is then reflected forward, and the opening into the middle ear enlarged for better exposure by burring away some of the mastoid cortex. The middle ear can now be cleaned out. A mastoidectomy is then performed, leaving a bridge of bone behind the ear canal.

Both the middle ear and mastoid having been cleaned, and repair of the ossicular chain having been carried out if necessary, the tympanic cavity is then packed with Gelfoam, and overlayed with a strip of temporalis fascia that had been exposed in the initial incision.

As shown in Plate X, the skin of the posterior ear canal is brought back into place, the position of the fascia adjusted, and the incision closed.

Chronic Adhesive Otitis Media

While the incidence of chronic otitis media simplex has been reduced by the use of antibiotics, chronic adhesive otitis media seems to be more prevalent, so that one now sees chronic otitis media in all its forms just as often as was formerly the case, before antibiotics were given.

This adhesive form of otitis media often starts with the serous otitis media which has been previously discussed (page 53). If the serous otitis media is not treated successfully, the drum becomes progressively retracted by an apparent negative pressure in the middle ear.

The fault seems to lie in loss of function of the eustachian tube. Normally this tube opens periodically to allow for equalization of pressure on the two sides of the drum. However, where the eustachian tube is no longer functioning, air in the middle ear is absorbed, producing a partial vacuum. The presence of this partial vacuum results in thinning and stretching of the drum until eventually it is seen to be draped over the ossicles and stapedius tendon and plastered against the medial wall, plainly outlining the promontory and the niche of the round window.

The posterosuperior portion of the drum, the pars flaccida, or Shrapnell's membrane, is quite thin, consisting of only two layers instead of the three layers present in the rest of the drum. In addition, the pars flaccida overlies the ossicular chain in the attic. Therefore, this portion of the drum, as it is drawn in by the negative pressure, tends to form pockets lined with squamous epithelium — the start of the most dangerous complication of adhesive otitis media, cholesteatoma.

Treatment: There is at present no satisfactory treatment for this condition. Where allergy is present, it should be treated, and upper respiratory infections should be avoided as far as possible. However, the main fault lies in the eustachian tube. Politzer inflation gives only transient relief.

Intubation of the eustachian tube in the hope of aerating the middle ear has been abandoned. Instead a small plastic tube is inserted through the anterior portion of the drum. This will permit aeration, and the drum, if not adherent to the promontory, may retract and pull

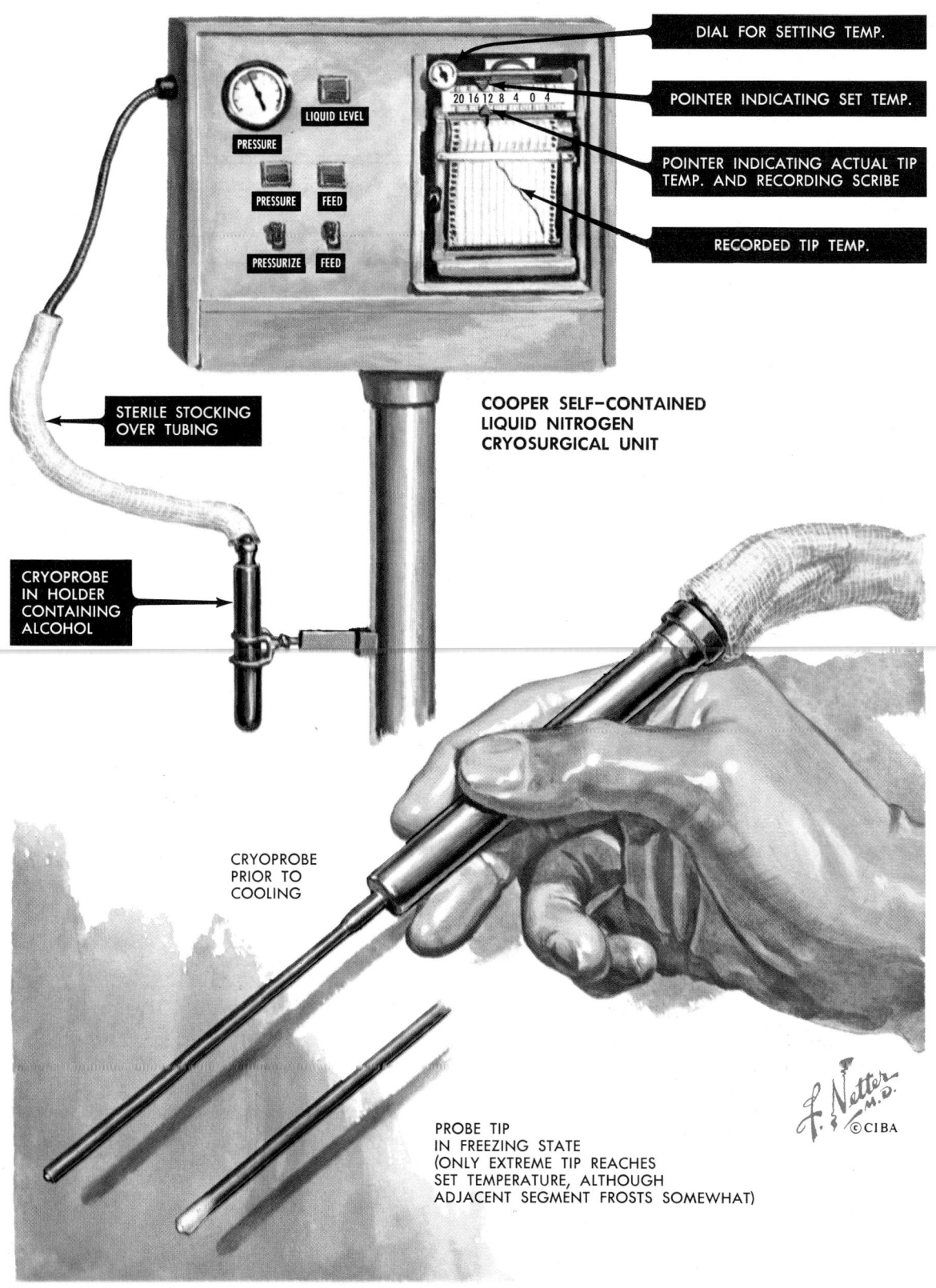

DIAL FOR SETTING TEMP.

POINTER INDICATING SET TEMP.

POINTER INDICATING ACTUAL TIP TEMP. AND RECORDING SCRIBE

RECORDED TIP TEMP.

LIQUID LEVEL

PRESSURE

PRESSURE

PRESSURE FEED

PRESSURIZE FEED

20 16 12 8 4 0 4

COOPER SELF-CONTAINED LIQUID NITROGEN CRYOSURGICAL UNIT

STERILE STOCKING OVER TUBING

CRYOPROBE IN HOLDER CONTAINING ALCOHOL

CRYOPROBE PRIOR TO COOLING

PROBE TIP IN FREEZING STATE (ONLY EXTREME TIP REACHES SET TEMPERATURE, ALTHOUGH ADJACENT SEGMENT FROSTS SOMEWHAT)

PLATE XI   CRYOSURGICAL APPARATUS

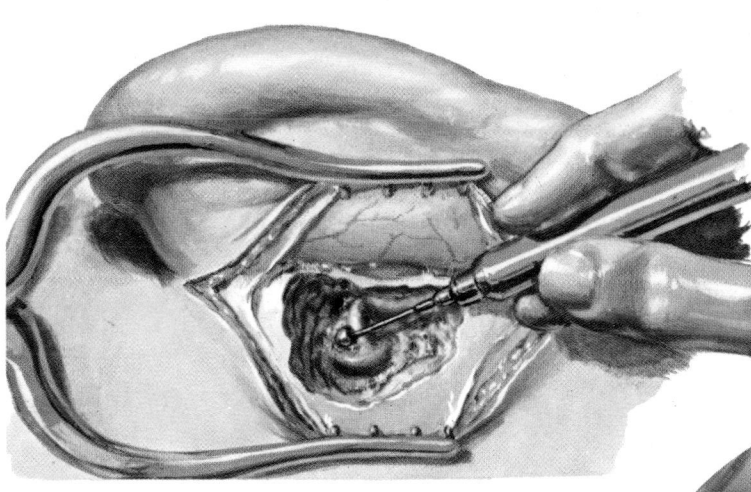

POSTAURICULAR INCISION; PERI-
OSTEUM ELEVATED AND RETRACTED
WITH SKIN AND FASCIA; MASTOID
CORTEX AND AIR CELLS BURRED
AWAY WITH DENTAL DRILL UNTIL
BONY HORIZONTAL SEMICIRCULAR
CANAL IS EXPOSED (OFTEN INCI-
DENTALLY EXPOSING THE INCUS
AND POSTERIOR SEMICIRCULAR CANAL)

INCUS

PROMINENCE
OF FACIAL
NERVE CANAL

BONY HORIZONTAL SEMICIRCULAR CANAL

BONY POSTERIOR SEMICIRCULAR CANAL

PROMINENCE OF SIGMOID SINUS

BONY WALL OF HORIZONTAL CANAL IS THINNED
UNTIL BLUISH–WHITE REFLEX IS SEEN

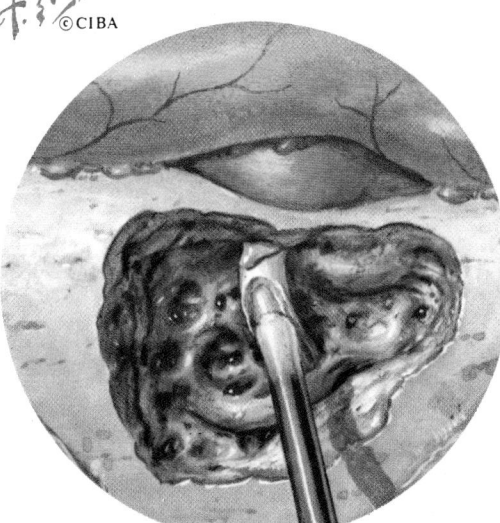

THE CRYOPROBE IS APPLIED TO THINNED
AREA OF HORIZONTAL CANAL. TIP
TEMPERATURE IS QUICKLY REDUCED FAR
BELOW FREEZING. SINCE PROBE FREEZES
TO CANAL, IT MUST BE ALLOWED TO
THAW FREE BEFORE REMOVAL.

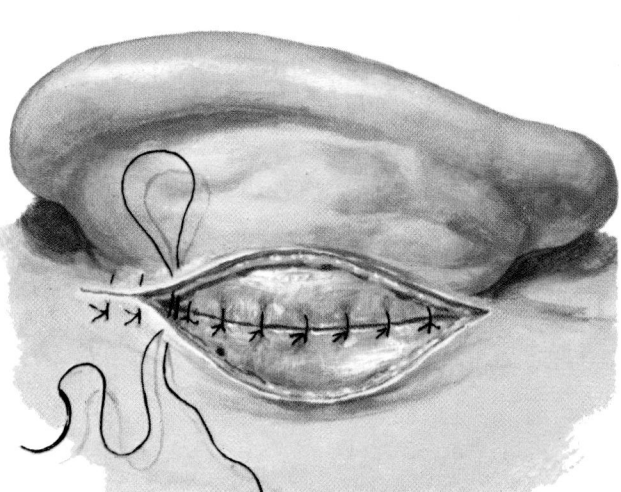

FASCIA SUTURED WITH INTERRUPTED STITCHES AND
SKIN CLOSED WITH MATTRESS SUTURES WITHOUT DRAINAGE

PLATE XII

CRYOSURGERY FOR MENIERE'S DISEASE

away. Where the eustachian tube remains closed, this tube must remain in place indefinitely. Unless complicated by cholesteatoma, tympanoplasty should not be attempted because no permanent relief can be expected. The new graft will have the same fate as the original drum, if indeed the persistent negative pressure allows it to take at all. At present, therefore, the best treatment consists of prophylaxis — the treatment of the preceding serous otitis media.

Chronic Otitis Media with Cholesteatoma

A cholesteatoma is a sac containing a silvery white debris of keratin, which is shed by the perfectly normal-appearing squamous epithelial lining. Often the epithelial lining is present in layers of shed skin, like the layers of an onion. As the lining of epithelium sheds and desquamates, the false tumor has to expand. In doing so, it erodes surrounding tissues, including bone. This erosive tendency can hardly be ascribed to pressure necrosis alone. Therefore, it has been attributed to some enzymatic action related to the presence of the cholesteatoma.

It is this erosive power of the cholesteatoma that converts a safe though annoying ear into a dangerous ear, prone to serious complications.

The formation of a cholesteatoma in an ear showing adhesive otitis media has already been referred to. In addition, while a perforation in the pars tensa of the drum rarely leads to cholesteatoma, a perforation in the pars flaccida, or Shrapnell's membrane, is quite prone to develop this condition. Thus, an ear with a perforation in Shrapnell's membrane is a potentially dangerous ear because of the tendency for cholesteatoma formation.

Complications of Cholesteatoma: Erosion of the bony wall of the horizontal portion of the canal of the facial nerve may cause facial paralysis. Bony erosion elsewhere can cause meningitis, labyrinthitis, epidural abscess, and lateral sinus thrombosis. The appearance of any of these complications demands immediate emergency surgery.

Diagnosis: Where a perforation is present, the silvery white false tumor may be seen directly, and the contents may be removed by gentle aspiration. If a probe is inserted, it will seem to fall into the soft cavity of the tumor before meeting resistance.

Treatment: Cholesteatoma is neither self-limiting nor spontaneously cured. Rather it is insidiously progressive and prone to serious complication.

Fortunately, the microsurgical techniques that have been developed provide an opportunity to remove cholesteatomatous material under highly magnified direct vision, with conservation or even improvement of the hearing function. No one operation can be used in every case. Therefore, modifications of the technique are often necessary in order to cope with the various conditions of disease and the demands for ossicular chain repair presented in the individual case.

In some cases, postauricular tympanoplasty, as previously described, will be ample. Usually, however, the bridge of bone between the external canal and mastoid cavity must be removed, creating a large cavity formed by the mastoid bowl and the external ear canal.

In closing this cavity, the front wall is formed by the anterior wall of the ear canal. The skin of the posterior wall of the ear canal is used as a tympanomeatal flap, temporalis fascia being used to seal the middle ear area after reconstruction.

The posterior skin of the concha is sutured to the periosteum of the mastoid cortex, widening of the external meatus being accomplished by two incisions in the conchal skin to form a flap.

MENIERE'S DISEASE

This condition, which we have discussed

in greater detail in "Vertigo" (CLINICAL SYMPOSIA, 17:99, 1965), is due to increased pressure of the endolymph. The disease usually has its onset between the ages of 30 and 60 years. It affects both sexes equally. The characteristic triad of symptoms are: 1. tinnitus, 2. deafness, and 3. acute attacks of vertigo.

The *tinnitus*, in the early stages, may be intermittent, occurring primarily when the patient is having an attack of vertigo. Within a short time, however, the tinnitus becomes constant, but increases in intensity during the attacks. The type of noise the patient hears may vary. Most frequently, it is described as a low-pitched roaring or rumbling sound, much like the ocean's surf. High-pitched whistling or hissing occurs less frequently. Often the tinnitus is only a minor annoyance, and it may not be mentioned unless the patient is questioned.

The *hearing loss,* which is usually unilateral, may occur simultaneously with the first vertigo attack, or it may precede the vertigo by many months. Each attack of vertigo tends to increase the loss of hearing. In the early stages, the hearing tends to fluctuate. However, as the disease continues, the loss becomes more persistent and pronounced. In spite of the impaired hearing, the patient is often less tolerant of loud sounds in the deafened ear than in a normal ear.

The chief symptom is *vertigo*. The attacks are acute in onset and produce a frightening and incapacitating experience. The patient feels that the room is spinning or that he is rolling about in a stationary room. Therefore, he is forced to lie quietly and avoid any movements of the head which tend to increase the sensation of vertigo. Pallor, sweating, nausea, and vomiting are usually present during the attack. The more severe the attack, the more prominent are these symptoms.

Attacks vary widely in frequency and severity. They may last for only a few minutes or may persist for many hours.

The usual duration is four to eight hours.

Diagnosis

A characteristic sign is the presence of *nystagmus*. This is present only during the acute attack of vertigo. During a period of remission, the caloric test (water 30°C or even ice water introduced into the external ear canal) is utilized to test labyrinthine function. Usually one finds a hypofunctioning labyrinth, however at times it may be normal.

Audiologic studies show characteristic findings, which are essential to make the diagnosis. There will be a flat or low-tone nerve deafness in the affected ear. "Recruitment" will be present. This term refers to an abnormal increase in sensitivity to sound once the threshold is reached. Sounds of low intensity may not be heard at all in the affected ear, but once the threshold is reached, small increases in intensity make the sound seem very loud or even painful. In addition, the same tone will sound differently pitched when comparing the sound heard in the normal and in the affected ear.

When testing the clarity of the hearing by means of a speech discrimination test, one finds that even when speech is made comfortably loud in the deafened ear, the ability of the patient to repeat simple words becomes markedly impaired because of the distorted perception of speech. Usually the involved ear is able to discriminate or understand less than 70% of the words presented to it even though these words are presented at a level well above the patient's depressed threshold.

Medical Treatment

Although not completely satisfactory, medical treatment will control symptoms sufficiently well to avoid surgery in about 85% of cases. Treatment of the acute attack of vertigo is symptomatic and supportive. It consists primarily of bed rest, sedation, antiemetics, antimotion sickness drugs, and reassurance that the attack will soon

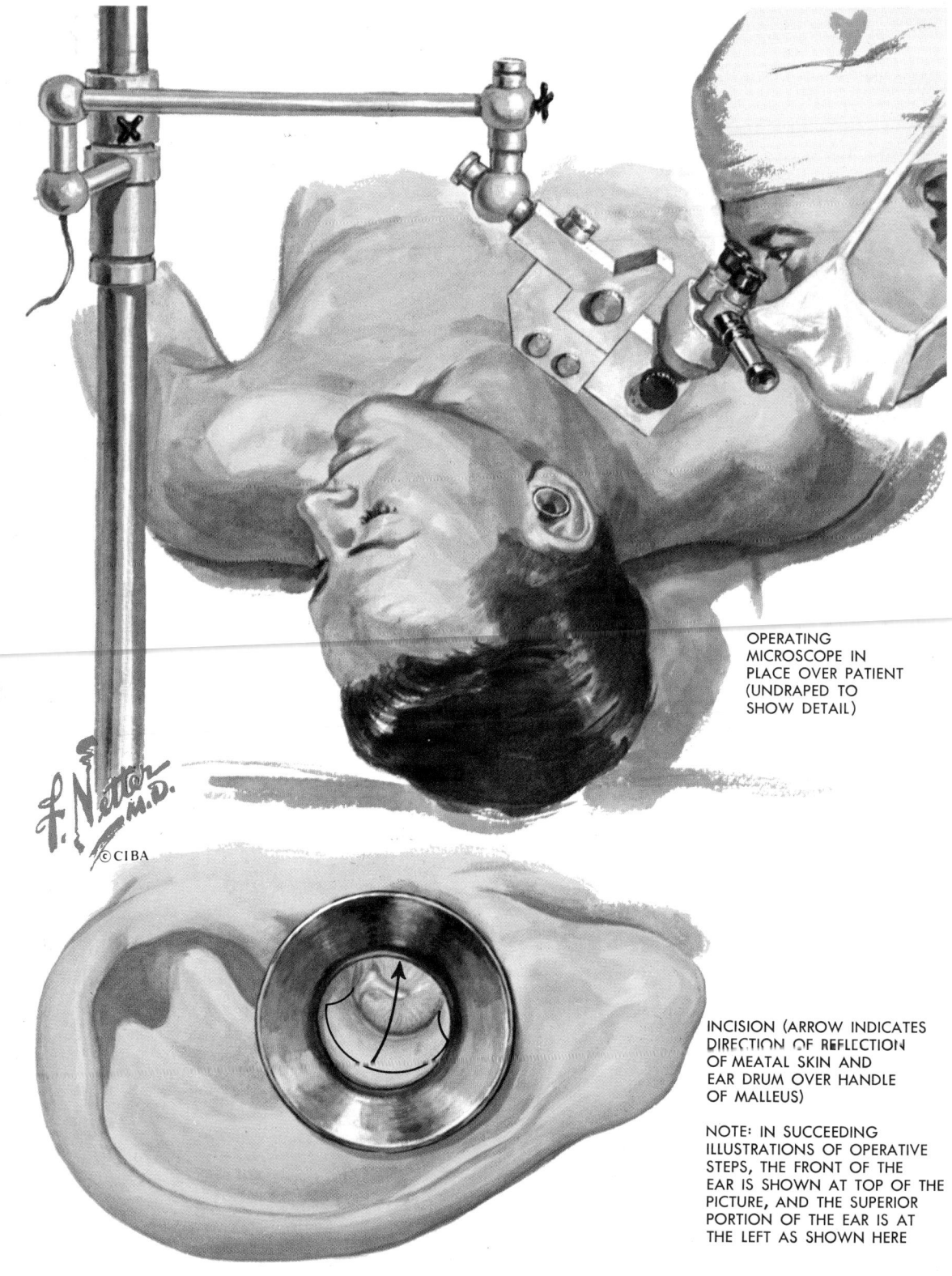

OPERATING
MICROSCOPE IN
PLACE OVER PATIENT
(UNDRAPED TO
SHOW DETAIL)

INCISION (ARROW INDICATES
DIRECTION OF REFLECTION
OF MEATAL SKIN AND
EAR DRUM OVER HANDLE
OF MALLEUS)

NOTE: IN SUCCEEDING
ILLUSTRATIONS OF OPERATIVE
STEPS, THE FRONT OF THE
EAR IS SHOWN AT TOP OF THE
PICTURE, AND THE SUPERIOR
PORTION OF THE EAR IS AT
THE LEFT AS SHOWN HERE

PLATE XIII   OPERATING MICROSCOPE AND LINE OF MEATAL INCISION FOR STAPEDECTOMY

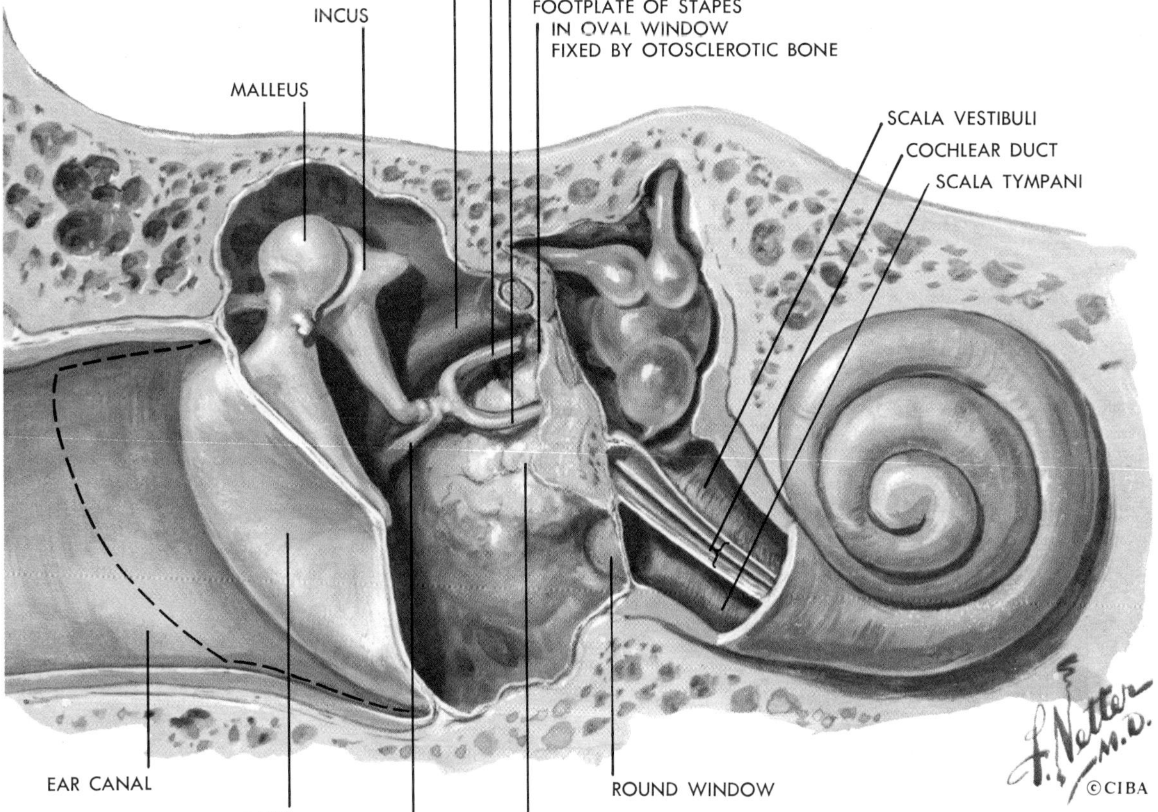

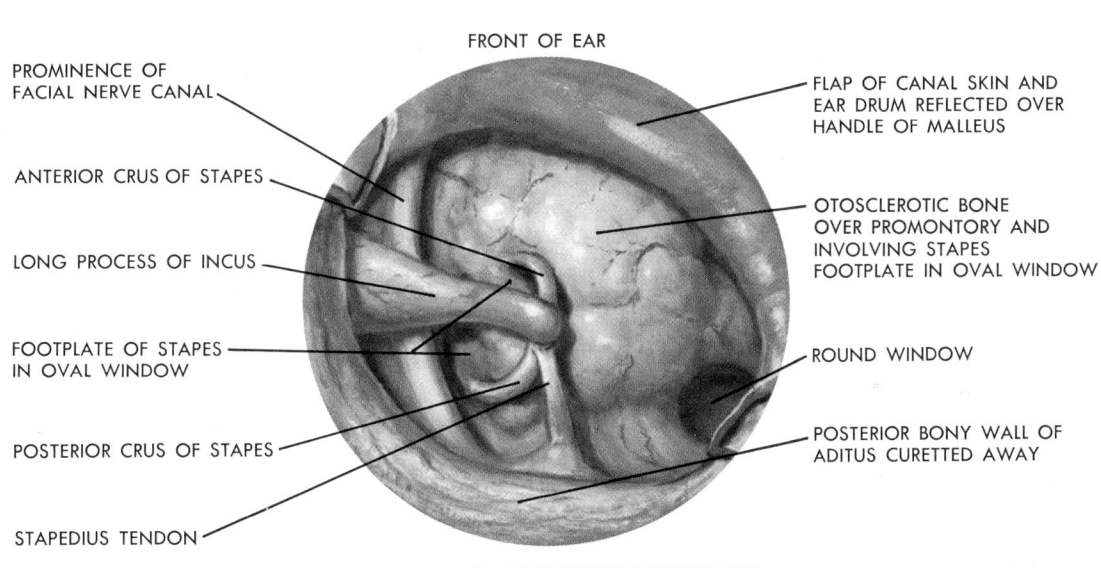

FACIAL NERVE CANAL

POSTERIOR CRUS OF STAPES

ANTERIOR CRUS OF STAPES

FOOTPLATE OF STAPES IN OVAL WINDOW FIXED BY OTOSCLEROTIC BONE

INCUS

MALLEUS

SCALA VESTIBULI

COCHLEAR DUCT

SCALA TYMPANI

EAR CANAL

EAR DRUM

STAPEDIUS TENDON

OTOSCLEROTIC BONE

ROUND WINDOW

FRONT OF EAR

PROMINENCE OF FACIAL NERVE CANAL

FLAP OF CANAL SKIN AND EAR DRUM REFLECTED OVER HANDLE OF MALLEUS

ANTERIOR CRUS OF STAPES

OTOSCLEROTIC BONE OVER PROMONTORY AND INVOLVING STAPES FOOTPLATE IN OVAL WINDOW

LONG PROCESS OF INCUS

FOOTPLATE OF STAPES IN OVAL WINDOW

ROUND WINDOW

POSTERIOR CRUS OF STAPES

POSTERIOR BONY WALL OF ADITUS CURETTED AWAY

STAPEDIUS TENDON

1. EXPOSURE OF OTOSCLEROTIC MIDDLE EAR. TOP OF EAR IS AT LEFT OF ILLUSTRATION

PLATE XIV

FIXATION OF STAPES BY OTOSCLEROSIS

subside, and that the vertigo does not indicate a serious, life-threatening situation.

Between attacks, prophylactic treatment is required to modify or forestall future attacks. The patient should have a low salt diet with moderate fluid restriction and receive maintenance doses of vasodilators. Diuretics, antihistamines, and supplementary vitamins, although difficult to evaluate, may be of additional help.

Surgical Treatment

Surgery is indicated primarily in those individuals who are seriously handicapped by the recurrent attacks of vertigo. The patient may be so handicapped that he is unable to care for the household, maintain a job, or pursue a normal social life. In some cases a severe psychological problem is created by the fear and anticipation of future attacks of vertigo.

The type of surgery to be recommended will depend upon the degree of hearing loss.

Surgical Destruction of the Labyrinth

This will cure the vertigo in practically every case, but will destroy the hearing at the same time. Therefore, it is indicated only in those in whom:

1. Involvement is unilateral and has been present for more than two years. (In the 10% of cases in which Meniere's disease is bilateral, the second ear usually becomes involved within two years.)

2. The hearing in the involved ear is so poor as to serve no useful purpose. This is indicated by pure-tone loss of at least 60 dB, with speech discrimination of 50% or less.

Cryosurgery of the Labyrinth

This consists of applying intense cold ($-160°C$) to the horizontal semicircular canal, as illustrated in Plates XI and XII. By this technique, the sensitivity of the vestibular apparatus is reduced so that an increase of pressure (hydrops) will not so easily initiate an attack of vertigo. This reduced sensitivity can be demonstrated objectively by caloric testing.

Indications

These consist of:

1. Unilateral involvement with pure-tone deficit less than 60 dB and speech discrimination better than 50%.

2. Bilateral involvement regardless of the hearing deficit.

3. Post-traumatic vertigo with a hypofunctioning labyrinth, but relatively good hearing.

Technique

Under general anesthesia, access to the horizontal semicircular canal is gained through a retroauricular simple mastoidectomy. The bony wall of the horizontal canal is thinned with a burr until a bluish-white reflex in seen (Plate XII). The cryogenic probe is then applied for a total of six minutes using three applications of two minutes each. The skin and fascia are then closed without drainage.

Postoperative Course

This is much smoother than in total destruction of the labyrinth. However, the patient is moderately dizzy for the first 2 days. Unsteadiness then persists from a few days to two or three weeks. The patient remains in the hospital for six days. He can usually resume employment by the third or fourth week.

Results

In the first 100 cases carried out since one of us (RJW) introduced this technique in 1966, 80% have had excellent results. Hearing has been unimpaired and attacks of vertigo have ceased or been replaced by only an occasional unsteadiness.

ACOUSTIC (VASCULAR) ACCIDENTS

Another type of deafness that may respond to medical treatment is the sudden loss of hearing (usually unilateral) which is due to vascular spasm, or a clot in one of the vessels supplying the inner ear. This sudden hearing loss usually is accompanied by tinnitus and vertigo.

Treatment: Immediate hospitalization with heparinization, corticosteroid therapy, and histamine intravenously will often produce a dramatic improvement. Delay of only a week will markedly reduce the effectiveness of treatment. However, even in patients seen late in the disease, medical therapy is still worthy of a trial.

OTOSCLEROSIS

This is one of the most important causes of hearing impairment in adults because of:

1. Its relatively high incidence which we would estimate as involving about 4 percent of the total population or 35 to 40 percent of those who are acoustically handicapped, and

2. The fact that it is usually correctible, either with a properly selected hearing aid or by modern methods of microsurgery.

Pathology

This disease of bone is unique to the human otic capsule. It may begin at any time in life but appears most frequently after puberty, during pregnancy, the puerperium, or menopause. The process begins by resorption of bone, starting in one or more minute foci which gradually extend until they coalesce. Sometimes the entire capsule is involved, including the walls of the semicircular canals and both labyrinthine windows. The resorbed bone is replaced by new bone laid down in irregular patterns of mosaic design. Not only is normal bone replaced by sclerotic bone, but a pronounced overgrowth of pathologic bone develops which progressively obliterates the oval window. By invading the footplate, the pathologic bone increasingly immobilizes the stapes, thus further reducing the transmission of vibrations.

Many advanced cases also develop a permanent sensorineural hearing loss, due perhaps to pressure of otosclerotic bone on the eighth nerve, atrophy or rupture of the basilar membrane by otosclerotic lesions of the bony capsule, or secondary inflammation which produces changes in the organ of Corti.

Symptoms

Normally we begin life with a greater degree of hearing acuity than we need, and it is only when we approach 30 decibels of hearing loss that impairment is actually noticed. The first thing observed is the inability to hear a whisper or to understand someone speaking from a distance. Most people so affected seem to blame everyone but themselves for their disability. If in high school, they say the teacher mumbles; at work, the boss mumbles. Thus, unable to fully comprehend instructions, a good scholar becomes a poor one, and a previously good worker appears indifferent and slipshod.

At least in earlier stages, the bone conduction by which we hear our own voices remains relatively unaffected. Therefore, to the otosclerotic, his own voice sounds unusually loud. To compensate, he pitches his voice lower and lower until he can scarcely be understood.

Because of this relative increase in bone conduction, the sounds of chewing seem intensified. Therefore, the otosclerotic hears even more poorly at the dinner table, which is an important focal point of social and family life. Unable to understand the conversation and jokes going on about him and tired of asking his relatives and friends to repeat, he withdraws further and further within himself. At the same time, family and friends, tired of talking loudly for his benefit, are glad to ignore him in their conversation. Thus, gradually but inescapably the otosclerotic may become a neurotic, emotionally crippled recluse.

Because bone conduction is relatively

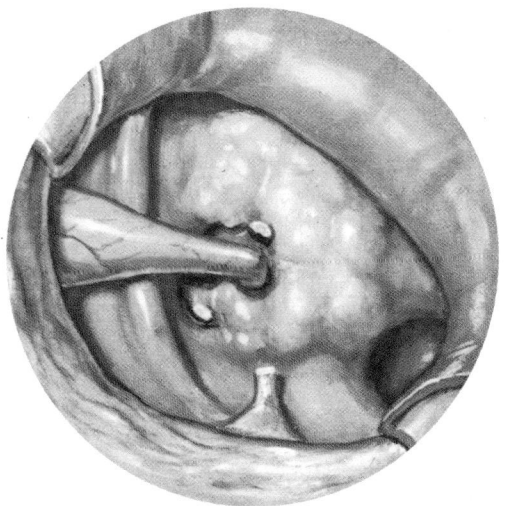

2. STAPEDIUS TENDON DIVIDED; CRURA AND HEAD OF STAPES REMOVED

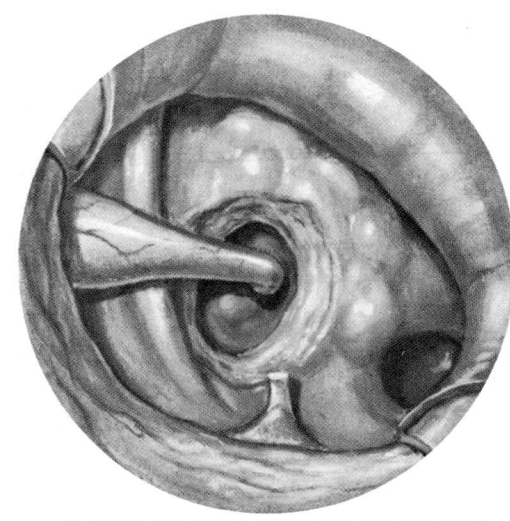

3. OVAL WINDOW RECREATED BY REMOVAL OF STAPES FOOT PLATE AND OTOSCLEROTIC PROMONTORY SAUCERIZED (SACCULE VISIBLE THROUGH OVAL WINDOW)

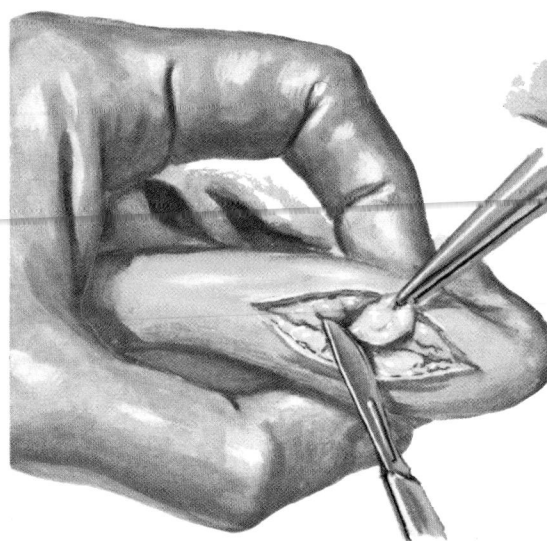

5. EAR WOUND SUTURED

4. LOBULE OF FAT REMOVED VIA LONGITUDINAL INCISION IN MARGIN OF EAR LOBE

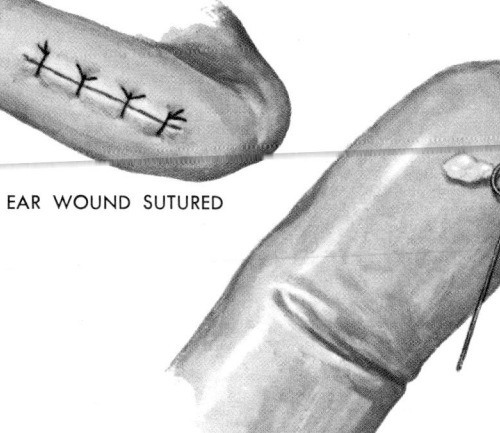

6. FAT LOBULE TRIMMED TO SIZE; LOOP OF STAINLESS STEEL WIRE SLIPPED OVER FAT AND DRAWN TIGHT

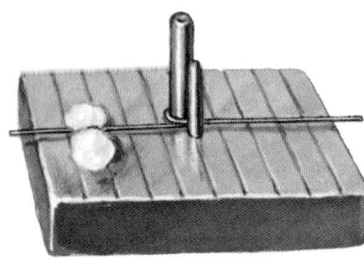

7. WIRE LOOPED AROUND LARGE POST OF SCHUKNECHT WIRE–BENDING DIE; FAT LOBULE AT 4 mm MARK

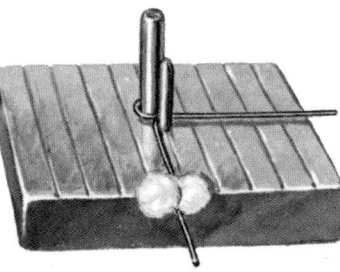

8. LEFT END OF WIRE WITH FAT LOBULE DRAWN FORWARD AGAINST SMALLER POST

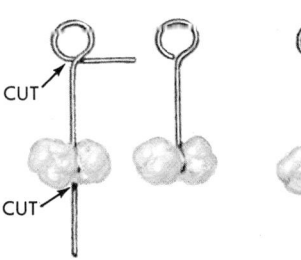

CUT

CUT

9. WIRE TRIMMED AND LOOP OPENED TO SLIP OVER LONG CRUS OF INCUS

PLATE XV

STAPEDECTOMY—CONTINUED

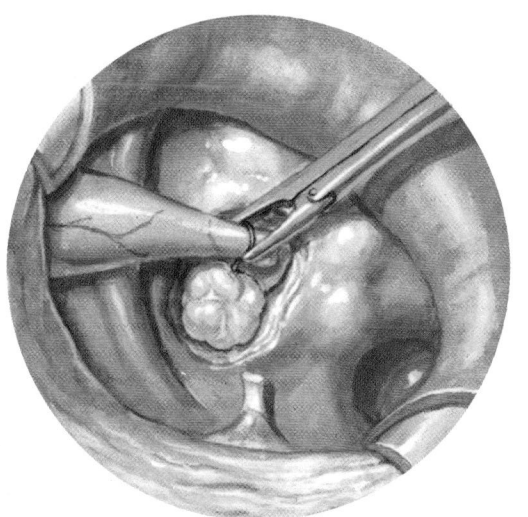

10. WIRE SLIPPED OVER LONG CRUS OF INCUS AND CRIMPED IN PLACE BY McGEE WIRE CLOSURE FORCEPS; FAT LOBULE LIES IN OVAL WINDOW

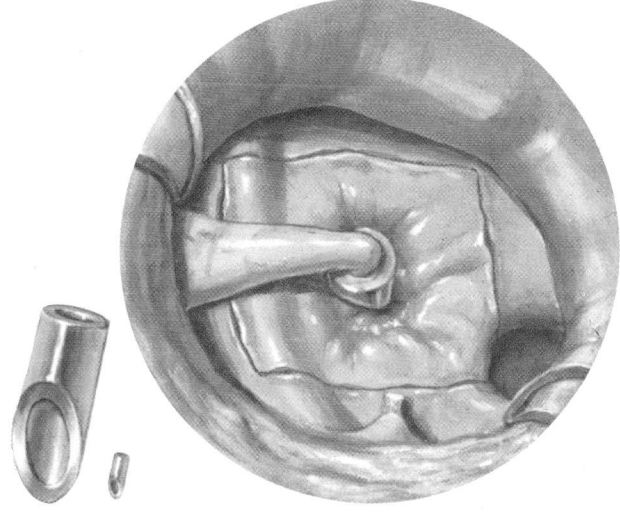

IN ORIGINAL OPERATION, STILL EMPLOYED BY SOME, A TUBULAR PLASTIC PROSTHESIS (SHOWN ENLARGED AND ACTUAL SIZE AT LEFT) WAS APPLIED TO LENTICULAR PROCESS OF INCUS AND A VEIN GRAFT EMPLOYED TO CLOSE THE OVAL WINDOW AS ILLUSTRATED ABOVE

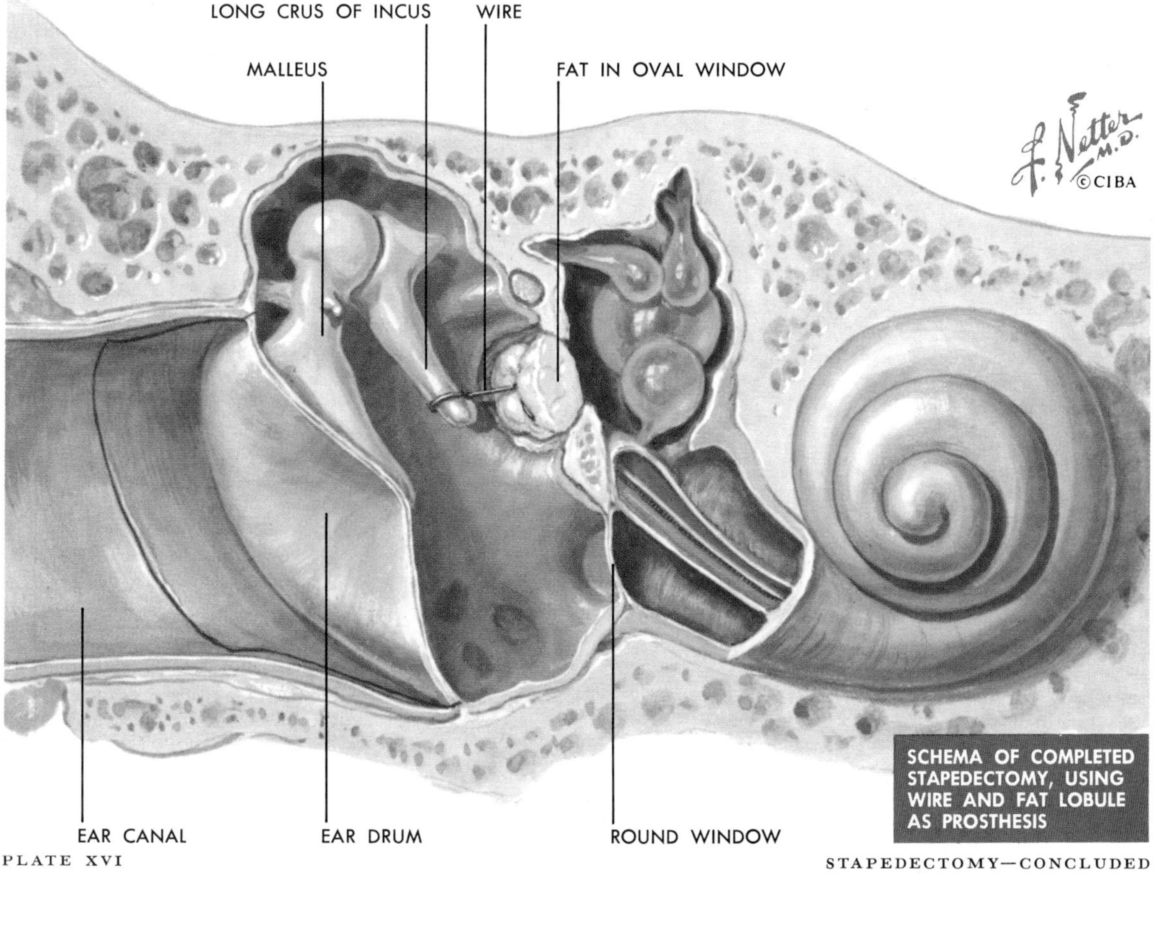

LONG CRUS OF INCUS   WIRE

MALLEUS   FAT IN OVAL WINDOW

EAR CANAL   EAR DRUM   ROUND WINDOW

SCHEMA OF COMPLETED STAPEDECTOMY, USING WIRE AND FAT LOBULE AS PROSTHESIS

PLATE XVI

STAPEDECTOMY—CONCLUDED

unimpaired, these people usually hear fairly well on the telephone which provides an amplified signal. They hear much better in noisy places, such as a subway train, where people must talk above surrounding noises.

Diagnosis

Tuning fork tests will indicate a hearing loss that is primarily conductive. In addition, careful audiometric studies should be carried out for the following reasons:

1. To guide in the proper selection of a hearing aid. In simple otosclerosis, the patient needs adequate amplification and a hearing aid that will not decrease speech perception. But where there is a concomitant sensorineural loss, most often affecting the higher frequencies, a special instrument may be required. When a decrease in speech perception exists, a training program may be necessary for acoustic and emotional rehabilitation.

2. To properly select cases for surgery. At best surgery can do no more than close the gap between air conduction and bone conduction. With an audiogram like Figure 2 on page 41, a moderate degree of high-tone deafness would be inescapable, even with successful surgery. On the other hand, considerable improvement would result if the audiogram were similar to Figure 3, and a great deal of improvement could be anticipated if there were practically normal bone conduction as shown in the Figure 4 audiogram.

All of this demonstrates that if surgery is to be carried out at all, it should be performed *before,* rather than after, a secondary sensorineural hearing loss has developed.

Treatment

Selection of hearing aids has been discussed on page 49. With regard to surgery, the otologic surgeon now has at his disposal a variety of techniques that can be adapted to the individual case. Of the two most frequently used, one employs a plastic prosthesis for the stapes and a vein graft to cover the oval window as developed by Dr. John J. Shea of Memphis (see Plate XVI). At times wire may be substituted for the plastic prosthesis. The other method, introduced by Dr. Harold Schuknecht of Boston, utilizes a fat and wire prosthesis.

At the present time, we prefer the fat and wire technique of Schuknecht. In our hands this prosthesis has the following advantages: 1. The fat is easy to obtain and prepare, having been gotten from the ear lobe adjacent to the operative site. 2. It is less difficult to handle and place in the middle ear. 3. Histologic examination of the temporal bone of a patient who died of cardiac arrest one year postoperatively, showed that the fat graft had become a strong covering of fibroareolar tissue over the endosteum of the oval window. 4. Use of this technique over a number of years in many hundreds of cases has given a high percentage of good results with a minimum of early or late complications.

Anesthesia: The operation is conducted under local anesthesia. The entire circumference of the meatus is injected with an anesthetic solution, thus permitting use of a much larger speculum without discomfort. With the speculum in place, the auditory meatus adjacent to the ear drum is injected with anesthetic.

Operative Technique: Using 10-power magnification provided by the operating microscope shown in Plate XIII, the posterior wall of the meatus is incised, as indicated in Plates XIII and XIV. The incision must be carried anteriorly and superiorly as far as the short process of the malleus and inferiorly to the midportion of the canal, so that the thinned skin flap can be folded forward to lie on the tympanic membrane. This provides wide exposure of the posterior portion of the tympanic cavity. Still better visibility is then obtained by dissection of the outer aditus wall with sharp curettes or surgical cutting burrs. This will bring the stapes footplate into view and accessible to manipulation.

The stapes tendon is then removed and the stapes separated from the incus, taking care not to damage the knob on the lenticular process of the latter bone. Firm pressure on the head of the stapes will then fracture the crura flush with the footplate so that all of the bone except the footplate can be removed.

Next the mucosa is excised in order to provide a bed for the graft. Since it is most important that blood does not seep into the fenestrated oval window, Gelfoam sponges soaked in 1:1000 epinephrine are placed over the denuded area and left in place until ready for the graft.

While these sponges are in place, the fat, which had previously been obtained from the ear lobe, is fashioned to fit the oval window (about 3 by 5 mm in size) and attached to a 35-gauge stainless steel wire as shown in Plate XV.

When preparation of this prosthesis is complete, the footplate of the stapes is removed from the oval window and replaced with the fat. The wire is crimped around the crus of the incus. (When vein is used, it is stripped of areolar and adipose tissue, split to expose its intimal surface and then trimmed for exact fit.)

Generally, the patient's hearing is improved when the footplate is removed. An additional increase of sensitivity occurs when the prosthesis is put in place.

Postoperative Course: If a minimal amount of manipulation has been done in the fossa ovalis, and if perilymph has not been removed by aspiration, the patient will experience little, if any, reaction. Labyrinthine reactions are usually mild and easily controlled with an intravenous antihistamine. Patients complain of transient unsteadiness rather than vertigo, and this may be controlled by an antimotion drug such as Dramamine. More serious degrees of nausea, vomiting, or vertigo have been experienced by only a few in our series of over 1,500 patients.

After operation the patient lies on the unaffected side for 24 hours. Then he may be out of bed but is cautioned against making sudden movements which might bring on giddiness. On the fourth or fifth postoperative day, the patient may return home, where he should remain on reduced activity for seven to ten days. Once the surgical incision has healed, the patient can bathe and swim as before, without worrying about getting water in the ear as is the case with lateral fenestration.

Results of Operation

The acuity of hearing postoperatively will depend upon the preoperative bone conduction, since we can do no better than close the air-bone gap. However, even in those cases of otosclerosis with serious nerve deafness, the degree of improvement, which is obtained in 85% of cases, is a considerable achievement from a practical standpoint.

For example, a patient with a 90 dB loss of air conduction cannot hear at all, because sound of this loudness is painful. However, if the hearing of such a patient can be improved to the level of his bone conduction, even if it be only 60 dB, he can then get along with a hearing aid. Where the air-bone gap can be closed to the 40 or 50 dB level, the patient will be able to hear loud conversation unaided; and with a hearing aid, he can listen comfortably to perfectly normal conversation. Where the bone conduction is normal or no worse than 30 dB, the patient will have normal hearing postoperatively.

Our experience with stapedectomy, embracing a period of 13 years, indicates that about 70% will have normal hearing postoperatively. Although about 5% are not benefited, less than 1% will have their hearing made worse due to labyrinthitis, or some other cause. Thus, microsurgery can offer a very high degree of salvage and rehabilitation with a minimum risk to those whose deafness is due to otosclerosis.